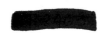
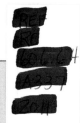
Injury & Trauma Sourcebook

Learning Disabilities Sourcebook, 3rd Edition

Leukemia Sourcebook

Liver Disorders Sourcebook

Medical Tests Sourcebook, 4th Edition

Men's Health Concerns Sourcebook, 3rd Edition

Mental Health Disorders Sourcebook, 4th Edition

Mental Retardation Sourcebook

Movement Disorders Sourcebook, 2nd Edition

Multiple Sclerosis Sourcebook

Muscular Dystrophy Sourcebook

Obesity Sourcebook

Osteoporosis Sourcebook

Pain Sourcebook, 3rd Edition

Pediatric Cancer Sourcebook

Physical & Mental Issues in Aging Sourcebook

Podiatry Sourcebook, 2nd Edition

Pregnancy & Birth Sourcebook, 3rd Edition

Prostate & Urological Disorders Sourcebook

Prostate Cancer Sourcebook

Rehabilitation Sourcebook

Respiratory Disorders Sourcebook, 2nd Edition

Sexually Transmitted Diseases Sourcebook, 4th Edition

Sleep Disorders Sourcebook, 3rd Edition

Smoking Concerns Sourcebook

Sports Injuries Sourcebook, 4th Edition

Stress-Related Disorders Sourcebook, 2nd Edition

Stroke Sourcebook, 2nd Edition

Surgery Sourcebook, 2nd Edition

Thyroid Disorders Sourcebook

Transplantation Sourcebook

Traveler's Health Sourcebook

Urinary Tract & Kidney Diseases & Disorders Sourcebook, 2nd Edition

Vegetarian Sourcebook

Women's Health Concerns Sourcebook, 3rd Edition

Workplace Health & Safety Sourcebook

Worldwide Health Sourcebook

Teen Health Series

Abuse & Violence Information for Teens

Accident & Safety Information for Teens

Alcohol Information for Teens, 2nd Edition

Allergy Information for Teens

Asthma Information for Teens, 2nd Edition

Body Information for Teens

Cancer Information for Teens, 2nd Edition

Complementary & Alternative Medicine Information for Teens

Diabetes Information for Teens, 2nd Edition

Diet Information for Teens, 3rd Edition

Drug Information for Teens, 3rd Edition

Eating Disorders Information for Teens, 2nd Edition

Fitness Information for Teens, 2nd Edition

Learning Disabilities Information for Teens

Mental Health Information for Teens, 3rd Edition

Pregnancy Information for Teens, 2nd Edition

Sexual Health Information for Teens, 3rd Edition

Skin Health Information for Teens, 2nd Edition

Sleep Information for Teens

Sports Injuries Information for Teens, 2nd Edition

Stress Information for Teens

Suicide Information for Teens, 2nd Edition

Tobacco Information for Teens, 2nd Edition

W9-BSY-841

AIDS
SOURCEBOOK

Fifth Edition

Health Reference Series

Fifth Edition

AIDS
SOURCEBOOK

Basic Consumer Health Information about the Human Immunodeficiency Virus (HIV) and Acquired Immunodeficiency Syndrome (AIDS), Including Facts about Its Origins, Stages, Types, Transmission, Risk Factors, and Prevention, and Featuring Details about Diagnostic Testing, Antiretroviral Treatments, and Co-Occurring Infections, Such As Cytomegalovirus, Mycobacterium Avium Complex, Pneumocystis Carinii Pneumonia, and Toxoplasmosis

Along with Tips for Living with HIV/AIDS, Updated Statistics, Reports on Current Research Initiatives, a Glossary of Related Terms, and a List of Resources for Additional Help and Information

Edited by
Sandra J. Judd

Omnigraphics

P.O. Box 31-1640, Detroit, MI 48231

Bibliographic Note

Because this page cannot legibly accommodate all the copyright notices, the Bibliographic Note portion of the Preface constitutes an extension of the copyright notice.

Edited by Sandra J. Judd

Health Reference Series

Karen Bellenir, *Managing Editor*
David A. Cooke, MD, FACP, *Medical Consultant*
Elizabeth Collins, *Research and Permissions Coordinator*
Cherry Edwards, *Permissions Assistant*
EdIndex, Services for Publishers, *Indexers*

* * *

Omnigraphics, Inc.

Matthew P. Barbour, *Senior Vice President*
Kevin M. Hayes, *Operations Manager*

* * *

Peter E. Ruffner, *Publisher*

Copyright © 2011 Omnigraphics, Inc.

ISBN 978-0-7808-1147-8

Library of Congress Cataloging-in-Publication Data

AIDS sourcebook : basic consumer health information about the human immunodeficiency virus (HIV) and acquired immunodeficiency syndrome (AIDS), including facts about its origins, stages, types, transmission, risk factors, and prevention, and featuring details about diagnostic testing, antiretroviral treatments, and co-occurring infections, such as cytomegalovirus, mycobacterium avium complex, Pneumocystis carinii pneumonia, and toxoplasmosis; along with tips for living with HIV/AIDS, updated statistics, reports on current research initiatives, a glossary of related terms, and a list of resources for additional help and information / edited by Sandra J. Judd. -- 5th ed.
    p. cm.
  Includes bibliographical references and index.
  Summary: "Provides basic consumer health information about transmission, testing, and treatment of human immunodeficiency virus (HIV), related complications, and tips for living with HIV/AIDS. Includes index, glossary of related terms and directory of resources"-- Provided by publisher.
  ISBN 978-0-7808-1147-8 (hardcover : alk. paper) 1. AIDS (Disease)--Popular works. I. Judd, Sandra J.
  RC606.64.A337 2011
  362.196'9792--dc22

                                                            2011013086

Table of Contents

Visit www.healthreferenceseries.com to view *A Contents Guide to the Health Reference Series*, a listing of more than 15,000 topics and the volumes in which they are covered.

Part II: HIV/AIDS Transmission, Risk Factors, and Prevention

Part V: Common Co-Occurring Infections and Complications of HIV/AIDS

Part VI: Living with HIV Infection

Preface

About This Book

According to the Centers for Disease Control and Prevention, more than one million Americans are living with human immunodeficiency virus (HIV) infection. Fifty-six thousand people in the United States were newly infected with HIV in 2008, the most recent year for which statistics are available. This devastating disease attacks the immune system and affects all parts of the body, eventually leading to acquired immunodeficiency syndrome (AIDS), its most deadly and advanced stage, for which there is currently no cure. Yet there is hope for the many Americans living with HIV infection or AIDS. Researchers are developing new and more effective drug combinations, and scientists are growing ever closer to a vaccine. Improvements in medication and earlier diagnosis mean that those infected with HIV are living longer, healthier, and more productive lives. Still, many Americans are unaware of even the basic facts about HIV—how it is transmitted, how HIV progresses to AIDS, and how HIV and AIDS are treated.

AIDS Sourcebook, Fifth Edition, provides basic consumer information about the human immunodeficiency virus (HIV) and acquired immunodeficiency syndrome (AIDS), including information about the stages and types of the disease and about how it is transmitted. It includes guidelines for preventing disease transmission and details about how it is diagnosed and the various drug regimens used in its treatment. Information on co-occurring infections, complications, and tips for living with HIV infection are also included. The book concludes with a glossary of related terms and a list of resources for additional help and information.

How to Use This Book

This book is divided into parts and chapters. Parts focus on broad areas of interest. Chapters are devoted to single topics within a part.

Part I: Basic Information about Human Immunodeficiency Virus / Acquired Immunodeficiency Syndrome (HIV / AIDS) defines HIV and AIDS and explains what is known about the origin of the virus. It describes the life cycle, stages, and types of HIV infection and explains how HIV causes AIDS. It also includes a brief discussion of the prevalence and incidence of HIV and AIDS in the United States and around the world.

Part II: HIV / AIDS Transmission, Risk Factors, and Prevention presents the facts about the transmission of the human immunodeficiency virus and debunks some of the rumors about how this infection is transmitted. It explains the factors that put people at risk for HIV and provides tips for avoiding these risks.

Part III: Receiving an HIV / AIDS Diagnosis describes the different types of HIV testing and explains consumer rights regarding confidentiality and counseling. It provides a detailed explanation of what the test results mean and how to determine if you have AIDS. Finally, it provides tips for choosing a provider and navigating the healthcare system.

Part IV: Treatment and Therapies for HIV / AIDS details the antiretroviral treatment process, describes the common side effects and complications of this treatment, and explains how the effectiveness of treatment is monitored and what to do in the event of treatment failure. It also discusses complementary and alternative HIV/AIDS treatments, other treatments currently being developed, and how treatment varies in the special cases of children and pregnant women.

Part V: Common Co-Occurring Infections and Complications of HIV / AIDS describes the bacterial, fungal, parasitic, and viral infections that often accompany HIV and AIDS. It also offers tips on how to avoid these infections and explains how they are treated when they do occur. In addition, AIDS-related cancer, wasting syndrome, AIDS dementia complex, and other AIDS-related health concerns are discussed.

Part VI: Living with HIV Infection offers advice on coping with an HIV/AIDS diagnosis and explains how diet and exercise can help maintain health. It discusses legal responsibility for disclosure and provides tips for telling a spouse or sexual partners, family and friends, co-workers, and healthcare providers about HIV status. The part concludes with a discussion about laws that apply to people with HIV and a description of the public benefits, insurance, and housing options available, including information about providing home care for someone with AIDS.

Part VII: Additional Help and Information includes a glossary of terms related to AIDS and HIV and a directory of resources for additional help and support.

Bibliographic Note

This volume contains documents and excerpts from the following U.S. government agencies: AIDS.gov and AidsInfo.gov, services of the U.S. Department of Health and Human Services; Centers for Disease Control and Prevention; National Cancer Institute; National Institute of Allergy and Infectious Diseases; National Institute of Neurological Disorders and Stroke; National Institutes of Health; Social Security Administration; U.S. Department of Justice; U.S. Department of Veterans Affairs; and the U.S. Food and Drug Association.

In addition, this volume contains copyrighted documents from the following organizations: A.D.A.M., Inc.; AIDS InfoNet; Aidsmeds.com; American Academy of Family Physicians; American Association for Clinical Chemistry; American Civil Liberties Union Foundation; AVERT; TheBody.com; Canadian Federation for Sexual Health; Center for AIDS; Center for AIDS Prevention Studies–University of California at San Francisco; HealthDay/Scout News LLC; Johns Hopkins Medicine Office of Corporate Communications; Immunization Action Coalition; International Center for Alcohol Policies; Kaiser Family Foundation; Marijuana Policy Project; New Zealand Dermatological Society; Project Inform; Tufts University School of Medicine–Public Health and Community Medicine; and The Well Project.

Acknowledgements

Thanks go to the many organizations, agencies, and individuals who have contributed materials for this *Sourcebook* and to medical consultant Dr. David Cooke and prepress services provider WhimsyInk. Special thanks go to managing editor Karen Bellenir and permissions coordinator Liz Collins for their help and support.

About the Health Reference Series

The *Health Reference Series* is designed to provide basic medical information for patients, families, caregivers, and the general public. Each volume takes a particular topic and provides comprehensive coverage. This is especially important for people who may be dealing with a newly diagnosed disease or a chronic disorder in themselves or in a family member. People looking for preventive guidance, information about disease warning signs, medical statistics, and risk factors for health problems will also find answers to their questions in the *Health Reference Series*. The *Series*, however, is not intended to serve as a tool for diagnosing illness, in prescribing treatments, or as a substitute for the physician/patient relationship. All people concerned about medical symptoms or the possibility of disease are encouraged to seek professional care from an appropriate healthcare provider.

A Note about Spelling and Style

Health Reference Series editors use *Stedman's Medical Dictionary* as an authority for questions related to the spelling of medical terms and the *Chicago Manual of Style* for questions related to grammatical structures, punctuation, and other editorial concerns. Consistent adherence is not always possible, however, because the individual volumes within the *Series* include many documents from a wide variety of different producers and copyright holders, and the editor's primary goal is to present material from each source as accurately as is possible following the terms specified by each document's producer. This sometimes means that information in different chapters or sections may follow other guidelines and alternate spelling authorities. For example, occasionally a copyright holder may require that eponymous terms be shown in possessive forms (Crohn's disease *vs.* Crohn disease) or that British spelling norms be retained (leukaemia *vs.* leukemia).

Locating Information within the Health Reference Series

The *Health Reference Series* contains a wealth of information about a wide variety of medical topics. Ensuring easy access to all the fact sheets, research reports, in-depth discussions, and other material contained within the individual books of the series remains one of our highest priorities. As the *Series* continues to grow in size and scope, however, locating the precise information needed by a reader may become more challenging.

A Contents Guide to the Health Reference Series was developed to direct readers to the specific volumes that address their concerns. It presents an extensive list of diseases, treatments, and other topics of general interest compiled from the Tables of Contents and major index headings. To access *A Contents Guide to the Health Reference Series*, visit www.healthreferenceseries.com.

Medical Consultant

Medical consultation services are provided to the *Health Reference Series* editors by David A. Cooke, MD, FACP. Dr. Cooke is a graduate of Brandeis University, and he received his M.D. degree from the University of Michigan. He completed residency training at the University of Wisconsin Hospital and Clinics. He is board-certified in Internal Medicine. Dr. Cooke currently works as part of the University of Michigan Health System and practices in Ann Arbor, MI. In his free time, he enjoys writing, science fiction, and spending time with his family.

Our Advisory Board

We would like to thank the following board members for providing guidance to the development of this series:

Dr. Lynda Baker, Associate Professor of Library and Information Science, Wayne State University, Detroit, MI

Nancy Bulgarelli, William Beaumont Hospital Library, Royal Oak, MI

Karen Imarisio, Bloomfield Township Public Library, Bloomfield Township, MI

Karen Morgan, Mardigian Library, University of Michigan-Dearborn, Dearborn, MI

Rosemary Orlando, St. Clair Shores Public Library, St. Clair Shores, MI

Health Reference Series Update Policy

The inaugural book in the *Health Reference Series* was the first edition of *Cancer Sourcebook* published in 1989. Since then, the *Series* has been enthusiastically received by librarians and in the medical community. In order to maintain the standard of providing high-quality health information for the layperson the editorial staff at Omnigraphics felt it was necessary to implement a policy of updating volumes when warranted.

Medical researchers have been making tremendous strides, and it is the purpose of the *Health Reference Series* to stay current with the most recent advances. Each decision to update a volume is made on an individual basis. Some of the considerations include how much new information is available and the feedback we receive from people who use the books. If there is a topic you would like to see added to the update list, or an area of medical concern you feel has not been adequately addressed, please write to:

Editor
Health Reference Series
Omnigraphics, Inc.
P.O. Box 31-1640
Detroit, MI 48231
E-mail: editorial@omnigraphics.com

Part One

Basic Information about Human Immunodeficiency Virus/ Acquired Immunodeficiency Syndrome (HIV/AIDS)

Chapter 1

Definition and Origin of HIV and AIDS

What is HIV?

HIV is the human immunodeficiency virus. It is the virus that can lead to acquired immune deficiency syndrome, or AIDS. The Centers for Disease Control and Prevention (CDC) estimates that about fifty-six thousand people in the United States contracted HIV in 2010, and that more than 1.2 million people in the United States are currently living with HIV infection.

HIV damages a person's body by destroying specific blood cells, called CD4+ T cells, which are crucial to helping the body fight diseases.

HIV is spread primarily by the following means:

- Not using a condom when having sex with a person who has HIV. All unprotected sex with someone who has HIV contains some risk. However, unprotected anal sex is riskier than unprotected vaginal sex, and among men who have sex with other men, unprotected receptive anal sex is riskier than unprotected insertive anal sex.

- Having multiple sex partners or the presence of other sexually transmitted diseases (STDs) can increase the risk of infection during sex. Unprotected oral sex can also be a risk for HIV transmission, but it is a much lower risk than anal or vaginal sex.

Excerpted from "HIV/AIDS Basics," Centers for Disease Control and Prevention, November 6, 2006. Updated by David A. Cooke, MD, FACP, November 2010.

- Sharing needles, syringes, rinse water, or other equipment used to prepare illicit drugs for injection.

- Being born to an infected mother. HIV can be passed from mother to child during pregnancy, birth, or breast-feeding.

Where did HIV come from?

The earliest known case of infection with HIV-1 in a human was detected in a blood sample collected in 1959 from a man in Kinshasa, Democratic Republic of the Congo. (How he became infected is not known.) Genetic analysis of this blood sample suggested that HIV-1 may have stemmed from a single virus in the late 1940s or early 1950s.

We know that the virus has existed in the United States since at least the mid- to late 1970s. From 1979 to 1981 rare types of pneumonia, cancer, and other illnesses were being reported by doctors in Los Angeles and New York among a number of male patients who had sex with other men. These were conditions not usually found in people with healthy immune systems.

In 1982 public health officials began to use the term "acquired immunodeficiency syndrome," or AIDS, to describe the occurrences of opportunistic infections, Kaposi sarcoma (a kind of cancer), and *Pneumocystis jiroveci* pneumonia in previously healthy people. Formal tracking (surveillance) of AIDS cases began that year in the United States.

In 1983, scientists discovered the virus that causes AIDS. The virus was at first named HTLV-III/LAV (human T-cell lymphotropic virus-type III/lymphadenopathy-associated virus) by an international scientific committee. This name was later changed to HIV (human immunodeficiency virus).

For many years scientists theorized as to the origins of HIV and how it appeared in the human population, most believing that HIV originated in other primates. Then in 1999, an international team of researchers reported that they had discovered the origins of HIV-1, the predominant strain of HIV in the developed world. A subspecies of chimpanzees native to west equatorial Africa had been identified as the original source of the virus. Many of these chimpanzees are infected with SIV (simian immunodeficiency virus). It is believed that mutant variants of this virus capable of infecting humans developed, and were introduced into the human population when hunters became exposed to infected blood. A rarer strain known as HIV-2 is believed to have similar origins to HIV-1, but probably originated in an African monkey species known as the sooty mangabey. Genetic studies suggest that both strains probably first spread across species during the first half of the twentieth century, but took considerably longer to spread outside remote areas.

What is AIDS?

AIDS stands for acquired immunodeficiency syndrome.

Acquired means that the disease is not hereditary but develops after birth from contact with a disease-causing agent (in this case, HIV).

Immunodeficiency means that the disease is characterized by a weakening of the immune system.

Syndrome refers to a group of symptoms that indicate or characterize a disease. In the case of AIDS, this can include the development of certain infections and/or cancers, as well as a decrease in the number of certain specific blood cells, called CD4+ T cells, which are crucial to helping the body fight disease.

Before the development of certain medications, people with HIV could progress to AIDS in just a few years. Currently, people can live much longer—even decades—with HIV before they develop AIDS. This is because of "highly active" combinations of medications that were introduced in the mid-1990s.

A diagnosis of AIDS is made by a physician using specific clinical or laboratory standards.

How long does it take for HIV to cause AIDS?

Prior to 1996, scientists estimated that about half the people with HIV would develop AIDS within ten years after becoming infected. This time varied greatly from person to person and depended on many factors, including a person's health status and their health-related behaviors.

Since 1996, the introduction of powerful antiretroviral therapies has dramatically changed the progression time between HIV infection and the development of AIDS. There are also other medical treatments that can prevent or cure some of the illnesses associated with AIDS, though the treatments do not cure AIDS itself. Because of these advances in drug therapies and other medical treatments, estimates of how many people will develop AIDS and how soon are being recalculated, revised, or are currently under study.

As with other diseases, early detection of infection allows for more options for treatment and preventative health care.

What is the evidence that HIV causes AIDS?

The epidemic of HIV and AIDS has attracted much attention both within and outside the medical and scientific communities. Much of this attention comes from the many social issues related to this disease such as sexuality, drug use, and poverty. Although the scientific evidence is overwhelming and compelling that HIV is the cause of AIDS, the disease process is still not completely understood. This incomplete understanding has led some persons to make statements that AIDS is not caused by an infectious agent or is caused by a virus that is not HIV. This is not only misleading, but may have dangerous consequences. Before the discovery of HIV, evidence from epidemiologic studies involving tracing of patients' sex partners and cases occurring in persons receiving transfusions of blood or blood clotting products had clearly indicated that the underlying cause of the condition was an infectious agent. Infection with HIV has been the sole common factor shared by AIDS cases throughout the world among men who have sex with men, transfusion recipients, persons with hemophilia, sex partners of infected persons, children born to infected women, and occupationally exposed healthcare workers.

The conclusion after more than twenty-eight years of scientific research is that people, if exposed to HIV through sexual contact or injecting drug use for example, may become infected with HIV. If they become infected, most will eventually develop AIDS.

Was HIV created in a lab?

No. HIV is a virus that has evolved over time and though it became a global pandemic only recently in human history, its origins are much older and found in nature.

Chapter 2

HIV Stages and Types

Chapter Contents

Section 2.1

The HIV Life Cycle

Excerpted from "The HIV Life Cycle," AIDSinfo.gov, May 2005.
Reviewed by David A. Cooke, MD, FACP, November 2010.

1. **Binding and Fusion:** The human immunodeficiency virus (HIV) begins its life cycle when it binds to a CD4 receptor and one of two co-receptors on the surface of a CD4+ T-lymphocyte. The virus then fuses with the host cell. After fusion, the virus releases ribonucleic acid (RNA), its genetic material, into the host cell.

2. **Reverse Transcription:** An HIV enzyme called reverse transcriptase converts the single-stranded HIV RNA to double-stranded HIV deoxyribonucleic acid (DNA).

3. **Integration:** The newly formed HIV DNA enters the host cell's nucleus, where an HIV enzyme called integrase "hides" the HIV DNA within the host cell's own DNA. The integrated HIV DNA is called provirus. The provirus may remain inactive for several years, producing few or no new copies of HIV.

4. **Transcription:** When the host cell receives a signal to become active, the provirus uses a host enzyme called RNA polymerase to create copies of the HIV genomic material, as well as shorter strands of RNA called messenger RNA (mRNA). The mRNA is used as a blueprint to make long chains of HIV proteins.

5. **Assembly:** An HIV enzyme called protease cuts the long chains of HIV proteins into smaller individual proteins. As the smaller HIV proteins come together with copies of HIV's RNA genetic material, a new virus particle is assembled.

6. **Budding:** The newly assembled virus pushes out ("buds") from the host cell. During budding, the new virus steals part of the cell's outer envelope. This envelope, which acts as a covering, is studded with protein/sugar combinations called HIV glycoproteins. These HIV glycoproteins are necessary for the

virus to bind CD4 and co- receptors. The new copies of HIV can now move on to infect other cells.

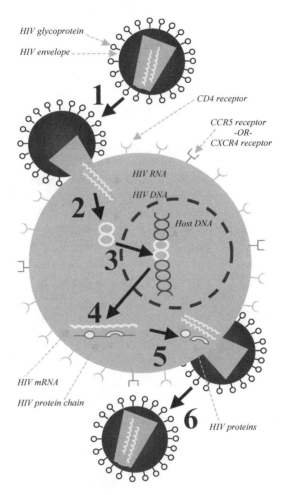

Figure 2.1. The HIV Life Cycle

Section 2.2

Stages of HIV Infection

Human immunodeficiency virus (HIV) infects cells in the immune system and the central nervous system. The main type of cell that HIV infects is the T helper lymphocyte. These cells play a crucial role in the immune system, by coordinating the actions of other immune system cells. A large reduction in the number of T helper cells seriously weakens the immune system.

HIV infects the T helper cell because it has the protein CD4 on its surface, which HIV uses to attach itself to the cell before gaining entry. This is why the T helper cell is sometimes referred to as a CD4+ lymphocyte. Once it has found its way into a cell, HIV produces new copies of itself, which can then go on to infect other cells.

Over time, HIV infection leads to a severe reduction in the number of T helper cells available to help fight disease. The process usually takes several years.

HIV infection can generally be broken down into four distinct stages: primary infection, clinically asymptomatic stage, symptomatic HIV infection, and progression from HIV to AIDS.

Stage 1: Primary HIV Infection

This stage of infection lasts for a few weeks and is often accompanied by a short flu-like illness. In up to about 20 percent of people the HIV symptoms are serious enough to consult a doctor, but the diagnosis of HIV infection is frequently missed.

During this stage there is a large amount of HIV in the peripheral blood and the immune system begins to respond to the virus by producing HIV antibodies and cytotoxic lymphocytes. This process is known as seroconversion. If an HIV antibody test is done before seroconversion is complete then it may not be positive.

Stage 2: Clinically Asymptomatic Stage

This stage lasts for an average of ten years and, as its name suggests, is free from major symptoms, although there may be swollen glands. The level of HIV in the peripheral blood drops to very low levels but people remain infectious and HIV antibodies are detectable in the blood, so antibody tests will show a positive result.

Research has shown that HIV is not dormant during this stage, but is very active in the lymph nodes. A test is available to measure the small amount of HIV that escapes the lymph nodes. This test, which measures HIV RNA (HIV genetic material), is referred to as the viral load test, and it has an important role in the treatment of HIV infection.

Stage 3: Symptomatic HIV Infection

Over time the immune system becomes severely damaged by HIV. This is thought to happen for three main reasons:

- The lymph nodes and tissues become damaged or "burnt out" because of the years of activity;
- HIV mutates and becomes more pathogenic, in other words stronger and more varied, leading to more T helper cell destruction;
- The body fails to keep up with replacing the T helper cells that are lost.

As the immune system fails, symptoms develop. Initially many of the symptoms are mild, but as the immune system deteriorates the symptoms worsen.

Symptomatic HIV infection is mainly caused by the emergence of opportunistic infections and cancers that the immune system would normally prevent. This stage of HIV infection is often characterized by multi-system disease and infections can occur in almost all body systems.

Treatment for the specific infection or cancer is often carried out, but the underlying cause is the action of HIV as it erodes the immune system. Unless HIV itself can be slowed down the symptoms of immune suppression will continue to worsen.

Stage 4: Progression from HIV to AIDS

As the immune system becomes more and more damaged the illnesses that occur become more and more severe, leading eventually to an acquired immunodeficiency syndrome (AIDS) diagnosis.

At present in the United Kingdom an AIDS diagnosis is confirmed if a person with HIV develops one or more of a specific number of severe opportunistic infections or cancers. In the United States, someone may also be diagnosed with AIDS if they have a very low count of T helper cells in their blood. It is possible for someone to be very ill with HIV but not have an AIDS diagnosis.

Examples of Opportunistic Infections and Cancers

Table 2.1 shows examples of common opportunistic infections and cancers and the body systems that they occur in.

Table 2.1. Common Opportunistic Infections and Where They Occur

System	Examples of Infection/Cancer
Respiratory system	*Pneumocystis jiroveci* pneumonia (PCP) Tuberculosis (TB) Kaposi sarcoma (KS)
Gastrointestinal system	Cryptosporidiosis Candida Cytomegalovirus (CMV) Isosporiasis Kaposi Sarcoma
Central/peripheral nervous system	Cytomegalovirus Toxoplasmosis Cryptococcosis Non-Hodgkin lymphoma Varicella Zoster Herpes simplex
Skin	Herpes simplex Kaposi sarcoma Varicella Zoster

World Health Organization Clinical Staging of HIV Disease in Adults and Adolescents (2006 Revision)

In resource-poor communities, medical facilities are sometimes poorly equipped, and it is not possible to use CD4 and viral load test results to determine the right time to begin antiretroviral treatment. The World Health Organization (WHO) has therefore developed a staging system for HIV disease based on clinical symptoms, which may be used to guide medical decision making.

Clinical Stage I

- Asymptomatic
- Persistent generalized lymphadenopathy

Clinical Stage II

- Moderate unexplained[1] weight loss (under 10 percent of presumed or measured body weight)[2]
- Recurrent respiratory tract infections (sinusitis, tonsillitis, otitis media, pharyngitis)
- Herpes zoster
- Angular cheilitis
- Recurrent oral ulceration
- Papular pruritic eruptions
- Seborrheic dermatitis
- Fungal nail infections

Clinical Stage III

- Unexplained[1] severe weight loss (over 10 percent of presumed or measured body weight)[2]
- Unexplained[1] chronic diarrhea for longer than one month
- Unexplained[1] persistent fever (intermittent or constant for longer than one month)
- Persistent oral candidiasis
- Oral hairy leukoplakia
- Pulmonary tuberculosis
- Severe bacterial infections (e.g. pneumonia, empyema, pyomyositis, bone or joint infection, meningitis, bacteremia)
- Acute necrotizing ulcerative stomatitis, gingivitis, or periodontitis
- Unexplained[1] anemia (below 8 g/dl), neutropenia (below 0.5 billion/l) and/or chronic thrombocytopenia (below 50 billion/l)

Clinical Stage IV[3]

- HIV wasting syndrome

- Pneumocystis pneumonia
- Recurrent severe bacterial pneumonia
- Chronic herpes simplex infection (orolabial, genital, or anorectal of more than one month's duration or visceral at any site)
- Esophageal candidiasis (or candidiasis of trachea, bronchi, or lungs)
- Extrapulmonary tuberculosis
- Kaposi sarcoma
- Cytomegalovirus infection retinitis or infection of other organs)
- Central nervous system toxoplasmosis
- HIV encephalopathy
- Extrapulmonary cryptococcosis including meningitis
- Disseminated non-tuberculous mycobacteria infection
- Progressive multifocal leukoencephalopathy
- Chronic cryptosporidiosis
- Chronic isosporiasis
- Disseminated mycosis (extrapulmonary histoplasmosis, coccidiomycosis)
- Recurrent septicemia (including non-typhoidal Salmonella)
- Lymphoma (cerebral or B cell non-Hodgkin)
- Invasive cervical carcinoma
- Atypical disseminated leishmaniasis
- Symptomatic HIV-associated nephropathy or HIV-associated cardiomyopathy

Notes

1. "Unexplained" refers to where the condition is not explained by other conditions.

2. Assessment of body weight among pregnant woman needs to consider the expected weight gain of pregnancy.

3. Some additional specific conditions can also be included in regional classifications (such as the reactivation of American trypanosomiasis [meningoencephalitis and/or myocarditis] in the WHO Region of the Americas and penicilliosis in Asia).

Sources

Centers for Disease Control and Prevention (18 December 1992), "1993 Revised Classification System for HIV Infection and Expanded Surveillance Case Definition for AIDS Among Adolescents and Adults" (http://www.cdc.gov/MMWR/preview/MMWRhtml/00018871,htm).

World Health Organization (7 August 2006), "WHO case definitions of HIV for surveillance and revised clinical staging and immunological classification of HIV-related disease in adults and children" (http://www.who.int/hiv/pub/guidelines/hivstaging/en/index.html).

Section 2.3

Acute HIV Infection

Acute HIV infection is caused by the human immunodeficiency virus (HIV), a virus that gradually destroys the immune system.

Causes

Primary or acute HIV infection occurs two to four weeks after infection with the human immunodeficiency virus (HIV). The virus is spread by:

- sexual contact;
- contaminated blood transfusions and blood products;
- injection drug use with contaminated needles and syringes;
- passing through the placenta from an infected, pregnant mother to the unborn baby;
- breastfeeding (rarely).

After someone is infected with HIV, blood tests can detect antibodies to the virus, even if they never had any symptoms of their infection. This is called HIV seroconversion (converting from HIV-negative to HIV-positive by blood testing), and usually occurs within three months of exposure, but on rare occasions can by delayed up to a year after infection.

Following the initial infection, there may be no further evidence of illness for the next ten years. This stage is called asymptomatic HIV infection.

Acute HIV infection can, but does not always, progress to early symptomatic HIV infection and to advanced HIV disease (acquired immunodeficiency syndrome [AIDS]). However, the vast majority of patients do ultimately progress to AIDS. To date there are a small number of people who have tested positive for HIV, but later no longer test positive and have no signs of disease. Although this is relatively rare, it provides evidence that the human body may be capable of removing the disease. These people are being carefully watched and studied.

HIV has spread throughout the world. Higher numbers of people with the disease are found in large metropolitan centers, inner cities, and among certain populations with high-risk behaviors.

Symptoms

Note: At the time of diagnosis with HIV, many people have not experienced any symptoms.

Acute HIV infection can appear like infectious mononucleosis, flu, or other viral illnesses. If symptoms occur, they are usually seen one to four weeks after becoming infected.

Any of the following symptoms can occur:

- decreased appetite;
- fatigue;
- fever;
- headache;
- malaise;
- muscle stiffness or aching;
- rash;
- sore throat;
- swollen lymph glands;
- ulcers of the mouth and esophagus.

These symptoms can last from a few days to four weeks, and then subside.

Exams and Tests

HIV enzyme-linked-immunosorbent serologic assay (ELISA)/Western blot test is usually negative or undetermined during the acute infection and will become positive over the next three months.

HIV ribonucleic acid (RNA) test ("viral load") is positive in patients with acute HIV infection.

Lower-than-normal CD4 (white blood cell) count may be a sign of a suppressed immune system. The CD4 count usually improves one to two months after acute infection.

White blood cell differential may show abnormalities.

Treatment

People with HIV infection need to be educated about the disease and its treatment so they can be active partners in making decisions with their healthcare provider.

There is still controversy about whether aggressive early treatment of HIV infection with anti-HIV medications (also called antiretroviral medications) will slow the long-term progression of disease. You should discuss this option with your healthcare provider.

Follow these healthy practices in the early stages of HIV infection:

- Avoid exposure to people with infectious illnesses.

- Avoid settings and situations that could lead to depression. Maintain positive social contacts, hobbies, interests, and pets.

- Eat a nutritious diet with enough calories.

- Get enough exercise, but don't wear yourself out.

- Keep stress to a minimum.

- Practice safer sex. The disease is highly transmissible, especially in the first months after infection.

Support Groups

You can often reduce the stress of illness by joining a support group where members share common experiences and problems.

Outlook (Prognosis)

There is no cure for HIV infection or AIDS. However, appropriate treatment can dramatically improve the length and quality of life for persons infected with HIV, and can delay the onset of AIDS.

Section 2.4

HIV Types, Subtypes, Groups, and Strains

Introduction to HIV Types, Groups, and Subtypes

Human immunodeficiency virus (HIV) is a highly variable virus which mutates very readily. This means there are many different strains of HIV, even within the body of a single infected person.

Based on genetic similarities, the numerous virus strains may be classified into types, groups, and subtypes.

What Is the Difference between HIV-1 and HIV-2?

There are two types of HIV: HIV-1 and HIV-2. Both types are transmitted by sexual contact, through blood, and from mother to child, and they appear to cause clinically indistinguishable AIDS. However, it seems that HIV-2 is less easily transmitted, and the period between initial infection and illness is longer in the case of HIV-2.

Worldwide, the predominant virus is HIV-1, and generally when people refer to HIV without specifying the type of virus they will be referring to HIV-1. The relatively uncommon HIV-2 type is concentrated in West Africa and is rarely found elsewhere.

How Many Subtypes of HIV-1 Are There?

The strains of HIV-1 can be classified into four groups: the "major" group M, the "outlier" group O, and two new groups, N and P. These four groups may represent four separate introductions of simian immunodeficiency virus into humans.

Group O appears to be restricted to west-central Africa and group N—a strain discovered in 1998 in Cameroon—is extremely rare. In 2009 a new strain closely relating to gorilla simian immunodeficiency virus was discovered in a Cameroonian woman. It was designated HIV-1 group P.[1] More than 90 percent of HIV-1 infections belong to

HIV-1 group M and, unless specified, the rest of this section will relate to HIV-1 group M only.

Within group M there are known to be at least nine genetically distinct subtypes (or clades) of HIV-1. These are subtypes A, B, C, D, F, G, H, J, and K.

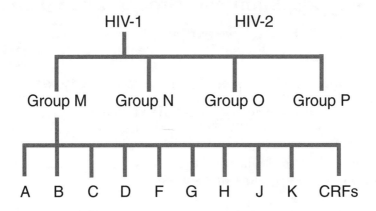

Figure 2.2. *The different levels of HIV classification*

Occasionally, two viruses of different subtypes can meet in the cell of an infected person and mix together their genetic material to create a new hybrid virus (a process similar to sexual reproduction, and sometimes called "viral sex").[2] Many of these new strains do not survive for long, but those that infect more than one person are known as "circulating recombinant forms" or CRFs. For example, the CRF A/B is a mixture of subtypes A and B.

The classification of HIV strains into subtypes and CRFs is a complex issue and the definitions are subject to change as new discoveries are made. Some scientists talk about subtypes A1, A2, A3, F1, and F2 instead of A and F, though others regard the former as sub-subtypes.

What about Subtypes E and I?

One of the CRFs is called A/E because it is thought to have resulted from hybridization between subtype A and some other "parent" subtype E. However, no one has ever found a pure form of subtype E. Confusingly, many people still refer to the CRF A/E as "subtype E" (in fact it is most correctly called CRF01_AE).[3]

A virus isolated in Cyprus was originally placed in a new subtype I, before being reclassified as a recombinant form A/G/I. It is now thought that this virus represents an even more complex CRF comprised of subtypes A, G, H, K, and unclassified regions. The designation "I" is no longer used.[4]

Where Are the Different Subtypes and CRFs Found?

The HIV-1 subtypes and CRFs are typically associated with certain geographical regions, with the most widespread being subtypes A and C. As studies have shown, individuals are increasingly presenting with subtypes not native to the country of diagnosis.[5][6] For example, a rise of non-B subtypes among men who have sex with men (MSM) in the United Kingdom has been identified.[7]

Subtype A and CRF A/G predominate in West and Central Africa, with subtype A possibly also causing much of the Russian epidemic.[8]

Historically, subtype B has been the most common subtype/CRF in Europe, the Americas, Japan, and Australia and is the predominant subtype found among MSM infected in Europe.[9] Although this remains the case, other subtypes are becoming more frequent and now account for at least 25 percent of new HIV infections in Europe.

Subtype C is predominant in Southern and East Africa, India, and Nepal. It has caused the world's worst HIV epidemics and is responsible for around half of all infections.

Subtype D is generally limited to East and Central Africa. CRF A/E is prevalent in Southeast Asia, but originated in Central Africa. Subtype F has been found in Central Africa, South America, and Eastern Europe. Subtype G and CRF A/G have been observed in West and East Africa and Central Europe.

Subtype H has only been found in Central Africa; J only in Central America; and K only in the Democratic Republic of Congo and Cameroon.

As a Belgium study highlighted, local epidemics can be better understood if subtypes, patient demographics, and transmission routes are recorded.[10] Furthermore, the availability of this data can be used to target risk groups more accurately and to improve the effectiveness of prevention strategies.

Are More Subtypes Likely to "Appear"?

It is almost certain that new HIV genetic subtypes and CRFs will be discovered in the future, and indeed that new ones will develop as virus recombination and mutation continue to occur. The current subtypes and CRFs will also continue to spread to new areas as the global epidemic continues.

The Implications of Variability

Does Subtype Affect Disease Progression?

A study presented in 2006 found that Ugandans infected with subtype D or recombinant strains incorporating subtype D developed AIDS sooner than those infected with subtype A, and also died sooner, if they did not receive antiretroviral treatment. The study's authors suggested that subtype D is more virulent because it is more effective at binding to immune cells.[11] This result was supported by another study presented in 2007, which found that Kenyan women infected with subtype D had more than twice the risk of death over six years compared with those infected with subtype A.[12] An earlier study of sex workers in Senegal, published in 1999, found that women infected with subtype C, D, or G were more likely to develop AIDS within five years of infection than those infected with subtype A.[13]

Several studies conducted in Thailand suggest that people infected with CRF A/E progress faster to AIDS and death than those infected with subtype B, if they do not receive antiretroviral treatment.[14]

Are There Differences in Transmission?

It has been observed that certain subtypes/CRFs are predominantly associated with specific modes of transmission. In particular, subtype B is spread mostly by homosexual contact and intravenous drug use (essentially via blood), while subtype C and CRF A/E tend to fuel heterosexual epidemics (via a mucosal route).

Whether there are biological causes for the observed differences in transmission routes remains the subject of debate. Some scientists, such as Dr. Max Essex of Harvard, believe such causes do exist. Among their claims are that subtype C and CRF A/E are transmitted much more efficiently during heterosexual sex than subtype B.[15,16] However, this theory has not been conclusively proven.[17,18]

More recent studies have looked for variation between subtypes in rates of mother-to-child transmission. One of these found that such transmission is more common with subtype D than subtype A.[19] Another reached the opposite conclusion (A worse than D), and also found that subtype C was more often transmitted that subtype D.[20] A third study concluded that subtype C is more transmissible than either D or A.[21] Other researchers have found no association between subtype and rates of mother-to-child transmission.[22,23,24,25]

Is It Possible to Be Infected More Than Once?

Until about 1994, it was generally thought that individuals do not become infected with multiple distinct HIV-1 strains. Since then, many cases of people co-infected with two or more strains have been documented.

All cases of co-infection were once assumed to be the result of people being exposed to the different strains more or less simultaneously, before their immune systems had had a chance to react. However, it is now thought that "superinfection" is also occurring. In these cases, the second infection occurred several months after the first. It would appear that the body's immune response to the first virus is sometimes not enough to prevent infection with a second strain, especially with a virus belonging to a different subtype. It is not yet known how commonly superinfection occurs, or whether it can take place only in special circumstances.[26,27]

Do HIV Antibody Tests Detect All Types, Groups, and Subtypes?

Initial tests for HIV are usually conducted using the enzyme immunoassay (EIA) or enzyme-linked-immunosorbent serologic assay (ELISA) antibody test or a rapid antibody test.

EIA tests which can detect either one or both types of HIV have been available for a number of years. According to the U.S. Centers for Disease Control and Prevention, current HIV-1 EIAs "can accurately identify infections with nearly all non-B subtypes and many infections with group O HIV subtypes."[28] However, because HIV-2 and group O infections are extremely rare in most countries, routine screening programs might not be designed to test for them. Anyone who believes they may have contracted HIV-2, HIV-1 group O, or one of the rarer subtypes of group M should seek expert advice.

Rapid tests—which can produce a result in less than an hour—are becoming increasingly popular. Most modern rapid HIV-1 tests are capable of detecting all the major subtypes of group M.[29] Rapid tests which can detect HIV-2 are also now available.[30]

What Are the Treatment Implications?

Although most current HIV-1 antiretroviral drugs were designed for use against subtype B, there is no compelling evidence that they are any less effective against other subtypes. Nevertheless, some subtypes may be more likely to develop resistance to certain drugs, and the types of mutations associated with resistance may vary. This is an important subject for future research.

The effectiveness of HIV-1 treatment is monitored using viral load tests. It has been demonstrated that some such tests are sensitive only to subtype B and can produce a significant underestimate of viral load if used to process other strains. The latest tests do claim to produce accurate results for most Group M subtypes, though not necessarily for Group O. It is important that health workers and patients are aware of the subtype/CRF they are testing for and of the limitations of the test they are applying.

Not all of the drugs used to treat HIV-1 infection are as effective against HIV-2. In particular, HIV-2 has a natural resistance to non-nucleoside reverse transcriptase inhibitor (NNRTI) antiretroviral drugs and they are therefore not recommended. As yet there is no Food and Drug Administration–licensed viral load test for HIV-2, and those designed for HIV-1 are not reliable for monitoring the other type. Instead, response to treatment may be monitored by following CD4+ T-cell counts and indicators of immune system deterioration. More research and clinical experience is needed to determine the most effective treatment for HIV-2.[31]

What Are the Implications For an AIDS Vaccine?

The development of an AIDS vaccine is affected by the range of virus subtypes as well as by the wide variety of human populations who need protection and who differ, for example, in their genetic make-up and their routes of exposure to HIV. In particular, the occurrence of superinfection indicates that an immune response triggered by a vaccine to prevent infection by one strain of HIV may not protect against all other strains. The increasing variety of subtypes found within countries suggests that the effectiveness of a vaccine is likely to vary between populations, unless an innovative method is developed which guards against many virus strains.[32]

Inevitably, different types of candidate vaccines will have to be tested against various viral strains in multiple vaccine trials, conducted in both high-income and developing countries.

References

1. Plantier, J.C. (2009) "A new human immunodeficiency virus derived from gorillas", *Nature Medicine*, 2nd August.

2. Burke DS (1997, September) "Recombination of HIV: An Important Viral Evolutionary Strategy" *Emerging Infectious Diseases* 3(3).

3. Los Alamos National Laboratory (2005–6) "The Circulating Recombinant Forms (CRFs)"

4. Gao F et. al (1998, December) "An Isolate of Human Immunodeficiency Virus Type 1 Originally Classified as Subtype I Represents a Complex Mosaic Comprising Three Different Group M Subtypes (A, G, and I)" *Journal of Virology* 72(12).

5. Le Vu S, et. al (2010, 9th September) "Population-based HIV-1 incidence in France, 2003–08: a modelling analysis" *The Lancet* 10.

6. Chalmet K, et. al (2010) "Epidemiological study of phylogenetic transmission clusters in a local HIV-1 epidemic reveals distinct differences between subtype B and non-B infections" *BMC Infectious Diseases* 10(262).

7. Fox J, et. al (2010) "Epidemiology of non-B clade forms of HIV-1 in men who have sex with men in the UK" *AIDS* 24.

8. Bobkov AF et. al (2004, October) "Temporal trends in the HIV-1 epidemic in Russia: predominance of subtype A" *J Med Virol* 74(2).

9. Le Vu S, et. al (2010, 9th September) "Population-based HIV-1 incidence in France, 2003–08: a modelling analysis" *The Lancet* 10.

10. Chalmet K, et. al (2010) "Epidemiological study of phylogenetic transmission clusters in a local HIV-1 epidemic reveals distinct differences between subtype B and non-B infections" *BMC Infectious Diseases* 10(262).

11. Laeyendecker O et. al (2006, February) "The Effect of HIV Subtype on Rapid Disease Progression in Rakai, Uganda" 13th Conference on Retroviruses and Opportunistic Infections (abstract no. 44LB).

12. Baeten D et. al (2007, 15th April) "HIV-1 subtype D infection is associated with faster disease progression than subtype A, in spite of similar HIV-1 plasma viral loads" *Journal of Infectious Disease* 195(8).

13. Kanki PJ et. al (1999, January) "Human Immunodeficiency Virus Type 1 Subtypes Differ in Disease Progression" *Journal of Infectious Diseases*, 179(1).

14. Nelson KE et. al (2007, November) "Survival of blood donors and their spouses with HIV-1 subtype E (CRF01 A_E) infection in northern Thailand, 1992–2007" *AIDS* 21(S6).

15. Bhoopat L et. al (2001, December) "In vivo identification of Langerhans and related dendritic cells infected with HIV-1 subtype E in vaginal mucosa of asymptomatic patients" *Modern Pathology* 14(12).

16. Essex M (1996, 20th March) "Retroviral vaccines: challenges for the developing world" *AIDS Res Hum Retroviruses*, 12(5).

17. Pope M et. al (1997, October) "Human immunodeficiency virus type 1 strains of subtypes B and E replicate in cutaneous dendritic cell-T-cell mixtures without displaying subtype-specific tropism" *J Virol* 71(10).

18. Dittmar MT et. al (1997, October) "Langerhans cell tropism of human immunodeficiency virus type 1 subtype A through F isolates derived from different transmission groups" *J Virol* 71(10).

19. Yang, Li et. al (2003, 25th July) "Genetic diversity of HIV-1 in western Kenya: subtype-specific differences in mother-to-child transmission" *AIDS* 17(11).

20. Blackard J T et. al (2001, 1st September) "HIV-1 LTR subtype and perinatal transmission" *J Virology*, 287(2).

21. Renjifo B et. al (2004, 20th August) "Preferential in-utero transmission of HIV-1 type C as compared to HIV-1 subtype A or D" *AIDS* 18(12).

22. Murray MC et. al (2000, February) "Effect of human immunodeficiency virus (HIV) type 1 viral genotype on mother-to-child transmission of HIV-1" *J Infect Dis* 181(2).

23. Tranchat C et. al (1999, November) "Maternal humoral factors associated with perinatal human immunodeficiency virus type-1 transmission in a cohort from Kigali, Rwanda, 1988–1994" *J Infect* 39(3).

24. Tapia N et. al (2003, March) "Influence of human immunodeficiency virus type 1 subtype on mother-to-child transmission" *Journal of General Virology* 84(Pt. 3).

25. Martinez AM et. al (2006, March) "Determinants of HIV-1 Mother-to-Child transmission in Southern Brazil" *Anais da Academia Brasileira de Ciencias*, 78(1).

26. Gross KL et. al (2004, 23rd July) "HIV-1 superinfection and viral diversity" *AIDS* 18(11).

27. Fultz PN (2004, 2nd January) "HIV-1 superinfections: omens for vaccine efficacy?" *AIDS* 18(1).

28. *Morbidity and Mortality Weekly Report* (2001, 9th November) "Revised Guidelines for HIV Counseling, Testing, and Referral" 50(RR19);1–58.

29. Phillips S et. al (2000, July) "Diagnosis of Human Immunodeficiency Virus Type 1 Infection with Different Subtypes Using Rapid Tests" *Clinical and Diagnostic Laboratory Immunology*, 7(4).

30. CDC (2004, 2nd November) "OraQuick Rapid HIV Test for Oral Fluid—Frequently Asked Questions."

31. CDC (2004, 23rd November) "Human Immunodeficiency Virus Type 2."

32. Fox J, et. al (2010) "Epidemiology of non-B clade forms of HIV-1 in men who have sex with men in the UK" *AIDS* 24.

Section 2.5

HIV Superinfection

"What Do We Know about HIV Superinfection?" Reprinted with permission from the Center for AIDS Prevention Studies (CAPS), University of California at San Francisco (www.caps.ucsf.edu). © 2006 Regents of the University of California. Reviewed by David A. Cooke, MD, FACP, November 2010.

What is dual infection, co-infection, superinfection?

Dual infection is when a person is infected with two or more strains of human immunodeficiency virus (HIV). That person may have acquired both strains simultaneously from a dually infected partner or from multiple partners. A different strain of the virus is one that can be genetically distinguished from the first in a "family" or phylogenetic tree.

Acquisition of different HIV strains from multiple partners is often called co-infection if all the virus strains were acquired prior to seroconversion, that is, very early before any HIV infection is recognized.

Acquisition of different HIV strains from multiple partners is called superinfection if the second virus is acquired after seroconversion when the first virus strain already has been established.[1] Superinfection and re-infection mean the same thing.

Dual infections can be sequentially expressed, which can make co-infection look like superinfection. Sequentially expressed dual infections (SEDI) may occur because immune responses against the predominant virus may allow other virus strains in the body to be expressed. Random shifts in evolving virus populations can also occur, which could look like superinfection even though dual infection was present from the beginning.

Why does superinfection matter?

Superinfection is a concern because it may be a way for someone who is HIV-positive to acquire drug resistance, and it may lead to more rapid disease progression.[2,3] Research on when superinfection may or may not occur could identify types of immune responses that may protect against infection. This could guide the development of HIV vaccines.

People who are HIV-positive and have HIV-positive partners often ask about superinfection. Public health officials need information about superinfection in order to craft messages that help people understand the possible risks of unprotected sexual intercourse among HIV-positive persons, without creating undue anxiety that could undermine rewarding relationships between HIV-positive persons and disclosure of HIV status with prospective new partners.

Does superinfection occur?

Many scientists believe that superinfection can occur. Research in monkeys has indicated that superinfection with viruses like HIV can occur.[4,5] Sixteen people with SEDI (apparent superinfection) have been reported in the scientific literature, including injection drug users in Asia, women in Africa, and men in Europe and the United States. Laboratory analysis in some of these reports suggested that the second virus that appeared in these individuals was not present earlier in the course of infection, which suggests superinfection. The sensitivity of these laboratory assays is limited, and source partners have not been identified, so there is no way to know for sure when the second virus was acquired.

Who is at highest risk?

Ninety-five percent of apparent superinfection cases have occurred during the first three years of infection. Studies have found evidence of superinfection in 2 to 5 percent of persons in the first year of infection.[6–9] Intermittent treatment in acute or recent HIV infection may prolong superinfection susceptibility.[10,11]

In contrast, studies in persons with longer term infection have found no evidence of superinfection. One study found no cases after 1,072 person-years of observation.[12] Another found none after 215 person-years of observation among intravenous drug users.[13] A third found none after 233 person-years and 20,859 exposures through unprotected sex.[14]

It is possible that people with very low viral load in their blood may be more susceptible to superinfection. Low viral load in the blood can occur during combination antiretroviral therapy or in "healthy non-progressors." Antiviral immune responses and viral interference are lower in persons with low viral load, so superinfection may occur more frequently.[15] More research is needed to know for sure.

Is it bad to have more than one virus?

Dual infection can have a harmful effect on the health of HIV-positive persons. Superinfected individuals may have higher viral loads and lower CD4 counts, which causes more rapid disease progression.[2,3] Disease progression can accelerate after a second virus appears.[1]

Superinfection may also affect treatment of HIV, as it increases the likelihood of drug resistance.[16] HIV-positive persons with dual infection may not respond as well to available antiretroviral medication due to resistant strains.

What don't we know?

There is a lot we still do not know about superinfection. First of all, we need to be more sure whether superinfection actually occurs between HIV-positive persons. A definitive case of superinfection has not been documented, which would require that the timing of the second infection be traced to initiation of a relationship with a new sexual partner.

Second, we need to understand how and when superinfection occurs. Among researchers some consensus is developing about the idea that HIV-positive persons in early infection—and particularly the first year of infection—may be at higher risk for superinfection than HIV-positive persons with chronic infection.[17] We also should determine whether persons with suppressed viral load on treatment are susceptible to superinfection.

Third, we need to know how to protect against superinfection. If superinfection is rare, or if it only happens in recent infection, it is important to determine what mechanisms make an HIV-positive person immune to acquiring a second virus. It would be important to know if exposure to different viral strains may provide protective immunity against superinfection.[18]

Lastly, we must continue to provide up-to-date scientific data on superinfection, its causes and consequences to HIV-positive persons and healthcare professionals who work with them.

What can we recommend right now?

Counseling about superinfection should be based on understanding the individual's sexual relationships. Before providing advice about superinfection, the counselor should know whether the individual is in a continuing relationship with another HIV-positive partner, whether the person routinely seeks out other HIV-positive partners for unprotected sex, and whether there is disclosure of HIV status with prospective partners. This background should inform the discussion about the risks and benefits of sex among HIV-positive partners. If the counselor does not have time to consider these personal issues, it would probably be best to simply say that "There is not enough information available about superinfection. If superinfection occurs at all, it probably occurs in the first few years after infection. After that, it may be rare."

Even less is known about superinfection as a result of sharing needles, although it is reasonable to expect that the same pattern of initial high risk followed by low risk during chronic infection may occur. However, because intravenous drug users are at high risk of hepatitis C infections from sharing needles, efforts to obtain clean needles through needle exchange should always be emphasized.

Interested persons should be referred to ongoing research studies so that important gaps in information can be filled.[19]

People with multiple sexual partners, or partners with multiple partners, should be counseled regarding the risks of other sexually transmitted infections. Vaccination for hepatitis B and periodic testing for syphilis is warranted.

Says who?

1. Smith DM, Richman DD, Little SJ. HIV superinfection. *Journal of Infectious Diseases*. 2005;192:438–44.

2. Gottlieb GS, Nickle DC, Jensen MA, et al. Dual HIV-1 infection associated with rapid disease progression. *The Lancet*. 2004;363:610–22.

3. Grobler J, Gray CM, Rademeyer C, et al. Incidence of HIV-1 dual infection and its association with increased viral load set point in a cohort of HIV-1 subtype c-infected female sex workers. *Journal of Infectious Diseases*. 2004;190:1355–59.

4. Otten RA, Ellenberger DL, Adams DR, et al. Identification of a window period for susceptibility to dual infection with two distinct human immunodeficiency virus type 2 isolates in a Macaca nemestrina model. *Journal of Infectious Diseases*. 1999;180:673–84.

5. Fultz PN, Srinivasan A, Greene CR, et al. Superinfection of a chimpanzee with a second strain of human immunodeficiency virus. *Journal of Virology*. 1987;61:4026–29.

6. Angel JB, Hu YW, Kravcik S, et al. Virological evaluation of the "Ottawa case" indicates no evidence for HIV-1 superinfection. *AIDS*. 2004;18:331–34.

7. Smith DM, Wong JK, Hightower GK, et al. Incidence of HIV superinfection following primary infection. *Journal of the American Medical Association*. 2004;292:1177–78.

8. Hu DJ, Subbarao S, Vanichseni S, et al. Frequency of HIV-1 dual subtype infections, including intersubtype superinfections, among injection drug users in Bangkok, Thailand. *AIDS*. 2005;19:303–8.

9. Grant R, McConnell J, Marcus J, et al. High frequency of apparent HIV-1 superinfection in a seroconverter cohort. 12th Conference on Retroviruses and Opportunistic Infections. 2005. Abst #287.

10. Altfeld M, Allen TM, Yu XG, et al. HIV-1 superinfection despite broad CD8+ T-cell responses containing replication of the primary virus. *Nature*. 2002;420:434–39.

11. Jost S, Bernard M, Kaiser L, et al. A patient with HIV-1 superinfection. *New England Journal of Medicine*. 2002;347:731–36.

12. Gonzales MJ, Delwart E, Rhee SY, et al. Lack of detectable human immunodeficiency virus type 1 superinfection during 1,072 person-years of observation. *Journal of Infectious Diseases*. 2003;188:397–405.

13. Tsui R, Herring BL, Barbour JD, et al. Human immunodeficiency virus type 1 superinfection was not detected following 215 years of injection drug user exposure. *Journal of Virology*. 2004;78:94–103.

14. Grant R, McConnell J, Herring B, et al. No superinfection among seroconcordant couples after well-defined exposure. International Conference on AIDS, Bangkok, Thailand, 2004. Abst #ThPeA6949.

15. Marcus J, McConnell J, Liegler T, et al. Highly divergent viral lineages in blood DNA appear frequently during suppressive therapy in persons exposed to superinfection. 13th Conference on Retroviruses and Opportunistic Infections. 2006. Abst #297.

16. Smith DM, Wong JK, High-tower GK, et al. HIV drug resistance acquired through superinfection. *AIDS*. 2005;19:1251–56.

17. Gross KL, Porco TC, Grant RM. HIV-1 superinfection and viral diversity. *AIDS*. 2004;18:1513–20.

18. McConnell J, Liu Y, Kreis C, et al. Broad neutralization of HIV-1 variants in couples without evidence of systemic super-infection. 13th Conference on Retroviruses and Opportunistic Infections. 2006. Abst #92.

19. HIV+ persons who have HIV+ partners residing or visiting San Francisco can call the Positive Partners Study 1-415-734-4878.

Chapter 3

How HIV Causes AIDS

Human immunodeficiency virus (HIV) destroys CD4-positive (CD4+) T cells, which are white blood cells crucial to maintaining the function of the human immune system. As HIV attacks these cells, the person infected with the virus is less equipped to fight off infection and disease, ultimately resulting in the development of acquired immunodeficiency syndrome (AIDS).

Most people who are infected with HIV can carry the virus for years before developing any serious symptoms. But over time, HIV levels increase in the blood while the number of CD4+ T cells declines. Antiretroviral medicines can help reduce the amount of virus in the body, preserve CD4+ T cells, and dramatically slow the destruction of the immune system.

People who are not infected with HIV and generally are in good health have roughly 800 to 1,200 CD4+ T cells per cubic millimeter (mm^3) of blood. Some people who have been diagnosed with AIDS have fewer than 50 CD4+ T cells in their entire body.

More on How HIV Causes AIDS

A significant component of the research effort of the National Institute of Allergy and Infectious Diseases (NIAID) is devoted to the pathogenesis of HIV disease. Studies on pathogenesis address the com-

Reprinted from "How HIV Causes AIDS," April 2009, and "More on How HIV Causes AIDS," January 2009, National Institute of Allergy and Infectious Diseases, National Institutes of Health.

plex mechanisms that result in the destruction of the immune system of an HIV-infected person. A detailed understanding of HIV and how it establishes infection and causes AIDS is crucial to identifying and developing effective drugs and vaccines to fight HIV and AIDS. This chapter summarizes the state of knowledge in this area.

Overview

Untreated HIV disease is characterized by a gradual deterioration of immune function. Most notably, crucial immune cells called CD4-positive (CD4+) T cells are disabled and killed during the typical course of infection. These cells, sometimes called "T-helper cells," play a central role in the immune response, signaling other cells in the immune system to perform their special functions.

A healthy, uninfected person usually has 800 to 1,200 CD4+ T cells per cubic millimeter (mm^3) of blood. During untreated HIV infection, the number of these cells in a person's blood progressively declines. When the CD4+ T cell count falls below $200/mm^3$, a person becomes particularly vulnerable to the opportunistic infections and cancers that typify AIDS, the end stage of HIV disease. People with AIDS often suffer infections of the lungs, intestinal tract, brain, eyes, and other organs, as well as debilitating weight loss, diarrhea, neurologic conditions, and cancers such as Kaposi sarcoma and certain types of lymphomas.

Most scientists think that HIV causes AIDS by directly inducing the death of CD4+ T cells or interfering with their normal function, and by triggering other events that weaken a person's immune function. For example, the network of signaling molecules that normally regulates a person's immune response is disrupted during HIV disease, impairing a person's ability to fight other infections. The HIV-mediated destruction of the lymph nodes and related immunologic organs also plays a major role in causing the immunosuppression seen in people with AIDS. Immunosuppression by HIV is confirmed by the fact that medicines, which interfere with the HIV life cycle, preserve CD4+ T cells and immune function as well as delay clinical illness.

Scope of the HIV Epidemic

Although HIV was first identified in 1983, studies of previously stored blood samples indicate that the virus entered the U.S. population sometime in the late 1970s. In the United States, 886,575 cases of AIDS, and 501,669 deaths among people with AIDS had been reported to the Centers for Disease Control and Prevention (CDC) by the end of 2002. Approximately 40,000 new HIV infections occur each year in the

United States, 70 percent of them among men and 30 percent among women. Of the new infections, approximately 40 percent are from male-to-male contact, 30 percent from heterosexual contact, and 25 percent from injection drug use. Minority groups in the United States have also been disproportionately affected by the epidemic.

Worldwide, an estimated 38 million people were living with HIV/AIDS as of December 2003, according to the Joint United Nations Programme on HIV/AIDS (UNAIDS). Through 2003, cumulative AIDS-associated deaths worldwide numbered more than 20 million. Globally, approximately 5 million new HIV infections and approximately 3 million AIDS-related deaths, including an estimated 490,000 children under fifteen years old, occurred in the year 2003 alone.

HIV Is a Retrovirus

HIV belongs to a class of viruses called retroviruses. Retroviruses are RNA (ribonucleic acid) viruses, and in order to replicate (duplicate). they must make a DNA (deoxyribonucleic acid) copy of their RNA. It is the DNA genes that allow the virus to replicate.

Like all viruses, HIV can replicate only inside cells, commandeering the cell's machinery to reproduce. Only HIV and other retroviruses, however, once inside a cell, use an enzyme called reverse transcriptase to convert their RNA into DNA, which can be incorporated into the host cell's genes.

Slow Viruses

HIV belongs to a subgroup of retroviruses known as lentiviruses, or "slow" viruses. The course of infection with these viruses is characterized by a long interval between initial infection and the onset of serious symptoms.

Other lentiviruses infect nonhuman species. For example, the feline immunodeficiency virus (FIV) infects cats and the simian immunodeficiency virus (SIV) infects monkeys and other nonhuman primates. Like HIV in humans, these animal viruses primarily infect immune system cells, often causing immune deficiency and AIDS-like symptoms. These viruses and their hosts have provided researchers with useful, albeit imperfect, models of the HIV disease process in people.

Structure of HIV

The viral envelope. HIV has a diameter of 1/10,000 of a millimeter and is spherical in shape. The outer coat of the virus, known as the viral envelope, is composed of two layers of fatty molecules called lipids, taken from the membrane of a human cell when a newly formed virus particle buds from the cell. Evidence from NIAID-supported research indicates that HIV may enter and exit cells through special areas of the cell membrane known as "lipid rafts." These rafts are high in cholesterol and glycolipids and may provide a new target for blocking HIV.

Embedded in the viral envelope are proteins from the host cell, as well as seventy-two copies (on average) of a complex HIV protein (frequently called "spikes") that protrudes through the surface of the virus particle (virion). This protein, known as Env, consists of a cap made of three molecules called glycoprotein (gp) 120, and a stem consisting of three gp41 molecules that anchor the structure in the viral envelope. Much of the research to develop a vaccine against HIV has focused on these envelope proteins.

The viral core. Within the envelope of a mature HIV particle is a bullet-shaped core or capsid, made of two thousand copies of another viral protein, p24. The capsid surrounds two single strands of HIV RNA, each of which has a copy of the virus's nine genes. Three of these genes, gag, pol, and env, contain information needed to make structural proteins for new virus particles. The env gene, for example, codes for a protein called gp160 that is broken down by a viral enzyme to form gp120 and gp41, the components of Env.

Six regulatory genes, tat, rev, nef, vif, vpr, and vpu, contain information necessary to produce proteins that control the ability of HIV to infect a cell, produce new copies of virus, or cause disease. The protein encoded by nef, for instance, appears necessary for the virus to replicate efficiently, and the vpu-encoded protein influences the release of new virus particles from infected cells. Recently, researchers discovered that Vif (the protein encoded by the vif gene) interacts with an antiviral defense protein in host cells (APOBEC3G), causing inactivation of the antiviral effect and enhancing HIV replication. This interaction may serve as a new target for antiviral drugs.

The ends of each strand of HIV RNA contain an RNA sequence called the long terminal repeat (LTR). Regions in the LTR act as switches to control production of new viruses and can be triggered by proteins from either HIV or the host cell.

The core of HIV also includes a protein called p7, the HIV nucleocapsid protein. Three enzymes carry out later steps in the virus's life cycle: reverse transcriptase, integrase, and protease. Another HIV protein called p17, or the HIV matrix protein, lies between the viral core and the viral envelope.

Replication Cycle of HIV

Entry of HIV into cells. Infection typically begins when an HIV particle, which contains two copies of the HIV RNA, encounters a cell with a surface molecule called cluster designation 4 (CD4). Cells carrying this molecule are known as CD4+ cells.

One or more of the virus's gp120 molecules binds tightly to CD4 molecule(s) on the cell's surface. The binding of gp120 to CD4 results in a conformational change in the gp120 molecule allowing it to bind to a second molecule on the cell surface known as a co-receptor. The envelope of the virus and the cell membrane then fuse, leading to entry of the virus into the cell. The gp41 of the envelope is critical to the fusion process. Drugs that block either the binding or the fusion process are being developed and tested in clinical trials. The Food and Drug Administration (FDA) has approved one of the so-called fusion inhibitors, T20, for use in HIV-infected people.

Studies have identified multiple co-receptors for different types of HIV strains. These co-receptors are promising targets for new anti-HIV drugs, some of which are now being tested in preclinical and clinical studies. Agents that block the co-receptors are showing particular promise as potential microbicides that could be used in gels or creams to prevent HIV transmission. In the early stage of HIV disease, most people harbor viruses that use, in addition to CD4, a receptor called CCR5 to enter their target cells. With disease progression, the spectrum of co-receptor usage expands in approximately 50 percent of patients to include other receptors, notably a molecule called CXCR4. Virus that uses CCR5 is called R5 HIV and virus that uses CXCR4 is called X4 HIV.

Although CD4+ T cells appear to be the main targets of HIV, other immune system cells with and without CD4 molecules on their surfaces are infected as well. Among these are long-lived cells called monocytes and macrophages, which apparently can harbor large quantities of the virus without being killed, thus acting as reservoirs of HIV. CD4+ T cells also serve as important reservoirs of HIV; a small proportion of these cells harbor HIV in a stable, inactive form. Normal immune processes may activate these cells, resulting in the production of new HIV virions.

Cell-to-cell spread of HIV also can occur through the CD4-mediated fusion of an infected cell with an uninfected cell.

Reverse transcription. In the cytoplasm of the cell, HIV reverse transcriptase converts viral RNA into DNA, the nucleic acid form in which the cell carries its genes. Fifteen of the twenty-six antiviral drugs approved in the United States for treating people with HIV infection work by interfering with this stage of the viral life cycle.

Integration. The newly made HIV DNA moves to the cell's nucleus, where it is spliced into the host's DNA with the help of HIV integrase. HIV DNA that enters the DNA of the cell is called a provirus. Several drugs that target the integrase enzyme are in the early stages of development and are being investigated for their potential as antiretroviral agents.

Transcription. For a provirus to produce new viruses, RNA copies must be made that can be read by the host cell's protein-making machinery. These copies are called messenger RNA (mRNA), and production of mRNA is called transcription, a process that involves the host cell's own enzymes. Viral genes in concert with the cellular machinery control this process; the tat gene, for example, encodes a protein that accelerates transcription. Genomic RNA is also transcribed for later incorporation in the budding virion.

Cytokines, proteins involved in the normal regulation of the immune response, also may regulate transcription. Molecules such as tumor necrosis factor (TNF)-alpha and interleukin (IL)-6, secreted in elevated levels by the cells of HIV-infected people, may help to activate HIV proviruses. Other infections, by organisms such as *Mycobacterium tuberculosis*, also may enhance transcription by inducing the secretion of cytokines.

Translation. After HIV mRNA is processed in the cell's nucleus, it is transported to the cytoplasm. HIV proteins are critical to this process; for example, a protein encoded by the rev gene allows mRNA encoding HIV structural proteins to be transferred from the nucleus to the cytoplasm. Without the rev protein, structural proteins are not made. In the cytoplasm, the virus co-opts the cell's protein-making machinery—including structures called ribosomes—to make long chains of viral proteins and enzymes, using HIV mRNA as a template. This process is called translation.

Assembly and budding. Newly made HIV core proteins, enzymes, and genomic RNA gather inside the cell and an immature viral particle forms and buds off from the cell, acquiring an envelope that includes both cellular and HIV proteins from the cell membrane. During this part of the viral life cycle, the core of the virus is immature and the virus is not yet infectious. The long chains of proteins and enzymes that make up the immature viral core are now cut into smaller pieces by a viral enzyme called protease.

This step results in infectious viral particles. Drugs called protease inhibitors interfere with this step of the viral life cycle. The FDA has approved eight such drugs—saquinavir, ritonavir, indinavir, amprenavir, nelfinavir, fosamprenavir, atazanavir, and lopinavir—for marketing in the United States. Recently, an HIV inhibitor that targets a unique step in the viral life cycle, very late in the process of viral maturation, has been identified and is currently undergoing further development.

Recently, researchers have discovered that virus budding from the host cell is much more complex than previously thought. Binding between the HIV Gag protein and molecules in the cell directs the accumulation of HIV components in special intracellular sacks, called multivesicular bodies (MVB), that normally function to carry proteins out of the cell. In this way, HIV actively hitchhikes out of the cell in the MVB by hijacking normal cell machinery and mechanisms. Discovery of this budding pathway has revealed several potential points for intervening in the viral replication cycle.

Transmission of HIV

Among adults, HIV is spread most commonly during sexual intercourse with an infected partner. During intercourse, the virus can enter the body through the mucosal linings of the vagina, vulva, penis, or rectum or, rarely, via the mouth and possibly the upper gastrointestinal tract after oral sex. The likelihood of transmission is increased by factors that may damage these linings, especially other sexually transmitted infections that cause ulcers or inflammation.

Research suggests that immune system cells of the dendritic cell type, which live in the mucosa, may begin the infection process after sexual exposure by binding to and carrying the virus from the site of infection to the lymph nodes where other immune system cells become infected. A molecule on the surface of dendritic cells, DC-SIGN, may be critical for this transmission process.

HIV also can be transmitted by contact with infected blood, most often by the sharing of needles or syringes contaminated with minute quantities of blood containing the virus. The risk of acquiring HIV from blood transfusions is extremely small in the United States, as all blood products in this country are screened routinely for evidence of the virus.

Almost all HIV-infected children in the United States get the virus from their mothers before or during birth. In the United States, approximately 25 percent of pregnant HIV-infected women not receiving antiretroviral therapy have passed on the virus to their babies. In 1994, researchers showed that a specific regimen of the drug AZT (zidovudine) can reduce the risk of transmission of HIV from mother to baby by two-thirds. The use of combinations of antiretroviral drugs and simpler drug regimens has further reduced the rate of mother-to-child HIV transmission in the United States.

In developing countries, cheap and simple antiviral drug regimens have been proven to significantly reduce mother-to-child transmission at birth in resource-poor settings. Unfortunately, the virus also may be transmitted from an HIV-infected mother to her infant via breastfeeding. Moreover, due to the use of medicines to prevent transmission at delivery, breastfeeding may become the most common mode of HIV infection in infants. Thus, development of affordable alternatives to breastfeeding is greatly needed.

Early Events in HIV Infection

Once it enters the body, HIV infects a large number of CD4+ cells and replicates rapidly. During this acute or primary phase of infection, the blood contains many viral particles that spread throughout the body, seeding various organs, particularly the lymphoid organs.

Two to four weeks after exposure to the virus, up to 70 percent of HIV-infected people suffer flu-like symptoms related to the acute infection. Their immune system fights back with killer T cells (CD8+ T cells) and B-cell-produced antibodies, which dramatically reduce HIV levels. A person's CD4+ T cell count may rebound somewhat and even approach its original level. A person may then remain free of HIV-related symptoms for years despite continuous replication of HIV in the lymphoid organs that had been seeded during the acute phase of infection.

One reason that HIV is unique is the fact that despite the body's aggressive immune responses, which are sufficient to clear most viral infections, some HIV invariably escapes. This is due in large part to the high rate of mutations that occur during the process of HIV replication. Even when the virus does not avoid the immune system by mutating, the body's best soldiers in the fight against HIV—certain subsets of killer T cells that recognize HIV—may be depleted or become dysfunctional.

In addition, early in the course of HIV infection, people may lose HIV-specific CD4+ T cell responses that normally slow the replication of viruses. Such responses include the secretion of interferons and other antiviral factors, and the orchestration of CD8+ T cells.

42

Finally, the virus may hide within the chromosomes of an infected cell and be shielded from surveillance by the immune system. Such cells can be considered as a latent reservoir of the virus. Because the antiviral agents currently in our therapeutic arsenal attack actively replicating virus, they are not effective against hidden, inactive viral DNA (so-called provirus). New strategies to purge this latent reservoir of HIV have become one of the major goals for current research efforts.

Course of HIV Infection

Among people enrolled in large epidemiologic studies in Western countries, the median time from infection with HIV to the development of AIDS-related symptoms has been approximately ten to twelve years in the absence of antiretroviral therapy. Researchers, however, have observed a wide variation in disease progression. Approximately 10 percent of HIV-infected people in these studies have progressed to AIDS within the first two to three years following infection, while up to 5 percent of individuals in the studies have stable CD4+ T cell counts and no symptoms even after twelve or more years.

Factors such as age or genetic differences among individuals, the level of virulence of an individual strain of virus, and co-infection with other microbes may influence the rate and severity of disease progression. Drugs that fight the infections associated with AIDS have improved and prolonged the lives of HIV-infected people by preventing or treating conditions such as *Pneumocystis carinii* pneumonia, cytomegalovirus disease, and diseases caused by a number of fungi.

HIV co-receptors and disease progression. Recent research has shown that most infecting strains of HIV use a co-receptor molecule called CCR5, in addition to the CD4 molecule, to enter certain of its target cells. HIV-infected people with a specific mutation in one of their two copies of the gene for this receptor may have a slower disease course than people with two normal copies of the gene. Rare individuals with two mutant copies of the CCR5 gene appear, in most cases, to be completely protected from HIV infection. Mutations in the gene for other HIV co-receptors also may influence the rate of disease progression.

Viral burden and disease progression. Numerous studies show that people with high levels of HIV in their bloodstream are more likely to develop new AIDS-related symptoms or die than those with lower levels of virus. For instance, in the Multicenter AIDS Cohort Study (MACS), investigators showed that the level of HIV in an untreated person's plasma six months to a year after infection—the so-called viral set point—is highly predictive of the rate of disease progression; that is, patients with high levels of virus are much more likely to get sicker faster than those with low levels of virus. The MACS and other studies have provided the rationale for providing aggressive antiretroviral therapy to HIV-infected people, as well as for routinely using newly available blood tests to measure viral load when initiating, monitoring, and modifying anti-HIV therapy.

Potent combinations of three or more anti-HIV drugs known as highly active antiretroviral therapy, or HAART, can reduce a person's "viral burden" (amount of virus in the circulating blood) to very low levels and in many cases delay the progression of HIV disease for prolonged periods. Before the introduction of HAART therapy, 85 percent of patients survived an average of three years following AIDS diagnosis. Today, 95 percent of patients who start therapy before they get AIDS survive on average three years following their first AIDS diagnosis. For those who start HAART after their first AIDS event, survival is still very high at 85 percent averaging three years after AIDS diagnosis.

Antiretroviral regimens, however, have yet to completely and permanently suppress the virus in HIV-infected people. Recent studies have shown that, in addition to the latent HIV reservoir discussed above, HIV persists in a replication-competent form in resting CD4+ T cells even in people receiving aggressive antiretroviral therapy who have no readily detectable HIV in their blood. Investigators around the world are working to develop the next generation of anti-HIV drugs that can stop HIV, even in these biological scenarios.

A treatment goal, along with reduction of viral burden, is the reconstitution of the person's immune system, which may have become sufficiently damaged that it cannot replenish itself. Various strategies for assisting the immune system in this regard are being tested in clinical trials in tandem with HAART, such as the Evaluation of Subcutaneous Proleukin in a Randomized International Trial (ESPRIT) trial exploring the effects of the T cell growth factor, IL-2.

HIV Is Active in the Lymph Nodes

Although HIV-infected people often show an extended period of clinical latency with little evidence of disease, the virus is never truly completely latent although individual cells may be latently infected. Researchers have shown that even early in disease, HIV actively replicates within the lymph nodes and related organs, where large amounts of virus become trapped in networks of specialized cells with long, tentacle-like extensions. These cells are called follicular dendritic cells (FDCs). FDCs are located in hot spots of immune activity in lymphoid tissue called germinal centers. They act like flypaper, trapping invading pathogens (including HIV) and holding them until B cells come along to start an immune response.

Over a period of years, even when little virus is readily detectable in the blood, significant amounts of virus accumulate in the lymphoid tissue, both within infected cells and bound to FDCs. In and around the germinal centers, numerous CD4+ T cells are probably activated by the increased production of cytokines such as TNF-alpha and IL-6 by immune system cells within the lymphoid tissue. Activation allows uninfected cells to be more easily infected and increases replication of HIV in already infected cells.

While greater quantities of certain cytokines such as TNF-alpha and IL-6 are secreted during HIV infection, other cytokines with key roles in the regulation of normal immune function may be secreted in decreased amounts. For example, CD4+ T cells may lose their capacity to produce IL-2, a cytokine that enhances the growth of other T cells and helps to stimulate other cells' response to invaders. Infected cells also have low levels of receptors for IL-2, which may reduce their ability to respond to signals from other cells.

Breakdown of lymph node architecture. Ultimately, with chronic cell activation and secretion of inflammatory cytokines, the fine and complex inner structure of the lymph node breaks down and is replaced by scar tissue. Without this structure, cells in the lymph node cannot communicate and the immune system cannot function properly. Investigators also have reported recently that this scarring reduces the ability of the immune system to replenish itself following antiretroviral therapy that reduces the viral burden.

Role of CD8+ T Cells

CD8+ T cells are critically important in the immune response to HIV. These cells attack and kill infected cells that are producing virus. Thus, vaccine efforts are directed toward eliciting or enhancing these killer T cells, as well as eliciting antibodies that will neutralize the infectivity of HIV.

CD8+ T cells also appear to secrete soluble factors that suppress HIV replication. Several molecules, including RANTES (regulated on activation, normal T expressed and secreted), macrophage inflammatory protein (MIP)-1alpha, MIP-1beta, and myeloid dendritic cells

(MDC) appear to block HIV replication by occupying the co-receptors necessary for many strains of HIV to enter their target cells. There may be other immune system molecules—including the so-called CD8 anti-viral factor (CAF), the defensins (type of antimicrobials), and others yet undiscovered—that can suppress HIV replication to some degree.

Rapid Replication and Mutation of HIV

HIV replicates rapidly; several billion new virus particles may be produced every day. In addition, the HIV reverse transcriptase enzyme makes many mistakes while making DNA copies from HIV RNA. As a consequence, many variants or strains of HIV develop in a person, some of which may escape destruction by antibodies or killer T cells. Additionally, different strains of HIV can recombine to produce a wide range of variants.

During the course of HIV disease, viral strains emerge in an infected person that differ widely in their ability to infect and kill different cell types, as well as in their rate of replication. Scientists are investigating why strains of HIV from people with advanced disease appear to be more virulent and infect more cell types than strains obtained earlier from the same person. Part of the explanation may be the expanded ability of the virus to use other co-receptors, such as CXCR4.

Theories of Immune System Cell Loss in HIV Infection

Researchers around the world are studying how HIV destroys or disables CD4+ T cells, and many think that a number of mechanisms may occur simultaneously in an HIV-infected person. Data suggest that billions of CD4+ T cells may be destroyed every day, eventually overwhelming the immune system's capacity to regenerate.

Direct cell killing. Infected CD4+ T cells may be killed directly when large amounts of virus are produced and bud out from the cell surface, disrupting the cell membrane, or when viral proteins and nucleic acids collect inside the cell, interfering with cellular machinery.

Apoptosis. Infected CD4+ T cells may be killed when the regulation of cell function is distorted by HIV proteins, probably leading to cell suicide by a process known as programmed cell death or apoptosis. Recent reports indicate that apoptosis occurs to a greater extent in HIV-infected people, in both their bloodstream and their lymph nodes. Apoptosis is closely associated with the aberrant cellular activation seen in HIV disease.

Uninfected cells also may undergo apoptosis. Investigators have shown in cell cultures that the HIV envelope alone or bound to antibodies sends an inappropriate signal to CD4+ T cells causing them to undergo apoptosis, even if not infected by HIV.

Innocent bystanders. Uninfected cells may die in an innocent bystander scenario: HIV particles may bind to the cell surface, giving them the appearance of an infected cell and marking them for destruction by killer T cells after antibody attaches to the viral particle on the cell. This process is called antibody-dependent cellular cytotoxicity.

Killer T cells also may mistakenly destroy uninfected cells that have consumed HIV particles and that display HIV fragments on their surfaces. Alternatively, because HIV envelope proteins bear some resemblance to certain molecules that may appear on CD4+ T cells, the body's immune responses may mistakenly damage such cells as well.

Anergy. Researchers have shown in cell cultures that CD4+ T cells can be turned off by activation signals from HIV that leave them unable to respond to further immune stimulation. This inactivated state is known as anergy.

Damage to precursor cells. Studies suggest that HIV also destroys precursor cells that mature to have special immune functions, as well as the microenvironment of the bone marrow and the thymus needed for developing such cells. These organs probably lose the ability to regenerate, further compounding the suppression of the immune system.

Central Nervous System Damage

Although monocytes and macrophages can be infected by HIV, they appear to be relatively resistant to being killed by the virus. These cells, however, travel throughout the body and carry HIV to various organs, including the brain, which may serve as a hiding place or "reservoir" for the virus that may be relatively resistant to most anti-HIV drugs.

Neurologic manifestations of HIV disease are seen in up to 50 percent of HIV-infected people, to varying degrees of severity. People infected with HIV often experience the following:

- Cognitive symptoms, including impaired short-term memory, reduced concentration, and mental slowing

- Motor symptoms such as fine motor clumsiness or slowness, tremor, and leg weakness

- Behavioral symptoms including apathy, social withdrawal, irritability, depression, and personality change

47

More serious neurologic manifestations in HIV disease typically occur in patients with high viral loads, generally when a person has advanced HIV disease or AIDS.

Neurologic manifestations of HIV disease are the subject of many research projects. Current evidence suggests that although nerve cells do not become infected with HIV, supportive cells within the brain, such as astrocytes and microglia (as well as monocyte/macrophages that have migrated to the brain) can be infected with the virus. Researchers postulate that infection of these cells can cause a disruption of normal neurologic functions by altering cytokine levels, by delivering aberrant signals, and by causing the release of toxic products in the brain. The use of anti-HIV drugs frequently reduces the severity of neurologic symptoms, but in many cases does not, for reasons that are unclear. The impact of long-term therapy and long-term HIV disease on neurologic function is also unknown and under intensive study.

Role of Immune Activation in HIV Disease

During a normal immune response, many parts of the immune system are mobilized to fight an invader. CD4+ T cells, for instance, may quickly multiply and increase their cytokine secretion, thereby signaling other cells to perform their special functions. Scavenger cells called macrophages may double in size and develop numerous organelles, including lysosomes that contain digestive enzymes used to process ingested pathogens. Once the immune system clears the foreign antigen, it returns to a relative state of quiescence.

Paradoxically, although it ultimately causes immune deficiency, HIV disease for most of its course is characterized by immune system hyperactivation, which has negative consequences. As noted above, HIV replication and spread are much more efficient in activated CD4+ cells. Chronic immune system activation during HIV disease also may result in a massive stimulation of B cells, impairing the ability of these cells to make antibodies against other pathogens.

Chronic immune activation also can result in apoptosis, and an increased production of cytokines that not only may increase HIV replication but also have other deleterious effects. Increased levels of TNF-alpha, for example, may be at least partly responsible for the severe weight loss or wasting syndrome seen in many HIV-infected people.

The persistence of HIV and HIV replication plays an important role in the chronic state of immune activation seen in HIV-infected people. In addition, researchers have shown that infections with other organisms activate immune system cells and increase production of the virus in HIV-infected people. Chronic immune activation due to persistent infections, or the cumulative effects of multiple episodes of immune activation and bursts of virus production, likely contribute to the progression of HIV disease.

New Clinical Signs of HIV in the Era of HAART Therapy

The clinical spectrum of disease among people with HIV has changed dramatically in the era of HAART. NIAID and its grantees are actively studying the new clinical syndrome of disease among persons on long term-therapy. Research is concentrating on the impact of HIV over the long term, the toxicity of the medicines used to control HIV, and the effects of aging on HIV disease progression. People with HIV have a variety of conditions including diabetes, heart disease, neurocognitive decline, and cancers that may, or may not, be directly due to HIV or its treatment. Long-term studies of people with HIV in the United States and abroad are underway.

NIAID Research on the Pathogenesis of AIDS

NIAID-supported scientists conduct research on HIV pathogenesis in laboratories on the campus of the National Institutes of Health (NIH) in Bethesda, Maryland; at the Institute's Rocky Mountain Laboratories in Hamilton, Montana; and at universities and medical centers in the United States and abroad.

A NIAID-supported resource, the NIH AIDS Research and Reference Reagent Program, in collaboration with the World Health Organization, provides critically needed AIDS-related research materials free to qualified researchers around the world.

The NIH Centers for AIDS Research, supported by NIAID in collaboration with six other NIH Institutes, fosters and facilitates development of infrastructure and interdisciplinary collaboration of HIV researchers at major medical and research centers across the United States.

In addition, the institute convenes groups of investigators and advisory committees to exchange scientific information, clarify research priorities, and bring research needs and opportunities to the attention of the scientific community.

Chapter 4

HIV/AIDS:
A Statistical Overview

Chapter Contents

Section 4.1

HIV/AIDS Prevalence and Incidence in the United States and Worldwide

"Basic Statistics" is excerpted from Centers for Disease Control and Prevention, February 26, 2009. "Worldwide HIV/AIDS Statistics" is reprinted from "Worldwide HIV and AIDS Statistics," © 2009 AVERT (www.avert.org). All rights reserved. Reprinted with permission.

Basic Statistics

Definitions

- **AIDS:** This refers to persons diagnosed with acquired immuno-deficiency syndrome (AIDS), based on the Centers for Disease Control and Prevention (CDC) definition in adults and adolescents and children.

- **HIV/AIDS:** This refers to cases of human immunodeficiency virus (HIV) infection, regardless of whether they have progressed to AIDS from the thirty-nine areas (thirty-four states and five U.S. dependent areas) that have had confidential name-based HIV infection reporting long enough to monitor trends. According to the number of AIDS cases, these thirty-four states represent approximately 66 percent of the epidemic in the fifty states and the District of Columbia.

- **Dependent areas:** American Samoa, Guam, the Northern Mariana Islands, Puerto Rico, and the U.S. Virgin Islands.

- **Thirty-four states and five dependent areas with confidential name-based HIV infection reporting:** Alabama, Alaska, Arizona, Arkansas, Colorado, Florida, Georgia, Idaho, Indiana, Iowa, Kansas, Louisiana, Michigan, Minnesota, Mississippi, Missouri, Nebraska, Nevada, New Jersey, New Mexico, New York, North Carolina, North Dakota, Ohio, Oklahoma, South Carolina, South Dakota, Tennessee, Texas, Utah, Virginia, West Virginia, Wisconsin, Wyoming, American Samoa, Guam, the Northern Mariana Islands, Puerto Rico, and the U.S. Virgin Islands.

- **Transmission category:** The classification of a case that indicates the risk factor most likely to have been responsible for transmission. Cases are counted only once in a hierarchy of transmission categories. Persons with more than one reported risk factor for HIV infection are classified in the transmission category listed first in the hierarchy. The exception is men who report sexual contact with other men and injection drug use; this group makes up a separate transmission category.

- **HIV incidence:** The number of new HIV infections in a specific population during a specific period of time.

- **HIV prevalence:** The number of people living with HIV/AIDS in a given year.

HIV Prevalence Estimate

Prevalence is the number of people living with HIV infection at the end of a given year.

At the end of 2006, an estimated 1,106,400 persons (95 percent confidence interval 1,056,400–1,156,400) in the United States were living with HIV infection, with 21 percent undiagnosed.[1]

HIV Incidence Estimate

Incidence is the number of new HIV infections that occur during a given year.

In 2008, CDC estimated that approximately 56,300 people were newly infected with HIV in 2006[2] (the most recent year that data are available). Over half (53 percent) of these new infections occurred in gay and bisexual men. Black/African American men and women were also strongly affected and were estimated to have an incidence rate that was seven times as high as the incidence rate among whites.

AIDS Cases

In 2007, the estimated number of persons diagnosed with AIDS in the United States and dependent areas was 37,041. Of these, 35,962 were diagnosed in the fifty states and the District of Columbia and 812 were diagnosed in the dependent areas. In the fifty states and the District of Columbia, adult and adolescent AIDS cases totaled 35,934, with 26,355 cases in males and 9,579 cases in females, and 28 cases estimated in children under age thirteen years.

The cumulative estimated number of diagnoses of AIDS through 2007 in the United States and dependent areas was 1,051,875. Of these, 1,018,428 were diagnosed in the fifty states and the District of Columbia and 32,051 were diagnosed in the dependent areas. In the fifty states and the District of Columbia, adult and adolescent AIDS cases totaled 1,009,220, with 810,676 cases in males and 198,544 cases in females, and 9,209 cases estimated in children under age thirteen years.

These numbers do not represent reported case counts. Rather, these numbers are point estimates, which result from adjustments of reported case counts. The reported case counts have been adjusted for reporting delays and for redistribution of cases in persons initially reported without an identified risk factor, but not for incomplete reporting.

AIDS Cases by Age

Of the estimated number of persons diagnosed with AIDS in the fifty states and the District of Columbia, persons' ages at time of diagnosis were distributed as shown in Table 4.1.

Table 4.1. AIDS Cases by Age

Age (Years)	Estimated # of AIDS Cases in 2007	Cumulative Estimated # of AIDS Cases through 2007[a]
Under 13	28	9,209
Ages 13–14	80	1,169
Ages 15–19	455	6,089
Ages 20–24	1,927	38,175
Ages 25–29	3,380	120,464
Ages 30–34	4,187	201,906
Ages 35–39	5,888	219,601
Ages 40–44	6,813	177,250
Ages 45–49	5,749	112,896
Ages 50–54	3,636	63,408
Ages 55–59	2,040	34,160
Ages 60–64	980	18,249
Ages 65 or older	800	15,853

[a]Includes persons with a diagnosis of AIDS from the beginning of the epidemic through 2007.

AIDS Cases by Race/Ethnicity

CDC tracks HIV/AIDS information on six racial and ethnic groups: American Indian/Alaska Native; Asian; black/African American; Hispanic/Latino; Native Hawaiian/other Pacific Islander; and white.

Table 4.2. Estimated Numbers of AIDS Cases in the Fifty States and the District of Columbia, by Race or Ethnicity

Race or Ethnicity	Estimated # of AIDS Cases in 2007	Cumulative Estimated # of AIDS Cases through 2007[a]
American Indian/Alaska Native	158	3,492
Asian[b]	475	7,511
Black/African American	17,507	426,003
Hispanic/Latino[c]	6,921	169,138
Native Hawaiian/Other Pacific Islander	76	721
White	10,407	404,465

[a]Includes persons with a diagnosis of AIDS from the beginning of the epidemic through 2007.

[b]Includes Asian/Pacific Islander legacy cases.

[c]Hispanics/Latinos can be of any race.

AIDS Cases by Transmission Category

Six common transmission categories are male-to-male sexual contact, injection drug use, male-to-male sexual contact and injection drug use, high-risk heterosexual (male-female) contact, mother-to-child (perinatal) transmission, and other (includes blood transfusions and unknown cause).

Tables 4.3 and 4.4 show the distribution of the estimated number of cases of AIDS among adults and adolescents by transmission category in the fifty states and the District of Columbia. A breakdown by sex is provided where appropriate.

The distribution of the estimated number of cases of AIDS, among children* in the 50 states and the District of Columbia, by transmission categories is shown in Table 4.5.

Table 4.3. Estimated Number of AIDS Cases in 2007

Transmission Category	Adult and Adolescent Male	Adult and Adolescent Female	Total
Male-to-male sexual contact	16,749	–	16,749
Injection drug use	3,750	2,260	6,010
Male-to-male sexual contact and injection drug use	1,664	–	1,664
High-risk heterosexual contact[a]	4,011	7,100	11,111
Other[b]	181	220	401

[a]Heterosexual contact with a person known to have, or to be at high risk for, HIV infection.

[b]Includes hemophilia, blood transfusion, perinatal exposure, and risk not reported or not identified.

Table 4.4. Estimated Number of AIDS Cases through 2007

Transmission Category	Adult and Adolescent Male	Adult and Adolescent Female	Total
Male-to-male sexual contact	487,695	–	487,695
Injection drug use	175,704	80,155	255,859
Male-to-male sexual contact and injection drug use	71,242	–	71,242
High-risk heterosexual contact[a]	112,230	176,157	63,927
Other[b]	12,108	6,158	18,266

Note: Includes persons with a diagnosis of AIDS from the beginning of the epidemic through 2007.

[a]Heterosexual contact with a person known to have, or to be at high risk for, HIV infection.

[b]Includes hemophilia, blood transfusion, perinatal exposure, and risk not reported or not identified

Table 4.5. Estimated Number of AIDS Cases among Children

Transmission Category	Estimated # of AIDS Cases in 2007	Cumulative Estimated # of AIDS Cases Through 2007[a]
Perinatal	24	8,434
Other[b]	4	775

Note: The term "children" refers to persons under age thirteen years at the time of diagnosis.

[a]Includes persons with a diagnosis of AIDS from the beginning of the epidemic through 2007.

[b]Includes hemophilia, blood transfusion, and risk not reported or not identified.

AIDS Cases by Top Ten States/Dependent Areas

The 10 states or dependent areas reporting the highest number of AIDS cases are shown in Tables 4.6 and 4.7.

Table 4.6. States/Dependent Areas with Highest Incidence of AIDS

State/Dependent Area	# of AIDS Cases in 2007
California	4,952
New York	4,810
Florida	3,961
Texas	2,964
Georgia	1,877
Pennsylvania	1,750
Maryland	1,394
Illinois	1,348
New Jersey	1,164
North Carolina	1,024

Table 4.7. States/Dependent Areas with Highest Prevalence of AIDS

State/Dependent Area	# of Cumulative AIDS Cases Through 2007[a]		
	Adults or Adolescents	Children (<13)	Total
New York	179,116	2,345	181,461
California	148,274	675	148,949
Florida	107,980	1,544	109,524
Texas	72,434	394	72,828
New Jersey	49,907	787	50,694
Pennsylvania	35,120	369	35,489
Illinois	34,783	283	35,066
Georgia	33,607	240	33,847
Maryland	31,611	320	31,931
Puerto Rico	30,333	403	30,736

[a]Includes persons with a diagnosis of AIDS from the beginning of the epidemic through 2007.

Persons Living with AIDS

At the end of 2007, the estimated number of persons living with AIDS in the United States and dependent areas was 468,578. In the fifty states and the District of Columbia, this included 454,747 adults and adolescents and 889 children under age thirteen years.

Deaths of Persons with AIDS

In 2007, the estimated number of deaths of persons with AIDS in the United States and dependent areas was 14,561. In the fifty states and the District of Columbia, this included 14,105 adults and adolescents and 5 children under age thirteen years.

The cumulative estimated number of deaths of persons with AIDS in the United States and dependent areas, through 2007, was 583,298. In the fifty states and the District of Columbia, this included 557,902 adults and adolescents and 4,891 children under age thirteen years.

HIV/AIDS Cases

In 2007, the estimated number of cases of HIV/AIDS diagnosed in the thirty-four states and five dependent areas with confidential name-based HIV infection reporting was 44,084. Of these, 42,655 were in the thirty-four states and 1,429 were in the five dependent areas.

In the thirty-four states, adult and adolescent HIV/AIDS cases totaled 42,495, with 31,518 cases in males and 10,977 cases in females, and 159 cases estimated in children under age thirteen years.

These numbers do not represent reported case counts. Rather, these numbers are point estimates, which result from adjustments of reported case counts. The reported case counts have been adjusted for reporting delays and for redistribution of cases in persons initially reported without an identified risk factor, but not for incomplete reporting.

HIV/AIDS Cases by Age

Of the estimated number of HIV/AIDS cases diagnosed in the thirty-four states with confidential name-based HIV infection reporting, persons' ages at time of diagnosis were distributed as shown in Table 4.8.

HIV/AIDS Cases by Race/Ethnicity

CDC tracks HIV/AIDS information on six racial and ethnic groups: American Indian/Alaska Native; Asian; Black/African American; Hispanic/Latino; Native Hawaiian/other Pacific Islander; and white.

Table 4.8. Incidence of HIV/AIDS by Age

Age (Years)	Estimated Number of HIV/AIDS Cases in 2007
Under 13	159
Ages 13–14	40
Ages 15–19	1,703
Ages 20–24	4,907
Ages 25–29	5,771
Ages 30–34	5,089
Ages 35–39	6,088
Ages 40–44	6,554
Ages 45–49	5,172
Ages 50–54	3,489
Ages 55–59	1,938
Ages 60–64	942
Ages 65 or older	803

Estimated numbers of HIV/AIDS cases diagnosed in the thirty-four states with confidential name-based HIV infection reporting, by race or ethnicity are shown in Table 4.9.

Table 4.9. Incidence of HIV/AIDS by Race or Ethnicity

Race or Ethnicity	Estimated # of HIV/AIDS Cases in 2007
American Indian/Alaska Native	228
Asian[a]	455
Black/African American	21,549
Hispanic/Latino[b]	7,484
Native Hawaiian/Other Pacific Islander	46
White	12,556

[a]Includes Asian/Pacific Islander legacy cases.
[b]Hispanics/Latinos can be of any race.

HIV/AIDS Cases by Transmission Category

Six common transmission categories are male-to-male sexual contact, injection drug use, male-to-male sexual contact and injection drug use, high-risk heterosexual (male-female) contact, mother-to-child (perinatal) transmission, and other (includes blood transfusions and unknown cause).

Table 4.10 shows the distribution of the estimated number of cases of HIV/AIDS diagnosed among adults and adolescents in the thirty-four states with confidential name-based HIV infection reporting, by transmission category. A breakdown by sex is provided where appropriate.

The distribution of the estimated number of cases of HIV/AIDS diagnosed among children (under age 13 at the time of diagnosis) in the thirty-four states with confidential name-based HIV infection reporting, by transmission categories, is shown in Table 4.11.

Persons Living with HIV/AIDS

At the end of 2007, the estimated number of persons living with HIV/AIDS in the thirty-four states and five dependent areas with confidential name-based HIV/AIDS infection reporting was 571,378. In the thirty-four states only, this included 549,196 adults and adolescents and 2,736 children under age thirteen years.

These numbers do not represent reported case counts. Rather, these numbers are point estimates, which result from adjustments of reported case counts. The reported case counts have been adjusted for reporting delays.

Table 4.10. Incidence of HIV/AIDS Cases in 2007 by Transmission Category

Transmission Category	Adult and Adolescent Male	Adult and Adolescent Female	Total
Male-to-male sexual contact	22,472	–	22,472
Injection drug use	3,133	1,806	4,939
Male-to-male sexual contact and injection drug use	1,260	–	1,260
High-risk heterosexual contact[a]	4,551	9,076	13,627
Other[b]	102	96	198

[a]Heterosexual contact with a person known to have, or to be at high risk for, HIV infection.
[b]Includes hemophilia, blood transfusion, perinatal exposure, and risk not reported or not identified.

Table 4.11. Incidence of HIV/AIDS Cases among Children

Transmission Category	Estimated # of HIV/AIDS Cases in 2007
Perinatal	139
Other[a]	20

Note: The term "children" refers to persons under age thirteen years at the time of diagnosis.
[a]Includes hemophilia, blood transfusion, and risk not reported or not identified.

References

1. CDC. HIV Prevalence Estimates—United States, 2006. *MMWR* 2008;57(39):1073–76.

2. Hall HI, Ruiguang S, Rhodes P, et al. Estimation of HIV incidence in the United States. *JAMA*. 2008;300:520–29.

Worldwide HIV/AIDS Statistics

The latest statistics of global HIV and AIDS were published by UN-AIDS in November 2009, and refer to the end of 2008 [Table 4.12].

More than twenty-five million people have died of AIDS since 1981.

Africa has over fourteen million AIDS orphans.

At the end of 2008, women accounted for 50 percent of all adults living with HIV worldwide.

In developing and transitional countries, 9.5 million people are in immediate need of life-saving AIDS drugs; of these, only 4 million (42 percent) are receiving the drugs.

The number of people living with HIV has risen from around eight million in 1990 to thirty-three million today, and is still growing. Around 67 percent of people living with HIV are in sub-Saharan Africa.

During 2008 more than two and a half million adults and children became infected with HIV (human immunodeficiency virus), the virus that causes AIDS. By the end of the year, an estimated 33.4 million people worldwide were living with HIV/AIDS. The year also saw two million deaths from AIDS, despite recent improvements in access to antiretroviral treatment [Table 4.13].

Notes

Adults are defined as men and women aged fifteen or above, unless specified otherwise.

Children orphaned by AIDS are defined as people aged under eighteen who are alive and have lost one or both parents to AIDS.

All the statistics in this section should be interpreted with caution because they are estimates.

Table 4.12. Global HIV/AIDS Estimates, End of 2008

	Estimate	Range
People living with HIV/AIDS in 2008	33.4 million	31.1–35.8 million
Adults living with HIV/AIDS in 2008	31.3 million	29.2–33.7 million
Women living with HIV/AIDS in 2008	15.7 million	14.2–17.2 million
Children living with HIV/AIDS in 2008	2.1 million	1.2–2.9 million
People newly infected with HIV in 2008	2.7 million	2.4–3.0 million
Children newly infected with HIV in 2008	0.43 million	0.24–0.61 million
AIDS deaths in 2008	2.0 million	1.7–2.4 million
Child AIDS deaths in 2008	0.28 million	0.15–0.41 million

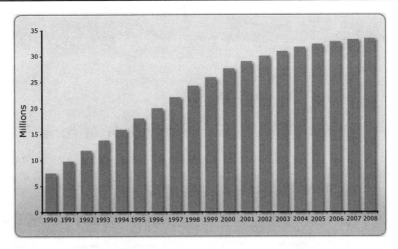

Figure 4.1. *Global Trends in HIV/AIDS Prevalence*

Table 4.13. Regional statistics for HIV & AIDS, End of 2008

Region	Adults & children living with HIV/AIDS	Adults & children newly infected	Adult prevalence[a]	Deaths of adults & children
Sub-Saharan Africa	22.4 million	1.9 million	5.2 percent	1.4 million
North Africa & Middle East	310,000	35,000	0.2 percent	20,000
South and South-East Asia	3.8 million	280,000	0.3 percent	270,000
East Asia	850,000	75,000	<0.1 percent	59,000
Oceania	59,000	3,900	0.3 percent	2,000
Latin America	2.0 million	170,000	0.6 percent	77,000
Caribbean	240,000	20,000	1.0 percent	12,000
Eastern Europe & Central Asia	1.5 million	110,000	0.7 percent	87,000
North America	1.4 million	55,000	0.4 percent	25,000
Western & Central Europe	850,000	30,000	0.3 percent	13,000
Global total	33.4 million	2.7 million	0.8 percent	2.0 million

[a]Proportion of adults aged fifteen to forty-nine who were living with HIV/AIDS.

Section 4.2

HIV/AIDS and Minority Populations

"Black Americans and HIV/AIDS" and "Latinos and HIV/AIDS," © 2009, are reprinted with permission from the Henry J. Kaiser Family Foundation. The Kaiser Family Foundation is a non-profit private operating foundation based in Menlo Park, California, dedicated to producing and communicating the best possible analysis and information on health issues. "HIV/AIDS among Asians and Pacific Islanders" and "HIV/AIDS among American Indians and Alaska Natives" are excerpted from the Centers for Disease Control and Prevention, August 3, 2008.

Black Americans and HIV/AIDS

Black Americans have been disproportionately affected by human immunodeficiency virus (HIV) and acquired immunodeficiency syndrome (AIDS) since the epidemic's beginning, and that disparity has deepened over time.[1,2] Blacks account for more new HIV infections, AIDS cases, people estimated to be living with HIV disease, and HIV-related deaths than any other racial/ethnic group in the United States.[1,3,4,5,6] The epidemic has also had a disproportionate impact on black women, youth, and gay and bisexual men, and its impact varies across the country. Moreover, blacks with HIV/AIDS may face greater barriers to accessing care than their white counterparts.[7,8,9] Today, there are approximately 1.1 million people living with HIV/AIDS in the United States, including more than 500,000 who are black.[5] Analysis of national household survey data found that 2 percent of blacks in the United States were HIV-positive, higher than any other group.[10]

Snapshot of the Epidemic

Although black Americans represent only 12 percent of the U.S. population,[11] they accounted for 45 percent of new HIV infections (see Figure 4.2) and 46 percent of people living with HIV disease in 2006.[3,4,5] Blacks also accounted for almost half of new AIDS diagnoses (49 percent) in 2007.[1,12]

The AIDS case rate per 100,000 among black adults/adolescents was nearly ten times that of whites in 2007 (see Figure 4.3).[1,13] The AIDS

64

case rate for black men (81.3) was the highest of any group, followed by black women (39.8). By comparison, the rate among white men was 10.6.[1,13] The rate of new infections is also highest among blacks and was seven times greater than the rate among whites in 2006.[3,4]

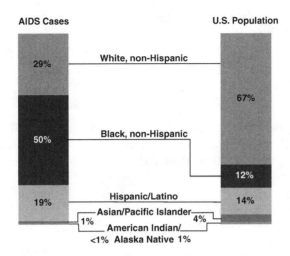

Figure 4.2. New HIV Infections and U.S. Population, by Race/Ethnicity, 2006

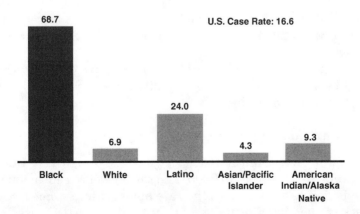

Figure 4.3. AIDS Case Rate per 100,000 Population, by Race/Ethnicity, for Adults/Adolescents, 2007

HIV-related deaths and HIV death rates are highest among blacks. Blacks accounted for 57 percent of deaths due to HIV in 2006[6] and their survival time after an AIDS diagnosis is lower on average than it is for most other racial/ethnic groups.[1] In 2006, black men had the highest HIV death rates per 100,000 men ages twenty-five to thirty-four and thirty-five to forty-four; the HIV death rates among black women in the same age groups were also the highest among women.[14]

HIV was the fourth leading cause of death for black men and third for black women, ages twenty-five to forty-four, in 2006, ranking higher than for their respective counterparts in any other racial/ethnic group.[15]

Key Trends and Current Cases

The number of new HIV infections per year among blacks is down from its peak in the late 1980s, but has exceeded the number of infections among whites since that time; new infections have remained stable in recent years.[4]

The share of AIDS diagnoses accounted for by blacks has risen over time, rising from 25 percent of cases diagnosed in 1985 to 49 percent in 2007; in recent years, this share also has remained relatively stable.[1,2]

A recent analysis of 1999–2006 data from a national household survey found that 2 percent of blacks in the United States (among those ages eighteen to forty-nine) were HIV-positive, significantly higher than whites (0.23 percent). Also, the prevalence of HIV was higher among black men (2.64 percent) than black women (1.49 percent).[10]

The number of black Americans living with AIDS increased by 24 percent between 2003 and 2007, compared to an 18 percent increase among whites.[1]

The number of deaths among both blacks and whites with AIDS declined between 2003 and 2007, by 20 percent respectively. Deaths among Latinos also declined.[1]

Women and Young People

Black women account for the largest share of new HIV infections among women (61 percent in 2006) and the incidence rate among black women is nearly fifteen times the rate among white women.[16]

Black women account for the majority of new AIDS cases among women (66 percent in 2007); white and Latina women account for 17 percent and 15 percent of new AIDS cases, respectively.[1,13]

Black women represent more than a third (36 percent) of AIDS cases diagnosed among blacks (black men and women combined) in 2007; by comparison, white women represent 15 percent of AIDS cases diagnosed among whites in 2007.[1,13]

Although black teens (ages thirteen to nineteen) represent only 15 percent of U.S. teenagers, they account for 68 percent of new AIDS cases reported among teens in 2007.[17] A similar impact can be seen among black children.[1]

Transmission

HIV transmission patterns among black men vary from those of white men. Although both groups are most likely to have been infected through sex with other men, white men are more likely to have been infected this way. Heterosexual transmission and injection drug use account for a greater share of infections among black men than white men.[1,16,18]

Black women are most likely to have been infected through heterosexual transmission, the most common transmission route for women overall. White women are more likely to have been infected through injection drug use than black women.[1,16]

Among gay and bisexual men, blacks have been disproportionately affected. A study in five major U.S. cities found that 46 percent of black gay and bisexual men in the study were infected with HIV, compared to 21 percent of white and 17 percent of Latino gay and bisexual men. Knowledge of HIV status among those already infected was also very low, particularly among blacks.[19,20] In addition, newly infected black gay and bisexual men are younger than their white counterparts with those ages thirteen to twenty-nine accounting for 52 percent of new infections among blacks compared to 25 percent among whites.[16]

Geography

Although AIDS cases among blacks have been reported throughout the country, the impact of the epidemic is not uniformly distributed:

- AIDS case rates per 100,000 among blacks are highest in the eastern part of the United States. The District of Columbia has the highest case rate for blacks (263.8) in the country.[13,21]

- The majority of blacks estimated to be living with AIDS and the majority of newly reported AIDS cases among blacks in 2007 occurred in the South; by comparison, blacks represent approximately 19 percent of the South's population.[21,22,23]

- Estimated AIDS prevalence among blacks is clustered in a handful of states, with ten states accounting for 71 percent of blacks estimated to be living with AIDS in 2007. New York, Florida, and Georgia top the list (see Figure 4.4).[21,22] Ten states also account for the majority of newly reported AIDS cases among blacks (68 percent in 2007).[21,22]

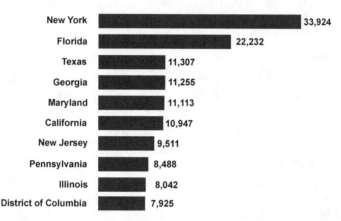

New York	33,924
Florida	22,232
Texas	11,307
Georgia	11,255
Maryland	11,113
California	10,947
New Jersey	9,511
Pennsylvania	8,488
Illinois	8,042
District of Columbia	7,925

Figure 4.4. Number of Black Americans Estimated to Be Living with AIDS, Top 10 States, 2007

Access to and Use of the Health Care System

The HIV Cost and Services Utilization Study (HCSUS), the only nationally representative study of people with HIV/AIDS receiving regular or ongoing medical care for HIV, found that blacks fared more poorly on several important measures of access and quality than whites; these differences diminished over time but were not completely eliminated.[7] HCSUS also found that blacks were more likely to report postponing medical care because they lacked transportation, were too sick to go to the doctor, or had other competing needs.[8]

An analysis of data from 2000 to 2002 in eleven HIV primary and specialty care sites in the United States found higher rates of hospitalization among blacks with HIV/AIDS, but differences in outpatient utilization were not significant.[9]

Health Insurance

Having health insurance, either public or private, improves access to care. Insurance coverage of those with HIV/AIDS varies by race/ethnicity, as it does for the U.S. population overall:

- According to HCSUS, blacks with HIV/AIDS were more likely to be publicly insured or uninsured than their white counterparts, with over half (59 percent) relying on Medicaid compared to 32 percent of whites. One-fifth of blacks with HIV/AIDS (22 percent) were uninsured compared to 17 percent of whites. Blacks were also much less likely to be privately insured than whites (14 percent compared to 44 percent).[24]

- Insurance status also varies at the time of HIV diagnosis. Analysis of data from twenty-five states between 1994 and 2000 found that blacks were less likely than whites to have private coverage and more likely to be covered by Medicaid, or uninsured, at the time of their HIV diagnoses.[25]

HIV Testing

Among the U.S. population overall, blacks are more likely than whites to report having been tested for HIV in the last twelve months (40 percent compared to 14 percent).[26]

Among those who are HIV-positive, CDC data indicate that 35 percent of blacks were tested for HIV late in their illness—that is, diagnosed with AIDS within one year of testing positive for HIV (in those states/areas with HIV name reporting); by comparison, 34 percent of whites and 41 percent of Latinos were tested late.[1]

Concern about HIV/AIDS

A recent survey found that black Americans express concern about HIV/AIDS. More than one in five black Americans surveyed named HIV/AIDS as the number one health problem in the United States and 40 percent say that HIV/AIDS is a more urgent problem in their community than it was a few years ago.[26]

Personal concern about becoming infected with HIV is highest among blacks, as is concern among black parents about their children becoming infected. However, the proportion of blacks saying they are personally concerned about becoming infected has declined since the mid-1990s.[26]

References

1. CDC. HIV/AIDS Surveillance Report, Vol.19; 2009.

2. CDC. Special Data Request; 2006.

3. Hall HI et al. "Estimation of HIV Incidence in the United States." *JAMA*, Vol. 300, No. 5; August 2008.

4. CDC. Fact Sheet: Estimates of New HIV Infections in the United States; August 2008.

5. CDC. *MMWR*, Vol. 57, No. 39; 2008.

6 NCHS. "Deaths: Final Data for 2006," *NVSR*, Vol. 57, No. 14; 2009.

7. Shapiro MF et al. "Variations in the Care of HIV-Infected Adults in the United States." *JAMA*, Vol. 281, No. 24; 1999.

8. Cunningham WE et al. "The Impact of Competing Subsistence Needs and Barriers to Access to Medical Care for Persons with Human Immunodeficiency Virus Receiving Care in the United States." *Medical Care*, Vol. 37, No. 12; 1999.

9. Fleishman JA et al. "Hospital and Outpatient Health Services Utilization Among HIV-Infected Adults in Care 2000–2002." *Medical Care*, Vol. 43, No. 9, Supplement; September 2005.

10. McQuillan GM et al. NCHS Data Brief, No. 4; January 2008.

11. U.S. Census Bureau. 2006 Population Estimates.

12. Calculations based only on cases for which race/ethnicity data were provided.

13. Includes estimated cases among those thirteen years of age and older. Estimates do not include U.S. dependencies, possessions, and associated nations, and cases of unknown residence.

14. CDC/NCHS. National Vital Statistics System, Deaths, Percent of Total Deaths, and Death Rates for the 15 Leading Causes of Death in 10-year Age Groups, by Hispanic Origin, Race for Non-Hispanic Population and Sex: United States, 2006 (LCWK5).

15. CDC. Slide Set: HIV Mortality (through 2006).

16. CDC. *MMWR*, Vol. 57, No. 36; 2008.

17. CDC. Slide Set: HIV/AIDS Surveillance in Adolescents and Young Adults (through 2007).

18. CDC. Slide Set: HIV/AIDS Surveillance by Race/Ethnicity (through 2007).

19. CDC. Fact Sheet: HIV/AIDS Among Men Who Have Sex with Men; June 2007.

20. CDC. *MMWR*, Vol. 54, No. 24; 2005.

21. The Kaiser Family Foundation, www.statehealthfacts.org. Data Source: Centers for Disease Control and Prevention, Division of HIV/AIDS Prevention-Surveillance and Epidemiology, Special Data Request; 2009.

22. Estimates include U.S. dependencies, possessions, and associated nations, and cases of unknown residence.

23. US Census Bureau. The Black Population: 2000; August 2001.

24. Fleishman JA. Personal Communication, Analysis of HCSUS Data; January 2002.

25. Kaiser Family Foundation analysis of CDC data.

26. Kaiser Family Foundation. Survey of Americans on HIV/AIDS; 2009.

Latinos and HIV/AIDS

Latinos in the United States continue to be heavily impacted by the HIV/AIDS epidemic, accounting for higher rates of new HIV infections, AIDS cases, and people living with HIV than their white counterparts.[1,2,3,4] The epidemic has also had a disproportionate impact on Latino young adults, and the impact varies across the country and by place of birth.[1,5] Moreover, studies have shown that Latinos with HIV/AIDS may face additional barriers to accessing care than whites.[6,7,8] Today, there are approximately 1.1 million people living with HIV/AIDS in the United States, including nearly 200,000 Latinos.[4] As the largest and fastest growing ethnic minority group in the United States, addressing the impact of HIV/AIDS in the Latino community takes on increased importance in efforts to improve the nation's health.

Snapshot of the Epidemic

Latinos accounted for 17 percent of new HIV infections and 18 percent of people living with HIV disease in 2006 (see Figure 4.2).[2,3,4] Latinos also accounted for 19 percent of new AIDS diagnoses in 2007.[1,10]

The AIDS case rate per 100,000 among Latino adults/adolescents was the third highest of any racial/ethnic group in the United States in 2007—about three times that of whites, but one-third that of blacks (see Figure 4.3).[1,11] The HIV incidence rate for Latinos follows a similar pattern.[3]

HIV was the sixth leading cause of death for Latino men and fifth for Latinas, ages twenty-five to forty-four, in 2006.[12]

Key Trends and Current Cases

The number of new infections among Latinos peaked in the late 1980s and has declined since then, and been fluctuating around ten thousand per year for most of the decade. Throughout the epidemic, the number of new HIV infections among Latinos has been lower than for whites and blacks.[3]

Latinos account for a growing share of AIDS diagnoses over the course of the epidemic, rising from 15 percent in 1985 to 19 percent in 2007; in recent years, this share has remained relatively stable.[1,13]

The number of Latinos living with AIDS has also increased over time, in part due to treatment advances but also due to the epidemic's continued impact on Latinos. Estimated AIDS prevalence among Latinos increased by 26 percent between 2003 and 2007, compared to an 18 percent increase among whites.[1]

The number of deaths among Latinos with AIDS declined between 2003 and 2007, although blacks and whites experienced more significant decreases.[1]

Women and Young People

Among women, Latinas account for 16 percent of new HIV infections and their HIV incidence rate is nearly four times the rate for white women, but about a quarter of the rate for black women.[14]

In looking at new AIDS cases in 2007 among women, Latinas similarly account for 15 percent of new cases; black women account for 66 percent and white women account for 17 percent.[1,10,11]

Latinas represented 21 percent of AIDS cases diagnosed among all Latinos (men and women combined) in 2007; by comparison, white women represented 15 percent of cases among whites, and black women represented 36 percent of cases diagnosed among blacks.[1,11]

The AIDS case rate per 100,000 among Latinas (8.9) is five times higher than the case rate for white women (1.8).[1,11]

Latino teens, ages thirteen to nineteen, account for 19 percent of AIDS cases among teens.[5] Latinos ages twenty to twenty-four account for 24 percent of new AIDS cases reported among young adults, but represent 18 percent of U.S. young adults, in 2007.[5]

Transmission

HIV transmission patterns among Latino men vary from those of white men. Both groups are most likely to be infected through sex with other men. Heterosexual transmission accounts for a greater share of infections among Latino men than white men.[1,14,15]

Latinas are somewhat more likely to have been infected through heterosexual transmission than white women, although this is the most common transmission route for both groups and for women overall. White women are somewhat more likely to have been infected through injection drug use than Latinas.[1,14]

Studies have found high HIV/AIDS prevalence among Latino gay and bisexual men.[16] A study in five major U.S. cities found that 17 percent of Latino gay and bisexual men in the study were infected with HIV. Prevalence among white gay and bisexual men was 21 percent and 46 percent among black gay and bisexual men, the highest of any group.[17] Knowledge of HIV status among those already infected is also very low.[16] In addition, newly infected Latino gay and bisexual men are younger than their white counterparts, with those ages thirteen to twenty-nine accounting for 43 percent of new infections among Latino gay and bisexual men compared to 25 percent among whites.[14]

Geography

Although AIDS cases among Latinos have been reported throughout the country, the impact of the epidemic is not uniformly distributed:

- AIDS case rates per 100,000 among Latinos are highest in the eastern part of the United States, particularly in the Northeast.[18]

- AIDS prevalence among Latinos is clustered in a handful of states, with ten states accounting for 88 percent of Latinos estimated to be living with AIDS in 2007. New York, California, and Puerto Rico top the list (see Figure 4.5). Ten states also account for the majority of newly reported AIDS cases among Latinos (83 percent in 2007).[18,19]

- AIDS cases among Latinos vary by place of birth. Latinos born in the United States accounted for 41 percent of estimated AIDS cases among Latinos in 2007, followed by Latinos born in Mexico (23 percent) and Puerto Rico (20 percent).[1,20] HIV transmission patterns among Latinos also vary by place of birth.[1]

Access to and Use of the Health Care System

The HIV Cost and Services Utilization Study (HCSUS), the only nationally representative study of people with HIV/AIDS receiving regular or ongoing medical care for HIV infection, found that Latinos fared more poorly on several important measures of access and quality, differences that diminished over time but were not completely eliminated.[6] In addition, HCSUS found that Latinos were more likely to report postponing medical care due to factors such as lack of transportation.[7] Latinos were also more likely than whites to delay care after their HIV diagnosis.[8]

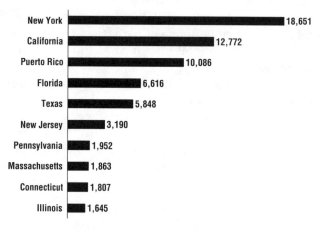

Note: Persons estimated to be living with AIDS as of the end of 2001.

Source: CDC, *HIV/AIDS Surveillance Supplemental Report*, Vol. 9, No. 2, 2003.

Figure 4.5. *Number of Latinos Estimated to Be Living with AIDS, Top Ten States/Areas, 2007*

Health Insurance

Having health insurance, either public or private, improves access to care. Insurance coverage of those with HIV/AIDS varies by race/ethnicity, as it does for the U.S. population overall:

- The HCSUS study found that Latinos with HIV/AIDS were more likely to be publicly insured or uninsured than their white counterparts, with half relying on Medicaid compared to 32 percent of whites. Approximately one quarter of Latinos with HIV/AIDS (24 percent) were uninsured compared to 17 percent of whites. Latinos were also about half as likely to be privately insured than whites (23 percent compared to 44 percent).[21]

- Insurance status also varies at the time of HIV diagnosis. Analysis of data from twenty-five states between 1994 and 2000 found that Latinos were less likely than whites to have private coverage and more likely to be covered by Medicaid at the time of their HIV diagnosis. A third of Latinos were uninsured at the time of their diagnosis, higher than other groups.[22]

HIV Testing

Among the U.S. population overall, Latinos are more likely than whites to report having been tested for HIV in the last twelve months (28 percent compared to 14 percent).[23]

Among those who are HIV-positive, CDC data indicate that four in ten Latinos (41 percent) were tested for HIV late in their illness—that is, diagnosed with AIDS within one year of testing positive (in those states/areas with HIV name reporting); by comparison, 35 percent of blacks and 34 percent of whites were tested late.[1]

Concern about HIV/AIDS

A recent survey found that Latinos express concern about HIV/AIDS. While only one in ten Latinos named it as the most urgent health problem facing the nation, more than one-third named it as a more urgent problem for their community than it was a few years ago.[23]

One in four Latinos say they are personally very concerned about becoming infected with HIV, a proportion that has declined since the mid-1990's. Latino parents are more concerned about a son or daughter becoming infected with HIV, with four in ten (39 percent) reporting they are very concerned.[23]

References

1. CDC. HIV/AIDS Surveillance Report, Vol. 19; 2009.

2. Hall HI et al. "Estimation of HIV Incidence in the United States." *JAMA*, Vol. 300, No. 5; August 2008.

3. CDC. Fact Sheet: Estimates of New HIV Infections in the United States; August 2008.

4. CDC. *MMWR*, Vol. 57, No. 39; 2008.

5. CDC. Slide Set: HIV/AIDS Surveillance in Adolescents and Young Adults (through 2007).

6. Shapiro MF et al. "Variations in the Care of HIV-Infected Adults in the United States." *JAMA*, Vol. 281, No. 24; 1999.

7. Cunningham WE et al. "The Impact of Competing Subsistence Needs and Barriers to Access to Medical Care for Persons with Human Immunodeficiency Virus Receiving Care in the United States." *Medical Care*, Vol. 37, No.12; 1999.

8. Turner BJ et al. "Delayed Medical Care After Diagnosis in a U.S. Probability Sample of Persons Infected with the Human Immuno-deficiency Virus." *Archives of Internal Medicine*, Vol. 160; 2000.

9. U.S. Census Bureau. 2006 Population Estimates.

10. Calculations based only on cases for which race/ethnicity data were provided.

11. Includes reported cases among those thirteen years of age and older. Estimates do not include cases from the U.S. dependencies, possessions, and associated nations, and cases of unknown residence.

12. CDC. Slide Set: HIV Mortality (through 2006).

13. CDC. Special Data Request; 2006.

14. CDC. *MMWR*, Vol. 57, No. 36; 2008.

15. CDC. Slide Set: HIV/AIDS Surveillance by Race/Ethnicity (through 2007).

16. CDC. Fact Sheet: HIV/AIDS Among Men Who Have Sex with Men; June 2007.

17. CDC. *MMWR*, Vol. 54, No. 24; 2005.

18. Kaiser Family Foundation, www.statehealthfacts.org. Data Source: Centers for Disease Control and Prevention, Division of HIV/AIDS Prevention-Surveillance and Epidemiology, Special Data Request; 2009.

19. Estimates include U.S. dependencies, possessions, and associated nations, and cases of unknown residence.

20. Calculations based only on cases for which data by place of birth were provided.

21. Fleishman JA. Personal Communication, Analysis of HCSUS Data; January 2002.

22. Kaiser Family Foundation analysis of CDC data.

23. Kaiser Family Foundation. Survey of Americans on HIV/AIDS; 2009.

HIV/AIDS among Asians and Pacific Islanders

In recent years, the number of AIDS diagnoses among Asians and Pacific Islanders has increased steadily. Although Asians and Pacific Islanders account for approximately 1 percent of the total number of

HIV/AIDS cases in the thirty-three states with long-term, confidential name-based HIV reporting, the Asian and Pacific Islander population in the United States is growing.[1]

Statistics

HIV/AIDS in 2005. An estimated 417 Asians and Pacific Islanders were given a diagnosis of HIV/AIDS, representing 1.1 percent of the 37,331 cases diagnosed that year.[2] Of the 475,220 persons living with HIV/AIDS, 2,996 (0.6 percent) were Asians and Pacific Islanders.[2] Of those given a diagnosis, 78 percent were men, 21 percent were women, and 1 percent were children (under thirteen years of age).[2] The numbers of HIV/AIDS cases may be larger than reported because of underreporting or misclassification of Asians and Pacific Islanders. (This data is based on data from the thirty-three states with long-term, confidential name-based HIV reporting.)

AIDS in 2005. Of the estimated 483 Asians and Pacific Islanders who received an AIDS diagnosis in 2005, 389 (81 percent) were men, and 92 (19 percent) were women. One Asian and Pacific Islander child (under thirteen years of age) received a diagnosis of AIDS.[2] The rate of AIDS diagnosis, by race/ethnicity, was lowest for Asians and Pacific Islanders (3.6 per 100,000 population), compared with 54.1 per 100,000 for blacks (including African Americans), 18.0 per 100,000 for Hispanics, 7.4 for American Indians and Alaska Natives, and 5.9 per 100,000 for whites.[2] An estimated 4,276 Asians and Pacific Islanders were living with AIDS, representing 1 percent of the 421,873 people known to be living with AIDS in the fifty states and the District of Columbia.[2] From the beginning of the epidemic through 2005, an estimated 7,659 Asians and Pacific Islanders were given a diagnosis of AIDS.[2] An estimated 97 Asians and Pacific Islanders with AIDS died in 2005. From the beginning of the epidemic through 2005, an estimated 3,383 Asians and Pacific Islanders with AIDS died, representing less than 1 percent of the 530,756 persons in the fifty states and the District of Columbia who died with AIDS.[2] Of persons given a diagnosis of AIDS during 1997–2004, 81 percent of Asians and Pacific Islanders were alive nine years after diagnosis, compared with 75 percent of whites, 74 percent of Hispanics, 67 percent of American Indians and Alaska Natives, and 66 percent of blacks.[2]

Risk Factors and Barriers to Prevention

Although the proportion of diagnoses of HIV infection and AIDS for Asian and Pacific Islander adults and adolescents remains small relative to other racial/ethnic groups, no evidence indicates significantly lower levels of risk behaviors among this group.[3,4] Asians and Pacific Islanders are likely to face challenges associated with the risk for HIV infection, especially in some regions of the country and for some specific ethnicities within the broader Asian and Pacific Islander group.

Sexual risk factors. Most of the Asians and Pacific Islanders who are infected with HIV are men who have sex with men (MSM).[2] A cause for concern is research that points to rising levels of risk behaviors among Asian and Pacific Islander MSM in certain areas of the country, for example, indications that an HIV epidemic is emerging among young Asian and Pacific Islander MSM in San Francisco.[5]

The findings of other studies support this concern. In a San Francisco study of 503 Asian and Pacific Islander MSM aged eighteen to twenty-nine years, the overall HIV prevalence was nearly 3 percent. This prevalence varied significantly by ethnicity, ranging from 0 percent for Vietnamese MSM to 13.6 percent for Thai MSM. Being of Thai ethnicity, having been born in the United States, being older, or having ever attended a circuit party or special MSM social event was associated with HIV infection. Of these 503 men, 48 percent reported having had unprotected anal intercourse during the past six months.[6] Another study conducted in San Francisco showed that the rates of unprotected anal intercourse and sexually transmitted diseases among young Asian and Pacific Islander MSM during 1999–2002 surpassed the rates for white MSM.[7]

High-risk heterosexual contact is the primary way Asian and Pacific Islander women become infected with HIV.[2] In focus groups, Asian and Pacific Islander women noted cultural taboos against discussing sexual topics and power differentials between genders as reasons for difficulty in getting their partners to use condoms. Domestic violence is also a concern, as is lack of knowledge about HIV/AIDS and lack of culturally and linguistically appropriate HIV prevention programs and materials.[8]

Substance use. The use of methamphetamines and other drugs has been shown to be an important factor associated with unprotected anal intercourse among Asian and Pacific Islander MSM. According to a study of Filipino American methamphetamine users in the San Francisco Bay Area, methamphetamine use was strongly associated with behavioral risk factors for HIV infection, including infrequent condom use, commercial sex activity, and low rates of HIV testing.[9] In a study of young Asian and Pacific Islander MSM, more than half used "party drugs," including

MDMA (3,4- methylenedioxymethamphetamine, or "ecstasy"), inhaled nitrates, hallucinogens, crack, and amphetamines. The use of drugs or alcohol was associated with unprotected anal intercourse.[10]

Low HIV testing rates. HIV testing is an important consideration for Asians and Pacific Islanders. Testing rates are lower for Asians and Pacific Islanders as a group, despite their risk factors for HIV infection. Data from an HIV testing survey in Seattle indicated that of the Asians and Pacific Islanders surveyed, 90 percent perceived themselves at some risk for HIV infection, yet only 47 percent had been tested during the past year[11] Also, CDC's Behavioral Risk Factor Surveillance System found that Asians and Pacific Islanders are significantly less likely than members of other races/ethnicities to report having been tested for HIV.[12]

Low HIV testing rates also affect the stage of HIV disease at which diagnosis is made. CDC surveillance shows that for many Asians and Pacific Islanders, the diagnosis of HIV infection is made late in the course of disease. In 2004, 44 percent of Asians and Pacific Islanders received an AIDS diagnosis within one year after their HIV infection was diagnosed. This is in comparison to 37 percent of whites, 40 percent of blacks, 41 percent of American Indians/Alaska Natives, and 43 percent of Hispanics.[2] Increasing the number of Asians and Pacific islanders who are tested will allow those who are infected to begin health-sustaining treatment and can help to reduce further transmission of the virus.

A study that showed an increase in testing (from 63 percent to 71 percent) between its first and fourth years (1999 to 2002) found that recent testing was most significantly and consistently associated with knowledge of testing sites to which respondents felt comfortable going.[13] This finding points to the importance of culturally and linguistically relevant health services.

Cultural and socioeconomic diversity. Among Asians and Pacific Islanders, there are many nationalities—Chinese, Filipinos, Koreans, Hawaiians, Indians, Japanese, Samoans, Vietnamese, and others—and more than one hundred languages and dialects. The subgroups differ in language, culture, and history. Because many Asians and Pacific Islanders living in the United States are foreign-born, they may experience cultural and language barriers to receiving public health messages. Additionally, many health surveys are administered only in English and perhaps Spanish, a situation that may cause miscommunication or exclude Asians and Pacific Islanders who do not speak English.

As a group, Asians and Pacific Islanders represent both extremes of socioeconomic and health issues. For example, although more than a million Asian Americans live at or below the federal poverty level ($20,650 for a family of four living in the forty-eight contiguous states or the District of Columbia), Asian American women have the longest life expectancy of any racial or ethnic group. Tailoring prevention interventions to meet the needs of this culturally and socioeconomically diverse population remains challenging.[14,15]

Data limitations. The low number of HIV cases among Asians and Pacific Islanders may not reflect the true burden of the epidemic on this population. Not all states with large Asian and Pacific Islander populations have been conducting HIV surveillance long enough to be included in CDC's surveillance. For example, California, where a large proportion of Asians and Pacific Islanders live, began HIV surveillance only during the past few years; thus, its HIV data are not included in CDC surveillance reports.

Additionally, race/ethnicity misclassification in medical records may contribute to the underreporting of HIV/AIDS among Asians and Pacific Islanders.[12]

Limited use of services. Because of language and cultural barriers, lack of access to care, and other issues, many Asians and Pacific Islanders underuse healthcare and prevention services. A study of the use of HIV services by 653 Asians and Pacific Islanders showed that a relatively high proportion had advanced disease and used hospital-based services. Few of them, however, used HIV case management services, housing assistance, substance use treatment, or health education services.[16]

Prevention

CDC estimates that 56,300 new HIV infections occurred in the United States in 2006.[17] Populations of minority races/ethnicities are disproportionately affected by the HIV epidemic. In the United States, Asians and Pacific Islanders are emerging as a group that is at risk for HIV infection.

To reduce the incidence of HIV, CDC released *Revised Recommendations for HIV Testing of Adults, Adolescents, and Pregnant Women in Health-Care Settings* in 2006. These recommendations advise routine HIV screening of adults, adolescents, and pregnant women in healthcare settings in the United States. They also address the need to reduce barriers to HIV testing. In 2003, CDC announced an initiative,

Advancing HIV Prevention. This initiative comprises four strategies: making HIV testing a routine part of medical care, implementing new models for diagnosing HIV infections outside medical settings, preventing new infections by working with HIV-infected persons and their partners, and further decreasing perinatal HIV transmission.

CDC, through the Minority AIDS Initiative, supports efforts to reduce the health disparities experienced in communities of persons of minority races/ethnicities who are at high risk for HIV infection. CDC provides funds to community-based organizations that focus primarily on Asians and Pacific Islanders and provides indirect funding through state, territorial, and local health departments to organizations serving this population. An example of CDC-funded projects focused on the Asian and Pacific Islander population is an organization in New York City that provides client services, education, training, and technical assistance to Asian and Pacific Islander MSM who are at high risk, female and transgender sex workers, and female sex partners of men who are HIV-positive or at high risk for HIV infection.

References

1. US Census Bureau. The Asian population: 2000. Census 2000 Brief. Available at http://www.census.gov/prod/ 2002pubs/ c2kbr01-16.pdf. Accessed April 30, 2007.

2. CDC. *HIV/AIDS Surveillance Report, 2005*. Vol. 17. Rev ed. Atlanta: US Department of Health and Human Services, CDC: 2007:1–46. Accessed June 28, 2007.

3. Hou S-I, Basen-Engquist K. Human immunodeficiency virus risk behavior among white and Asian/Pacific Islander high school students in the United States: does culture make a difference? *Journal of Adolescent Health* 1997;20:68–74.

4. Peterson JL, Bakeman R, Stokes J, and the Community Intervention Trial for Youth Study Team. Racial/ethnic patterns of HIV sexual risk behaviors among young men who have sex with men. *Journal of the Gay and Lesbian Medical Association* 2001;5:155–62.

5. Raymond HF, Chen S, Truong H-H, et al. Trends in sexually transmitted diseases, sexual risk behavior, and HIV infection among Asian/Pacific Islander men who have sex with men, San Francisco 1999–2005. *Sexually Transmitted Diseases*. Published online, August 28, 2006.

6. Choi K, McFarland W, Neilands TB, et al. Low HIV prevalence but high sexual risk among young Asian American men who have sex with men: HIV prevention opportunities. XIV International Conference on AIDS; July 2002; Barcelona, Spain. Abstract MoPeC3434.

7. McFarland W, Chen S, Weide D, Kohn R, Klausner J. Gay Asian men in San Francisco follow the international trend: increases in rates of unprotected anal intercourse and sexually transmitted diseases, 1999–2002. *AIDS Education and Prevention* 2004;16:13–18.

8. Jemmott LS, Maula EC, Bush E. Hearing our voices: assessing HIV prevention needs among Asian and Pacific Islander women. *Journal of Transcultural Nursing* 1999;10:102–11.

9. Nemoto T, Operario D, Soma T. Risk behaviors of Filipino methamphetamine users in San Francisco: implications for prevention and treatment of drug use and HIV. *Public Health Reports* 2002;117(suppl 1): S30–S38.

10. Choi K, McFarland W, Chu PL, et al. Heavy "party" drug and polydrug use and associated sexual risk for HIV among young Asian men who have sex with men. XIV International Conference on AIDS; July 2002; Barcelona, Spain. Abstract E10725.

11. Kahle EM, Freedman MS, Buskin SE. HIV risks and testing behavior among Asians and Pacific Islanders: results of the HIV Testing Survey, 2002–2003. *Journal of the National Medical Association* 2005;97:13S–18S.

12. Zaidi IF, Crepaz N, Song R, et al. Epidemiology of HIV/ AIDS among Asians and Pacific Islanders in the United States. *AIDS Education and Prevention* 2005;17: 405–17.

13. Do TD, Hudes ES, Proctor K, Han C-S, Choi K-H. HIV testing trends and correlates among young Asian and Pacific Islander men who have sex with men in two U.S. cities. *AIDS Education and Prevention* 2006;18:44–55.

14. CDC, Office of Minority Health. Asian American populations. Available at http://www.cdc.gov/omh/Populations/AsianAm/AsianAm.htm. Accessed April 30, 2007.

15. U.S. Department of Health and Human Services. The 2007 HHS poverty guidelines. Available at http://aspe.hhs.gov/poverty/07poverty.shtml. Accessed April 30, 2007.

16. Pounds MB, Conviser R, Ashman JJ, Bourassa V. Ryan White CARE Act service use by Asian/Pacific Islanders and other clients in three California metropolitan areas (1997–1998). *Journal of Community Health* 2002;27:403–17.

17. Hall HI, Ruiguang S, Rhodes P, et al. Estimation of HIV incidence in the United States. *JAMA*. 2008;300:520–29.

HIV/AIDS among American Indians and Alaska Natives

HIV/AIDS is a growing problem among American Indians and Alaska Natives.

Even though the numbers of HIV and AIDS diagnoses for American Indians and Alaska Natives represent less than 1 percent of the total number of HIV/AIDS cases reported to CDC's HIV/AIDS Reporting System, when population size is taken into account, American Indians and Alaska Natives in 2005 ranked third in rates of HIV/AIDS diagnosis, after blacks (including African Americans) and Hispanics.[1] American Indians and Alaska Natives make up 1.5 percent (4.1 million people) of the total U.S. population.[2] The rate of AIDS diagnosis for this group has been higher than that for whites since 1995.

Statistics

HIV/AIDS in 2005. HIV/AIDS was diagnosed for an estimated 195 American Indians and Alaska Natives (adults, adolescents, and children), representing 0.5 percent of the total number of HIV/AIDS diagnoses reported for that year.[1] The rate (per 100,000 persons) of HIV/AIDS diagnosis for American Indians and Alaska Natives was 10.4, compared with 71.3 for blacks, 27.8 for Hispanics, 8.8 for whites, and 7.4 for Asians and Pacific Islanders. Women accounted for 29 percent of the HIV/AIDS diagnoses among American Indians and Alaska Natives.[1] (This information refers to the thirty-three states with long-term, confidential name-based HIV reporting.)

AIDS in 2005. The estimated rate (per 100,000) of AIDS diagnosis for American Indian and Alaska Native adults and adolescents was 9.3, the third highest after the rates for black adults and adolescents (68.7) and Hispanic adults and adolescents (24.0). The estimated AIDS diagnosis rate was 6.9 for white adults and adolescents and 4.3 for Asian and Pacific Islander adults and adolescents.[1] AIDS was diagnosed for an estimated 182 American Indians and Alaska Natives, representing approximately 0.4 percent of all AIDS diagnoses in 2005.[1] These data include persons whose HIV infection had been diagnosed earlier. An estimated 1,581 American Indians and Alaska Natives were living with AIDS.[1] An estimated 81 American Indians and Alaska Natives with AIDS died in 2005, representing approximately 0.5 percent of all deaths of persons with AIDS for that year.[1] From the beginning of the epidemic through 2005, AIDS was diagnosed for an estimated 3,238 American Indians and Alaska Natives.[1] From the beginning of the epidemic through 2005, an estimated 1,657 American Indians and Alaska Natives with AIDS had died.[1] In comparison, 235,879 whites, 211,559 blacks, 77,125 Hispanics, and 3,383 Asians and Pacific Islanders with AIDS had died. Of persons who had received a diagnosis of AIDS during 1997– 2004, American Indians and Alaska Natives had survived for a shorter time than had Asians and Pacific Islanders, whites, or Hispanics. After nine years, 67 percent of American Indians and Alaska Natives were alive, compared with 66 percent of blacks, 74 percent of Hispanics, 75 percent of whites, and 81 percent of Asians and Pacific Islanders.[1] From the beginning of the epidemic through 2005, AIDS had been diagnosed for an estimated 32 American Indian and Alaska Native children (younger than thirteen years).[1]

Risk Factors and Barriers to Prevention

Race and ethnicity are not, by themselves, risk factors for HIV infection. However, American Indians and Alaska Natives are likely to face challenges associated with risk for HIV infection, including the following.

Sexual risk factors. The presence of a sexually transmitted disease can increase the chance of contracting or spreading HIV.[3] High rates of *Chlamydia trachomatis* infection, gonorrhea, and syphilis among American Indians and Alaska Natives suggest that the sexual behaviors that facilitate the spread of HIV are relatively common among American Indians and Alaska Natives. According to 2005 surveillance data by race/ethnicity, the second highest rates of gonorrhea and *Chlamydia trachomatis* infection were those for American Indians and Alaska Natives. The third highest rate of syphilis was that for American Indians and Alaska Natives.[4,5]

Substance use. Persons who use illicit drugs (casually or habitually) or who abuse alcohol are more likely to engage in risky behaviors, such as unprotected sex, when they are under the influence of drugs or alcohol.[6] Results of the 2005 National Survey on Drug Use and Health indicate that the rate of current illicit drug use was higher among American Indians and Alaska Natives (12.8 percent) than among persons of other races or ethnicities.[7]

Cultural diversity. To be effective, HIV/AIDS prevention interventions must be tailored to specific audiences. The American Indian and Alaska Native population makes up 562 federally recognized tribes plus at least 50 state-recognized tribes.[8] Because each tribe has its own culture, beliefs, and practices and these tribes may be subdivided into language groups, it can be challenging to create programs for each group. Therefore, prevention programs that can be adapted to individual tribal cultures and beliefs are critically important. Current programs emphasize traditional teachings and the importance of the community.

Socioeconomic issues. Issues related to poverty (for example, lower levels of education and poorer access to healthcare) may directly or indirectly increase the risk for HIV infection.[9] Socioeconomic factors, such as poverty, coexist with epidemiologic risk factors for HIV infection in American Indian and Alaska Native communities. During 2002–2004, approximately one quarter (24.3 percent) of American Indians and Alaska Natives about twice the national average (12.4 percent) were living in poverty.[10] The proportion of the American Indian and Alaska Native population with a high school diploma (66 percent) in 1990 was less than the national average (75 percent).[11]

Life expectancy for American Indians and Alaska Natives is shorter than that for persons of other races/ethnicities in the United States; the rates of many diseases, including diabetes, tuberculosis, and alcoholism, are higher; and access to healthcare is poorer.[12,13]

These indicators demonstrate the vulnerability of American Indians and Alaska Natives to additional health stress, including HIV infection.

HIV testing issues. Access to HIV testing and issues concerning confidentiality are important for many American Indians and Alaska Natives. For example, at the time of AIDS diagnosis, more American Indians and Alaska Natives, compared with persons of other races/ethnicities, resided in rural areas.[14] Those who live in rural areas may be less likely to be tested for HIV because of limited access to testing. Also, American Indians and Alaska Natives may be less likely to seek testing because of concerns about confidentiality in close-knit communities, where someone who seeks testing is likely to encounter a friend, a relative, or an acquaintance at the local healthcare facility.

During 1997–2000, 50.5 percent of American Indians and Alaska Natives who responded to the Behavioral Risk Factor Surveillance System survey reported that they had never been tested for HIV. This percentage was higher in the southwestern United States, where 58.1 percent of the American Indians and Alaska Natives reported never having been tested.[15]

Data limitations. Current data regarding HIV infection and AIDS among American Indians and Alaska Natives have limitations.

Surveillance data are incomplete. Not all states with large American Indian and Alaska Native populations have been conducting HIV surveillance. For example, California began HIV surveillance only during the past few years and thus is not included in these data.

Racial misclassification and underreporting is also a problem. Even though the numbers of diagnoses for American Indians and Alaska Natives are relatively low, these numbers may be affected by racial misclassification. Studies in Alaska and Los Angeles have shown that the degree of misclassification differs geographically. In Alaska, 3 percent of American Indians and Alaska Natives with HIV/AIDS were misclassified as being of another race; in Los Angeles, 56 percent of American Indians and Alaska Natives with AIDS were racially misclassified.[16,17]

Prevention

CDC estimates that 56,300 new HIV infections occurred in the United States in 2006.[18] Persons of minority races/ethnicities are disproportionately affected by the HIV epidemic. To reduce further the incidence of HIV infection, CDC announced Advancing HIV Prevention (AHP) in 2003. This initiative comprises four strategies: making HIV testing a routine part of medical care, implementing new models for diagnosing HIV infections outside medical settings, preventing new infections by working with HIV-infected persons and their partners, and further decreasing perinatal HIV transmission.

Through AHP, CDC conducted demonstration projects in American Indian and Alaska Native communities to examine ways to make voluntary HIV testing a routine part of medical care and to implement new models for diagnosing HIV infections outside medical settings. Preliminary data show that through these projects, over two thousand American Indians and Alaska Natives were tested for HIV. Demonstration projects were conducted at the following sites:

- Salt Lake City, Utah, where a community-based organization (CBO) partnered with the Indian Walk-In Center to offer routine testing—including rapid testing at some sites—to five tribal entities and eleven reservations.

- Phoenix, Arizona, where a CBO conducted routine HIV testing in nontraditional settings (e.g., health fairs, powwows) through local outreach.

- Sault Ste. Marie, Michigan, where the Sault Ste. Marie Tribe and the Chippewa Indian Sault Tribe Health Center conducted routine HIV testing for clients aged seventeen to forty-nine. Rapid testing was conducted simultaneously at one main health center and four satellite clinics as well as an urgent care clinic.

CDC, through the Minority AIDS Initiative, supports efforts to reduce the health disparities experienced in communities of persons of minority races/ethnicities who are at high risk for HIV. These funds are used to address high-priority HIV prevention needs in such communities. The following are some CDC-funded prevention programs that state and local health departments and CBOs provide for American Indians and Alaska Natives:

- Helping tribes develop or expand HIV prevention services and improve services for persons infected with, or affected by, HIV/AIDS

- Building and strengthening the capacity of tribal organizations and urban Indian health centers throughout the United States to develop effective HIV prevention through intertribal networking and collaboration

- Providing HIV prevention education in rural Alaska Native communities and implementing an evidence-based intervention, Community PROMISE, in the Yukon-Kuskokwim delta and Maniilaq regions.

References

1. CDC. *HIV/AIDS Surveillance Report, 2005*. Vol. 17. Rev ed. Atlanta: U.S. Department of Health and Human Services, CDC: 2007:1–46. Accessed June 28, 2007.

2. U.S. Census Bureau. *The American Indian and Alaska Native population: 2000*. Census 2000 Brief. February 2002.

3. Fleming DT, Wasserheit JN. From epidemiological synergy to public health policy and practice: the contribution of other sexually transmitted diseases to sexual transmission of HIV infection. *Sexually Transmitted Infections* 1999;75:3–17.

4. CDC. *Sexually Transmitted Disease Surveillance 2005*. Atlanta: U.S. Department of Health and Human Services, CDC; November 2006: Tables 10B, 20B, 32B.

5. McNaghten AD, Neal JJ, Li J, Fleming PL. Epidemiologic profile of HIV and AIDS among American Indians/Alaska Natives in the USA through 2000. *Ethnicity and Health* 2005;10:55–71.

6. Leigh B, Stall R. Substance use and risky sexual behavior for exposure to HIV: issues in methodology, interpretation, and prevention. *American Psychologist* 1993;48:1035–45.

7. Substance Abuse and Mental Health Services Administration. *Results from the 2005 National Survey on Drug Use and Health: National Findings*. Rockville, MD: Substance Abuse and Mental Health Services Administration; 2006. Office of Applied Studies, NSDUH Series H-30, DHHS Publication No. SMA 06-4195.

8. U.S. Department of the Interior, Bureau of Indian Affairs. Indian entities recognized and eligible to receive services from the United States Bureau of Indian Affairs. *Federal Register* 2003(December 5);68(234):68179–84.

9. Diaz T, Chu SY, Buehler JW, et al. Socioeconomic differences among people with AIDS: results from a multistate surveillance project. *American Journal of Preventive Medicine* 1994;10:217–22.

10. DeNavas-Walt C, Proctor BD, Lee CH. *Income, Poverty, and Health Insurance Coverage in the United States: 2004*. Washington, DC: US Government Printing Office; August 2005. Current Population Reports P60-229.

11. U.S. Census Bureau. *The American Indian, Eskimo, and Aleut population*. 2001.

12. Korenbrot CC, Ehlers S, Crouch JA. Disparities in hospitalizations of rural American Indians. *Medical Care* 2003;41:626–36.

13. Zuckerman S, Haley J, Roubideaux Y, Lillie-Blanton M. Health service access, use, and insurance coverage among American Indians/Alaska Natives and whites: what role does the Indian Health Service play? *American Journal of Public Health* 2004;94:53–59.

14. Bertolli J, McNaghten AD, Campsmith M, et al. Surveillance systems monitoring HIV/AIDS and HIV risk behaviors among

American Indians and Alaska Natives. *AIDS Education and Prevention* 2004;16:218–37.

15. CDC. Surveillance for health behaviors of American Indians and Alaska Natives: findings from the Behavioral Risk Factor Surveillance System 1997–2000. *MMWR* 2003;52(No. SS-07):1–13.

16. State of Alaska Health and Social Services, Section of Epidemiology. Accuracy of race/ethnicity data for HIV/AIDS cases among Alaska Natives. *State of Alaska Epidemiology Bulletin* 2003;No. 11(May 13).

17. Hu YW, Yu Harlan M, Frye DM. Racial misclassification among American Indians/Alaska Natives who were reported with AIDS in Los Angeles County, 1981–2002. National HIV Prevention Conference; August 2003; Atlanta. Abstract W0-B0703.

18. Hall HI, Ruiguang S, Rhodes P, et al. Estimation of HIV incidence in the United States. *JAMA*. 2008;300:520–29.

Part Two

HIV/AIDS Transmission, Risk Factors, and Prevention

Chapter 5

HIV and Its Transmission: An Overview

Research has revealed a great deal of valuable medical, scientific, and public health information about the human immunodeficiency virus (HIV) and acquired immunodeficiency syndrome (AIDS). The ways in which HIV can be transmitted have been clearly identified. Unfortunately, false information or statements that are not supported by scientific findings continue to be shared widely through the internet or popular press. It is hoped that this chapter will correct a few misperceptions about HIV.

How HIV Is Transmitted

HIV is spread by sexual contact with an infected person, by sharing needles and/or syringes (primarily for drug injection) with someone who is infected, or, less commonly (and now very rarely in countries where blood is screened for HIV antibodies), through transfusions of infected blood or blood clotting factors. Babies born to HIV-infected women may become infected before or during birth or through breast-feeding after birth.

In the healthcare setting, workers have been infected with HIV after being stuck with needles containing HIV-infected blood or, less frequently, after infected blood gets into a worker's open cut or a mucous membrane (for example, the eyes or inside of the nose). There has been only one instance of patients being infected by a healthcare worker in

Reprinted from the Centers for Disease Control and Prevention, March 8, 2007.

the United States; this involved HIV transmission from one infected dentist to six patients. Investigations have been completed involving more than twenty-two thousand patients of sixty-three HIV-infected physicians, surgeons, and dentists, and no other cases of this type of transmission have been identified in the United States.

Some people fear that HIV might be transmitted in other ways; however, no scientific evidence to support any of these fears has been found. If HIV were being transmitted through other routes (such as through air, water, or insects), the pattern of reported AIDS cases would be much different from what has been observed. For example, if mosquitoes could transmit HIV infection, many more young children and preadolescents would have been diagnosed with AIDS.

All reported cases suggesting new or potentially unknown routes of transmission are thoroughly investigated by state and local health departments with the assistance, guidance, and laboratory support from the Centers for Disease Control and Prevention (CDC). No additional routes of transmission have been recorded, despite a national sentinel system designed to detect just such an occurrence.

The following paragraphs specifically address some of the common misperceptions about HIV transmission.

HIV in the Environment

Scientists and medical authorities agree that HIV does not survive well in the environment, making the possibility of environmental transmission remote. HIV is found in varying concentrations or amounts in blood, semen, vaginal fluid, breast milk, saliva, and tears. To obtain data on the survival of HIV, laboratory studies have required the use of artificially high concentrations of laboratory-grown virus. Although these unnatural concentrations of HIV can be kept alive for days or even weeks under precisely controlled and limited laboratory conditions, CDC studies have shown that drying of even these high concentrations of HIV reduces the amount of infectious virus by 90 to 99 percent within several hours. Since the HIV concentrations used in laboratory studies are much higher than those actually found in blood or other specimens, drying of HIV-infected human blood or other body fluids reduces the theoretical risk of environmental transmission to that which has been observed—essentially zero. Incorrect interpretation of conclusions drawn from laboratory studies have unnecessarily alarmed some people.

Results from laboratory studies should not be used to assess specific personal risk of infection because the amount of virus studied is not found in human specimens or elsewhere in nature, and no one has been identified as infected with HIV due to contact with an environmental surface. Additionally, HIV is unable to reproduce outside its living host (unlike many bacteria or fungi, which may do so under suitable conditions), except under laboratory conditions, therefore, it does not spread or maintain infectiousness outside its host.

Households

Although HIV has been transmitted between family members in a household setting, this type of transmission is very rare. These transmissions are believed to have resulted from contact between skin or mucous membranes and infected blood. To prevent even such rare occurrences, precautions should be taken in all settings—including the home—to prevent exposures to the blood of persons who are HIV infected, at risk for HIV infection, or whose infection and risk status are unknown. For example:

- Gloves should be worn during contact with blood or other body fluids that could possibly contain visible blood, such as urine, feces, or vomit.

- Cuts, sores, or breaks on both the caregiver's and patient's exposed skin should be covered with bandages.

- Hands and other parts of the body should be washed immediately after contact with blood or other body fluids, and surfaces soiled with blood should be disinfected appropriately.

- Practices that increase the likelihood of blood contact, such as sharing of razors and toothbrushes, should be avoided.

- Needles and other sharp instruments should be used only when medically necessary and handled according to recommendations for healthcare settings. (Do not put caps back on needles by hand or remove needles from syringes. Dispose of needles in puncture-proof containers out of the reach of children and visitors.)

Businesses and Other Settings

There is no known risk of HIV transmission to co-workers, clients, or consumers from contact in industries such as food-service establishments. Food-service workers known to be infected with HIV need not be restricted from work unless they have other infections or illnesses (such as diarrhea or hepatitis A) for which any food-service worker, regardless of HIV infection status, should be restricted. CDC recommends that all food-service workers follow recommended standards and practices of good personal hygiene and food sanitation.

In 1985, CDC issued routine precautions that all personal-service workers (such as hairdressers, barbers, cosmetologists, and massage therapists) should follow, even though there is no evidence of transmission from a personal-service worker to a client or vice versa. Instruments that are intended to penetrate the skin (such as tattooing and acupuncture needles, ear piercing devices) should be used once and disposed of or thoroughly cleaned and sterilized. Instruments not intended to penetrate the skin but which may become contaminated with blood (for example, razors) should be used for only one client and disposed of or thoroughly cleaned and disinfected after each use. Personal-service workers can use the same cleaning procedures that are recommended for healthcare institutions.

CDC knows of no instances of HIV transmission through tattooing or body piercing, although hepatitis B virus has been transmitted during some of these practices. One case of HIV transmission from acupuncture has been documented. Body piercing (other than ear piercing) is relatively new in the United States, and the medical complications for body piercing appear to be greater than for tattoos. Healing of piercings generally will take weeks, and sometimes even months, and the pierced tissue could conceivably be abraded (torn or cut) or inflamed even after healing. Therefore, a theoretical HIV transmission risk does exist if the unhealed or abraded tissues come into contact with an infected person's blood or other infectious body fluid. Additionally, HIV could be transmitted if instruments contaminated with blood are not sterilized or disinfected between clients.

Kissing

Casual contact through closed-mouth or "social" kissing is not a risk for transmission of HIV. Because of the potential for contact with blood during "French" or open-mouth kissing, CDC recommends against engaging in this activity with a person known to be infected. However, the risk of acquiring HIV during open-mouth kissing is believed to be very low. CDC has investigated only one case of HIV infection that may be attributed to contact with blood during open-mouth kissing.

Biting

In 1997, CDC published findings from a state health department investigation of an incident that suggested blood-to-blood transmission of HIV by a human bite. There have been other reports in the medical literature in which HIV appeared to have been transmitted by a bite. Severe trauma with extensive tissue tearing and damage and presence of blood were reported in each of these instances. Biting is not a common way of transmitting HIV. In fact, there are numerous reports of bites that did not result in HIV infection.

Saliva, Tears, and Sweat

HIV has been found in saliva and tears in very low quantities from some AIDS patients. It is important to understand that finding a small amount of HIV in a body fluid does not necessarily mean that HIV can be transmitted by that body fluid. HIV has not been recovered from the sweat of HIV-infected persons. Contact with saliva, tears, or sweat has never been shown to result in transmission of HIV.

Insects

From the onset of the HIV epidemic, there has been concern about transmission of the virus by biting and bloodsucking insects. However, studies conducted by researchers at CDC and elsewhere have shown no evidence of HIV transmission through insects—even in areas where there are many cases of AIDS and large populations of insects such as mosquitoes. Lack of such outbreaks, despite intense efforts to detect them, supports the conclusion that HIV is not transmitted by insects.

The results of experiments and observations of insect biting behavior indicate that when an insect bites a person, it does not inject its own or a previously bitten person's or animal's blood into the next person bitten. Rather, it injects saliva, which acts as a lubricant or anticoagulant so the insect can feed efficiently. Such diseases as yellow fever and malaria are transmitted through the saliva of specific species of mosquitoes. However, HIV lives for only a short time inside an insect and, unlike organisms that are transmitted via insect bites, HIV does not reproduce (and does not survive) in insects. Thus, even if the virus enters a mosquito or another sucking or biting insect, the insect does not become infected and cannot transmit HIV to the next human it feeds on or bites. HIV is not found in insect feces.

There is also no reason to fear that a biting or bloodsucking insect, such as a mosquito, could transmit HIV from one person to another through HIV-infected blood left on its mouthparts. Two factors serve to explain why this is so—first, infected people do not have constant, high levels of HIV in their bloodstreams and, second, insect mouth parts do not retain large amounts of blood on their surfaces. Further, scientists who study insects have determined that biting insects normally do not travel from one person to the next immediately after ingesting blood. Rather, they fly to a resting place to digest this blood meal.

Effectiveness of Condoms

Condoms are classified as medical devices and are regulated by the Food and Drug Administration (FDA). Condom manufacturers in the United States test each latex condom for defects, including holes, before it is packaged. The proper and consistent use of latex or polyurethane (a type of plastic) condoms when engaging in sexual intercourse—vaginal, anal, or oral—can greatly reduce a person's risk of acquiring or transmitting sexually transmitted diseases, including HIV infection.

There are many different types and brands of condoms available—however, only latex or polyurethane condoms provide a highly effective mechanical barrier to HIV. In laboratories, viruses occasionally have been shown to pass through natural membrane ("skin" or lambskin) condoms, which may contain natural pores and are therefore not recommended for disease prevention (they are documented to be effective for contraception). Women may wish to consider using the female condom when a male condom cannot be used.

For condoms to provide maximum protection, they must be used consistently (every time) and correctly. Several studies of correct and consistent condom use clearly show that latex condom breakage rates in this country are less than 2 percent. Even when condoms do break, one study showed that more than half of such breaks occurred prior to ejaculation.

When condoms are used reliably, they have been shown to prevent pregnancy up to 98 percent of the time among couples using them as their only method of contraception. Similarly, numerous studies among sexually active people have demonstrated that a properly used latex condom provides a high degree of protection against a variety of sexually transmitted diseases, including HIV infection.

Chapter 6

Risky Behaviors and HIV

Chapter Contents

Section 6.1

Alcohol Use and HIV Risk

"HIV/AIDS Risk and Drinking Patterns," copyright © 1995–2010 by International Center for Alcohol Policies. Reproduced by permission of the International Center for Alcohol Policies. Originally published as: International Center for Alcohol Policies (2008). Module 24 HIV/AIDS Risks and Drinking Patterns. In *ICAP Blue Book: Practical Guides for Alcohol Policy and Prevention Approaches*, available online at http://www.icap.org/PolicyTools/ICAPBlueBook/BlueBookModules/24HIVAIDSRisksandDrinkingPatterns/

The spread of human immunodeficiency virus (HIV), the virus that causes acquired immunodeficiency syndrome (AIDS), is not only a challenge to public health but also to the social and economic wellbeing of individuals, families, communities, and countries.[1] With this in mind, one positive step toward reducing the transmission of HIV has included assessing the roles of risky behavioral patterns (e.g., risky drinking) in the spread of the disease. To that end, the intersection of risky drinking patterns with high-risk injection and/or sex-related practices—two major modes of HIV transmission—must be thoroughly examined.

HIV Risk-Taking Behaviors and Harmful Drinking Patterns

HIV is spread via unprotected sexual contact with an infected person, by direct blood contact through contaminated needles (primarily for illicit drug injection or in healthcare settings without proper sterilization procedures), during birth or breast-feeding (for infants born to HIV-infected mothers), or through transfusions of infected blood.[2] Unsafe sex, identified by the World Health Organization (WHO) as one of ten leading risk factors for harm globally, is the most common mode of HIV transmission (World Health Organization [WHO], 2002). "Unsafe sex" refers to sexual contact with partners of unknown HIV status without the use of condoms. Its toll is particularly great in developing countries that are characterized by high mortality rates, where unsafe sex is the second highest risk factor for harm, accounting for 10.2 percent of the total disease burden.[3]

There is much debate in the scientific literature about the relationship between certain risky drinking patterns and sexual risk-taking. It has been suggested that heavy drinking patterns may influence sexual risk-taking by affecting judgment and reducing inhibitions, thereby diminishing perceived risk or excusing behaviors otherwise considered socially unacceptable (National Institute on Alcohol Abuse and Alcoholism [NIAAA], 2002).

For example, a study undertaken by WHO in eight countries[4] found that inebriation was considered a culturally acceptable excuse for acting irresponsibly (including engaging in unsafe sexual activities) in Belarus, Kenya, Mexico, Romania, the Russian Federation, and South Africa. In Romania, this conceptualization was exclusive to men, implying that such behavior was correlated with an assertion of masculinity (WHO, 2005).

Research indicates that the relationship between alcohol and sexual conduct is context- and community-specific. Outcomes are likely to vary, depending on situation, gender, sexual and alcohol experiences, cultural norms and practices, drinking patterns, and individual physiological responses to alcohol (e.g., Cooper, 2002; Corte & Sommers, 2005; Markos, 2005; McNair, Carter, & Wlliams, 1998; Poulson, Eppler, Satterwaite, Wuensch, & Bass, 1998). Expectations surrounding the effects of alcohol (e.g., the perception that alcohol enhances sexual arousal and performance)[5] and personality traits associated with both drinking and sexual risk-taking (e.g., impulsive decision-making, stimulus- and sensation-seeking)[6] may also influence unsafe sexual practices. The WHO study supports this assertion, reporting that in the Russian Federation "there was a common misconception that a person without alcohol was incapable of engaging in sex" (WHO, 2005, p. 46).

These factors are, however, subjective and difficult to quantify. In addition, the important and multifaceted role alcohol plays in various cultures, traditions, and social contexts does not afford an easy comparative analysis across borders or even within a given country (e.g., Heath, 1995, 2000). A consistent methodology for measuring an association between drinking patterns and the transmission of HIV/AIDS has not yet been developed.

Multiple-Risk Groups and HIV/AIDS

Several studies have linked alcohol intoxication with greater injection drug risk behaviors, including the sharing of needles or other injection equipment (e.g., Robles et al., 2004; Stein, Charuvastra, Anderson, Sobota, & Friedmann, 2002; Stein, Hanna, et al., 2000). HIV transmission rates through sexual contact are also shown to be higher in the presence of harmful drinking patterns, especially among groups whose behaviors, context, or lifestyles already place them at risk of acquiring the virus. Therefore, many of those persons at risk of experiencing alcohol-related problems.

The intersection between alcohol misuse and HIV risk behaviors is particularly visible among populations disproportionately affected by poverty, inequality, discrimination, instability, insecurity, and limited opportunities, lacking social or institutional support. These factors may expose individuals to co-occurring risks such as sexual coercion and violence and/or contribute to the incidence of transactional sex for drugs, money, or shelter. For example, many young women around the globe (and, to a lesser extent, young men) encounter personal danger while trying to secure monetary or material resources for themselves and their families. This is especially the case in the context of extreme poverty, where many girls and young women are forced to trade sex as a means of survival (Gregson et al., 2002; UN Secretary General's Task Force on Women, Girls and HIV/AIDS in Southern Africa, 2004). A recent study of a refugee camp in Kakuma, Kenya, described the link between women brewing, selling, and consuming illegal forms of traditional alcohol and transactional sex (Adelekan, 2006). Sex work was frequently exchanged for money or alcohol, often in an inebriated state, with "lack of condom use being the rule rather than the exception" (Adelekan, 2006, p. 46). The report also detailed the increased vulnerability of women, while intoxicated, to forms of gender-based sexual violence and rape.

Some studies have also shown a higher rate of HIV infection among individuals with problem drinking, such as persons in alcohol abuse treatment. One such study based in San Francisco, California, identified HIV prevalence rates in alcohol treatment facilities to be several times higher than local published estimates, irrespective of injection drug use (Avins, Woods, Lindan, Hudes, Clark, & Hulley, 1994; see also Mahler et al., 1994, Petry, 1999). However, due to the concurrence of social, economic, and personality factors, this is likely to be a correlative, not causative, relationship. The potential link between sexual risk-taking and problem drinking in HIV-positive individuals could have significant implications for the spread of the virus (Parsons, Vicioso, Kutnick, Punzalan, Halkitis, & Velasquez, 2004, Kalichman et al., 2003, Bouhnik et al., 2007); therefore, dyadic interventions may prove most effective in mitigating harm.

High-Risk Settings and Sexual Networks

Understanding sexual networks is crucial to reducing transmission rates of HIV, as an individual's risk is greatly influenced by his or her location within a sexual network.[7] In drinking establishments where sexual networking is likely to occur, sexual contact may be facilitated by particular drinking patterns. Two studies in South Africa reported that 75 percent of respondents identified local drinking places as public venues where people went specifically to meet new sexual partners and with the intention to engage in sex (Morojele et al., 2006; Weir, Pailman, Mahlalela, Coetzee, Meidany, Boerma, 2003). Research participants reported that low lighting, seductive music, unisex toilets, and lack of condoms were conducive to sexual intercourse. When combined with heavy alcohol consumption, these factors were stated to contribute to the incidence of unsafe sex. In both studies, condoms were seen by the participants as less important or even forgettable when drinking, and alcohol was perceived by many male respondents to improve sexual performance. Further research conducted in sub-Saharan Africa has linked risky drinking places, sexual networking, and increased prevalence of HIV/AIDS. In Tanzania, for example, local brew sellers and female workers in bars, guesthouses, and restaurants were found to be at high risk for sexually transmitted infections (STI) and HIV exposure (Ao, Sam, Masenga, Seage, & Kapiga, 2006; Hoffman et al., 2004).

When assessing the nature and risks associated with drinking patterns and sexual networking, it is necessary to consider the influence of cultural beliefs and expectations surrounding drinking and sex. For example, certain ingrained gender norms about masculinity and cultural practices, such as intergenerational marriage, contribute to and even condone sexual coercion. One Ugandan study found that perceptions surrounding women's acceptance of drinks from men in a bar was viewed by men as signifying consent to sex and that refusal could then "justify" resorting to sexual coercion (Wolff, Busza, Bufumbo, & Whitworth, 2006). In this context, frequenting drinking venues may promote sexual risk for many young girls and women. Simply reducing alcohol misuse in and of itself—while helpful—would not address the underlying sociocultural context and therefore would be insufficient to lower sexual risks in all circumstances. As one study concluded, "heavy drinking seems to exacerbate rather than cause the sexual risk behaviors in question" (Morojele et al., 2006, p. 226).

Heavy Drinking and Progression of HIV/AIDS

Heavy alcohol use has been shown to negatively impact the body's immune function. By suppressing the normal responses that protect it from disease, alcohol misuse may decrease the body's ability to defend itself upon exposure to the HIV virus. Moreover, chronic heavy alcohol consumption and HIV infection each can compromise the immune system; in combination, they may also increase the risk of subsequent opportunistic infections and accelerate progression of HIV to AIDS (see Bryant, 2006).[8]

For individuals living with HIV, problem drinking may also contribute to delays in seeking treatment and deter adherence to antiretroviral (ARV) drugs.[9] A range of factors such as lack of housing, drug use, social stigma, and lack of support for infected individuals are known to deter compliance with HIV/AIDS treatments among problem drinkers (Berg, Demas, Howard, Schoenbaum, Gourevitch, & Arnsten, 2004). Patient noncompliance to ARV therapy not only results in poorer HIV treatment outcomes but can also lead to drug resistance (Lucas, Gebo, Chaisson, & Moore, 2002; Meyerhoff, 2001; Palepu, Raj, Horton, Tibbetts, Meli, & Samet, 2005). Treating HIV-positive individuals with a history of alcohol abuse calls for special attention to these patients' drinking problems and may require going beyond motivational interviewing to include supervised medication delivery or simplified dosing regiments to enhance adherence to treatment (e.g., Samet et al., 2005).

Implications for Policy and Prevention

In developing policies to address HIV/AIDS within a given society, it is vital to explore patterns of risky behavior. This is impossible without government commitment to and coordination of relevant political, economic, and social interventions. Unfortunately, governments in many countries are reluctant or even unwilling to address HIV/AIDS as a matter of urgency. While the private sector cannot compensate for a lack of political will in reforming specific national health and education frameworks and policies, it can contribute to prevention, treatment, and/or education within areas relevant to its core business interests and activities.

An open dialogue at both the national and local levels is essential in developing appropriate, responsive, sustainable, and robust policy change. By engaging various stakeholders—such as civil society groups, the private sector, municipal and/or national governments—local knowledge can be drawn from the community and assimilated into policy-making activities. In this context, successful programs that are focused on behavior modification require the approval and participation of local leaders and public figures influencing popular opinion (e.g., Kelly et al., 1992; Sikkema et al., 2000; Woelk, Fritz, Bassett, Todd, & Chingono, 2001; Sivaram et al., 2007). For instance, effecting behavioral change in the workplace (e.g., in convincing people to step forward for voluntary HIV testing) requires the buy-in of (local) management. Finding appropriate ways to expand successful workplace programs into surrounding communities to include customers, suppliers, and consumers is also desired, but may again be difficult unless all local leadership is enthusiastic about addressing such issues.

The beverage alcohol sector—defined broadly to include producers, retailers, sellers, distributors, and others—is particularly well placed to access multiple risk populations. Potential routes to prevention, education, and treatment exist within the sector's broad supply and transportation networks, its available skills and resources, and along its supply and production chains. These may include rural and urban communities, migrant labor/truckers and community-based employees, small and medium-sized businesses, management and staff divided by differing socioeconomic levels, and both male and female workers. Alcohol distribution points within communities, such as shebeens,[10] bars, hotels, and guesthouses, can often be fertile grounds for intervention programs based on community-specific patterns of alcohol purchases and drinking. In the Indian city of Chennai, for example, community-based HIV educational interventions led by local opinion leaders have targeted wine shops (Sivaram et al., 2007), a practice endorsed by other research, in order to address and reduce the role risky drinking plays in transmitting HIV (Weir et al., 2003).

The same India-based study emphasized the use of men as a target for HIV education interventions in risky drinking settings, underscoring the often dominant role men play in sexual partnerships (Sivaram et al., 2007). Men are important stakeholders in effective alcohol–HIV/AIDS interventions as concepts of masculinity generally afford them more social liberties with respect to alcohol use and sex (WHO, 2005). Community settings can also be utilized to provide social skills training for women, affecting their ability to negotiate condom use and increasing awareness of testing/counseling on alcohol and STI/HIV issues. For example in Mariakani, Kenya, the ROADS Project[11] is working through local women's groups to reach out to women who brew mnazi (an inexpensive and strong form of alcohol) in a program that focuses primary prevention measures for HIV and discusses the link between HIV transmission and alcohol abuse. The brewers are trained in addressing gender-based violence, to be peer leaders, to promote condoms in their informal establishments, and to refer customers and peers for HIV counseling, testing, care, and treatment. The project is also working to promote alternative economic activities for these women (Family Health International & USAID, 2007).

Innovative HIV/AIDS prevention and treatment programs can address the ramifications of intersecting patterns of risky behavior and, therefore, incorporate messages about alcohol misuse and its potential adverse outcomes to effect behavior change. In one such example, the Society to Help Rural Empowerment & Education (STHREE) in Andhra Pradesh, India, promotes behavioral change in remote rural communities, along the highways, and at truck stops (a particular source of HIV/AIDS infections in India), using various forms of traditional and interactive media including plays, songs, and folk dancing (Bedi, 2002). Through these culturally familiar media, STHREE delivers educational, consequential, and remedial information on HIV/AIDS, sexually transmitted infections (STIs), alcohol abuse, violence, and sexual coercion.

In complementary activities, educational and informational campaigns that are principally focused on responsible drinking can incorporate messages for the general public and targeted subgroups about the risks associated with unsafe sex. HIV/AIDS education and prevention programs implemented in alcohol treatment facilities also present a unique and multifaceted approach to mitigating harm in multiple-risk groups (Brems & Dewane, 2007). Though there is wider agreement about such programs, few have been executed, and more research is needed to confirm their efficacy (Palepu et al., 2005). Such multi-component interventions can help mitigate the complex intersection of problem alcohol consumption and HIV transmission. However, to be successful, policy and prevention strategies must also consider and address the broader underlying issues of poverty, culture, education, alcohol and sexual expectations, and inequality.

Conclusions

Risky patterns of drinking may overlap with other risky patterns of behavior to compound the spread of HIV/AIDS. According to WHO, "the synergy between sexual behavior and alcohol use enormously multiplies the potential negative consequences of the two behaviors separately" (WHO, 2005, p. vii). To tackle the relationship between problem drinking and HIV/AIDS, interventions must consider individual/group perceptions and expectations surrounding alcohol use and sex in the context of the broader socioeconomic conditions that simultaneously influence risk behaviors. Prevention initiatives must identify key patterns of alcohol misuse and sexual risk behaviors (e.g., the acceptance of alcohol as a facilitator for sex or conceptualizing drinking as an expression of masculinity) and address underlying notions of risk (e.g., unwanted pregnancy, STIs, losing a partner, economic loss, etc.) to foster behavior change (WHO, 2005).

Research-based interventions that target these overlapping behaviors can provide a unique opportunity to strengthen HIV/AIDS prevention activities. For example, prevention education in treatment facilities or high-risk sites such as bars, nightclubs, and guesthouses can address both problem drinking and risky sexual behaviors. More general educational programs will inform local communities about the potential intersection of alcohol and HIV/AIDS and the merit of responsible drinking, thereby reducing problem drinking behaviors.

References

Adelekan, M. (2006). Rapid assessment of substance use and HIV vulnerability in Kakuma refugee camp and surrounding community, Kakuma, Kenya. Unpublished paper, joint UNHCR/WHO project on rapid assessment of substance use in conflict-affected and displaced populations.

Ao, T., Sam, N., Masenga, E., Seage, G. 3rd., & Kapiga, S. (2006). Human immunodeficiency virus type 1 among bar and hotel workers in northern Tanzania: The role of alcohol, sexual behavior, and herpes simplex virus type 2. *Sexually Transmitted Diseases, 33*, 163–69.

Avins, A., Woods, W., Lindan, C., Hudes, E., Clark, W., & Hulley, S. (1994). HIV infection and risk behaviors among heterosexuals in alcohol treatment programs. *Journal of the American Medical Association 271*, 515–18.

Berg, K., Demas, P., Howard, A., Schoenbaum, E., Gourevitch, M., & Arnsten, J. (2004). Gender differences in factors associated with adherence to antiretroviral therapy. *Journal of General Internal Medicine, 19*, 1111–17.

Bouhnik, A., Préau, M., Lert, F., Peretti-Watel, P., Schiltz, M., Obadia, Y., et al. (2007). Unsafe sex in regular partnerships among heterosexual persons living with HIV: Evidence from a large representative sample of individuals attending outpatients service in France (ANRS-EN12-VESPA Study). *AIDS, 21*(Suppl. 1), S57–S62.

Brems, C., & Dewane, S. (2007). Hearing consumer voices: Planning HIV/sexually transmitted infection prevention in alcohol detoxification. *Journal of the Association of Nurses in AIDS Care, 18*, 12–24.

Bryant, K. (2006). Expanding research on the role of alcohol consumption and related risks in the prevention and treatment of HIV/AIDS. *Substance Use & Misuse, 41*, 1465–1507.

Cooper, M. (2002). Alcohol use and risky sexual behaviour among college students and youth: Evaluating the evidence. *Journal of Studies on Alcohol*, (Suppl. 14), 101–17.

Corte, C., & Sommers, M. (2005). Alcohol and risky behaviors. *Annual Review of Nursing Research*, 23, 327–60.

Family Health International & USAID. (2007). *Roads signs: Recent highlights from the ROADS project*. Nairobi, Kenya: Family Health International.

Gregson, S., Nyamukapa, C., Garnett, G., Mason, P., Zhuwau, T., Caraël, M., et al. (2002). Sexual mixing patterns and sex-differentials in teenage exposure to HIV infection in rural Zimbabwe. *The Lancet*, 359, 1896–1903.

Greig, F., & Koopman, C. (2003). Multilevel analysis of women's empowerment and HIV prevention: Qualitative survey. Results from a preliminary study in Botswana. *AIDS and Behavior*, 7, 195–208.

Haworth, A., & Simpson, R. (2004). *Moonshine markets: Issues in unrecorded alcohol beverage production and consumption*. Washington, DC: Brunner-Routledge.

Heath, D. B. (Ed.). (1995). *International handbook on alcohol and culture*. Westport, CT: Greenwood Press.

Heath, D. B. (2000). *Drinking occasions: Comparative perspectives on alcohol and culture*. Philadelphia: Brunner/Mazel.

Hoffmann, O., Zaba, B., Wolff, B., Sanga, E., Maboko, L., Mmbando, D., et al. (2004). Methodological lessons from a cohort study of high-risk women in Tanzania. *Sexually Transmitted Infections*, 80(Suppl. 2), ii69–ii73.

Kalichman, S., Cain, D., Zweben, A., & Swain, G. (2003). Sensation seeking, alcohol use and sexual risk behaviors among men receiving services at a clinic for sexually transmitted infections. *Journal of Studies on Alcohol*, 64, 564–69.

Kalichman, S., Simbayi, L., Kaufman, M., Cain, D., Cherry, C., Jooste, S., et al. (2005). Gender attitudes, sexual violence and HIV/AIDS risks among men and women in Cape Town, South Africa. *Journal of Sex Research*, 42, 299–305.

Kapiga, S., Sam, N., Shao, J., Masenga, E., Renjifo, B., Kiwelu, I., et al.(2003). Herpes simplex virus type 2 infection among bar and hotel workers in northern Tanzania: Prevalence and risk factors. *Sexually Transmitted Diseases*, 30, 187–92.

Kelly, J., St. Lawrence, J., Stevenson, Y., Hauth, A., Kalichman, S., Diaz, Y., et al. (1992). Community AIDS/HIV risk reduction: The effects of endorsements by popular people in three cities. *American Journal of Public Health*, 82, 1483–89.

Lucas, G., Gebo, K., Chaisson, R., & Moore, R. (2002). Longitudinal assessment of the effects of drug and alcohol abuse on HIV-1 treatment outcomes in an urban clinic. *AIDS*, 16, 767–74.

Mahler, J., Yi, D, Sacks, M., Dermatis, H., Stebinger, A., Card, C., et al. (1994). Undetected HIV infection among patients admitted to an alcohol rehabilitation unit. *American Journal of Psychiatry*, 151, 439–40.

Markos, A. (2005). Alcohol and sexual behavior. *International Journal of STD & AIDS*, 16, 123–27.

McNair, L., Carter, J., & Williams, M. (1998). Self-esteem, gender, and alcohol use: Relationships with HIV risk perception and behaviors in college students. *Journal of Sex and Marital Therapy*, 24, 29–36.

Meyerhoff, D. J. (2001). Effects of alcohol and HIV infection on the central nervous system. *Alcohol Research and Health*, 25, 288–98.

Morojele, N., Kachieng'a, M., Mokoko, E., Nkoko, M., Parry, C., Nkowane, A., et al. (2006). Alcohol use and sexual behaviour among risky drinkers and bar and shebeen patrons in Gauteng province, South Africa. *Social Science and Medicine*, 62, 217–27.

National Institute on Alcohol Abuse and Alcoholism (NIAAA). (2001). *Alcohol & AIDS: A guide to research issues and opportunities.* Retrieved June 27, 2007, from http://www.niaaa.nih.gov/ResearchInformation/ExtramuralResearch/NIAAAResearchAreas/contents.htm.

National Institute on Alcohol Abuse and Alcoholism (NIAAA). (2002, September). Alcohol and HIV/AIDS. *Alcohol Alert*, No. 57. Retrieved June 27, 2007, from http://pubs.niaaa.nih.gov/publications/aa57.htm.

Palepu, A., Raj, A., Horton, N., Tibbetts, N., Meli, S., & Samet, J. (2005). Substance abuse treatment and risk behaviors among HIV-infected persons with alcohol problems. *Journal of Substance Abuse Treatment*, 28, 3–9.

Parsons, J., Vicioso, K., Kutnick, A., Punzalan, J., Halkitis, P., & Velasquez, M. (2004). Alcohol use and stigmatized sexual practices of HIV seropositive gay and bisexual men. *Addictive Behaviors*, 29, 1045–51.

Petry, N. (1999). Alcohol use in HIV patients: What we don't know may hurt us. *International Journal of STD & AIDS*, 10, 561–70.

Poulson, R., Eppler, M., Satterwhite, T., Wuensch, K., & Bass, L. (1998). Alcohol consumption, strength of religious beliefs, and risky sexual behavior in college students. *Journal of American College Health*, 46, 227–32.

Robles, R., Matos, T., Colón, H., Reyes, J., Marrero, C., Sahai, H., et al. (2004). HIV risk behaviors and alcohol intoxication among injection drug users in Puerto Rico. *Drug and Alcohol Dependence*, 76, 229–34.

Samet, J., Horton, N., Meli, S., Dukes, K., Tripps, T., Sullivan, L., et al. (2005). A randomized controlled trial to enhance antiretroviral therapy adherence in patients with a history of alcohol problems. *Antiviral Therapy*, 10, 83–93.

Sikkema, K. J., Kelly, J. A., Winett, R. A., Solomon, L. J., Cargill, V. A., Roffman, R., et al. (2000). Outcomes of a randomized community-level HIV prevention intervention for women living in 18 low-income housing developments. *American Journal of Public Health*, 90, 57–63.

Sivaram, S., Johnson, S., Bentley, M., Srikrishnan, A., Latkin, C., Go, V., et al. (2007). Exploring "wine shops" as a venue for HIV prevention interventions in urban India. *Journal for Urban Health*, 84, 563–76.

Stein, M., Charuvastra, A., Anderson, B., Sobota, M., & Friedmann, P. (2002). Alcohol and HIV risk taking among intravenous drug users. *Addictive Behaviors*, 27, 727–36.

Stein, M., Hanna, L., Natarajan, R., Clarke, J., Marisi, M., Sobota, M., et al. (2000). Alcohol use patterns predict high-risk HIV behaviors among active injection drug users. *Journal of Substance Abuse Treatment*, 18, 359–63.

UN Secretary General's Task Force on Women, Girls and HIV/AIDS in Southern Africa. (2004). *Facing the future together: Report of the United Nations Secretary-General's Task Force on Women, Girls and HIV/AIDS in southern Africa*. New York: Author.

Weir, S., Pailman, C., Mahlalela, X., Coetzee, N., Meidany, F., & Boerma, J. (2003). From people to places: Focusing AIDS prevention efforts where it matters most. *AIDS*, 17, 895–903.

Wolff, B., Busza, J., Bufumbo, L., & Whitworth, J. (2006). Women who fall by the roadside: Gender, sexual risk and alcohol in rural Uganda. *Addiction*, 101, 1277–84.

Woelk, G., Fritz, K., Bassett, M., Todd, C., & Chingono, A. (2001). *A rapid assessment in relation to alcohol and other substance use and sexual behavior in Zimbabwe*. Harare, Zimbabwe: University of Zimbabwe.

World Health Organization (WHO). (2002). *The World Health Report 2002: Reducing risks, promoting healthy life.* Geneva, Switzerland: Author.

World Health Organization (WHO). (2005). *Alcohol use and sexual risk behaviour: A cross-cultural study in eight countries*. Geneva, Switzerland: Author.

Notes

1. Human immunodeficiency virus (HIV) causes acquired immunodeficiency syndrome (AIDS), a condition characterized by the depletion of the immune system, leading to life-threatening opportunistic infections.

2. For more information about HIV transmission channels, see the U.S. Centers for Disease Control and Prevention (CDC) at http://www.cdc.gov/hiv/pubs/facts/transmission.htm.

3. In developed countries, unsafe sex is ranked among the top ten risk factors, accounting for 0.8 percent of total disease burden (see WHO, 2002).

4. Belarus, India, Kenya, Mexico, Romania, the Russian Federation, South Africa, and Zambia.

5. See, for example, NIAAA (2002).

6. See, for example, Kalichman, Cain, Zweben, & Swain (2003).

7. A sexual network is a social network that connects individuals by their sexual relationships.

8. Immunosuppressed persons with advanced HIV are susceptible to infections and malignancies called "opportunistic infections," which take advantage of the body's weakened defenses.

9. Antiretroviral drugs are medications used for the treatment of HIV. A combination of several antiretroviral drugs is known as highly active anti-retroviral therapy (HAART).

10. A shebeen is an unlicensed drinking establishment.

11. The Regional Outreach Addressing AIDS through Development Strategies (ROADS) project is a five-year cooperative agreement managed by Family Health International and funded by USAID/East Africa.

12. K. Bedi (personal communication with ICAP, July 2007).

Section 6.2

Club Drug Use and HIV Risk

"How Do Club Drugs Impact HIV Prevention?" reprinted with permission from the Center for AIDS Prevention Studies (CAPS), University of California at San Francisco (www.caps.ucsf.edu). © 2004 Regents of the University of California. Reviewed by David A. Cooke, MD, FACP, November 2010.

What are club drugs?

Club drugs are illegal drugs that are often, although not exclusively, used at dance clubs, raves and circuit parties. Drugs often referred to as club drugs include: MDMA (methylenedioxy-n-methylamphetamine; ecstasy), methamphetamine (crystal meth, speed), GHB (gamma hydroxybutyrate; liquid X), ketamine (special K), and less often, Viagra and amyl nitrites (poppers).[1] These drugs also are often used outside of clubs and parties.

Raves are large parties featuring house or techno music and visual effects. Mostly younger people attend raves. Circuit parties are a series of large, predominantly gay parties lasting several days and nights in a row that are frequented mostly by younger and older middle-class white men. They occur annually in different cities.[2]

Some of the physical and psychological effects of club drugs include: elevated mood; increased empathy; altered vision, sensations, and emotions; increased alertness; decreased appetite; relaxation; increased physical energy and/or self-confidence. Many people use drugs recreationally with few or no immediate repercussions. Misuse of club drugs can lead to problems with toxicity (from the drugs themselves or from interactions with other drugs), with legal issues, and sometimes with addiction. Persons using one or more club drugs during sex often report engaging in extremely high human immunodeficiency virus (HIV) risk behaviors.[3]

Club drugs can cause a variety of non-HIV-related health risks. This section will focus on sexual and drug-using HIV risk behaviors that can occur with club drug use.

Who uses club drugs?

Most of the research on club drugs has been with gay men, mainly because HIV prevalence and risk of infection are high among gay men. Use of club drugs varies by different populations and by geography.[4]

A survey of gay male circuit party attenders in San Francisco found that 80 percent used ecstasy, 66 percent ketamine, 43 percent methamphetamines, 29 percent GHB, 14 percent Viagra, and 12 percent poppers during their most recent out-of-town weekend party. Half (53 percent) used four or more drugs.[5]

A study of rave attenders in Chicago found that 48.9 percent had used any club drugs, 29.8 percent used LSD (lysergic acid diethylamide), 27.7 percent ecstasy, and 8.5 percent methamphetamine. Rave attenders used club drugs with other drugs such as marijuana (87 percent), alcohol (65.2 percent) and cocaine/crack (26.1 percent).[6]

What is the risk?

There are many negative physical and psychological side effects of club drugs. The reason club drugs present a potential HIV risk is because they can lower inhibitions, impair judgment, increase sexual endurance, and encourage sexual risk-taking. With injected drugs, there is also a potential risk from sharing injection equipment.

The risk for HIV occurs mainly when drug use occurs during sexual activity. For example, methamphetamine is often used to initiate, enhance, and prolong sexual encounters, allowing individuals to have sexual intercourse with numerous partners. Poppers are used for receptive anal sex, to relax the anal sphincter. Speed is also dehydrating, which may make men and women more prone to tears in the anus, vagina, or mouth, and therefore more prone to HIV/STD (sexually transmitted disease) infections.[3,7]

In one study, HIV-negative heterosexual methamphetamine users reported an average of 9.4 sex partners over two months. The number of unprotected sexual acts in two months averaged 21.5 for vaginal sex, 6.3 for anal sex, and 41.7 for oral sex. Most users (86 percent) reported engaging in "marathon sex" while high on methamphetamine. Over one-third (37 percent) of users reported injecting, and of those, almost half had shared and/or borrowed needles.[7]

Unprotected sex with a partner whose HIV status is unknown is a high-risk activity. A survey of gay men found that 21 percent of HIV-positive and 9 percent of HIV-negative men reported unprotected anal sex with a partner of unknown status at their most recent circuit party.[5]

A study of gay men at raves in New York City found that about one-third (34 percent) used ecstasy at least once a month. Men who used ecstasy were more likely to report recent unprotected anal intercourse than men who used other drugs, including alcohol.[8]

Why do people use club drugs?

For many people, straight or gay, drug use and sex are a natural occurrence at raves and circuit parties, and one of the appeals of these parties. These parties are popular social activities for some groups of youth and gay men, and there can be strong peer pressure to use drugs and be sexually active.[9] While circuit parties and raves may not themselves cause drug use, they may attract persons who are more inclined to use drugs.[10]

People use club drugs for many reasons. Some people use club drugs to have fun, dance, and loosen inhibitions. Others use them to escape their problems and to counter feelings of depression or anxiety. Parental drug use, childhood sexual abuse, and depression are some of the factors that may lead to drug use.[4]

What's being done?

A drug treatment program for gay methamphetamine users in Los Angeles, California, sought to reduce drug use and HIV-related sexual risk behaviors. Treatment options included: (1) cognitive behavioral therapy, a ninety-minute group session delivered three times a week; (2) contingency management, a behavioral intervention that offered increasingly valuable vouchers for abstinence from drug use; and (3) cognitive behavioral therapy culturally tailored to gay issues. All men reduced their drug use, and those using contingency management reduced drug use longer. The highest reduction in sexual risk-taking occurred in men who used the culturally tailored program.[11]

DanceSafe promotes health and safety within the rave and night-club community, with local chapters throughout the United States and Canada. DanceSafe trains volunteers to be health educators and drug abuse prevention counselors at raves and nightclubs. They use a harm reduction approach and primarily target non-addicted, recreational drug users. DanceSafe offers information on drugs, safer sex, and staying healthy, and in some venues offers pill testing to make sure drugs do not contain harmful substitutes.[12]

Twelve-step programs such as Crystal Meth Anonymous (CMA), Narcotics Anonymous (NA), and Alcoholics Anonymous (AA) are for people for whom drug use has become a problem. Twelve-step advocates abstinence from crystal meth, alcohol, and other illicit drugs. Twelve-step meetings occur in many cities across the United States.[13]

The PROTECT project at the South Florida Regional Prevention Center aims to reduce club-drug use among young gay men. PROTECT trains police officers, teachers, and other community stakeholders on club drugs, particularly ecstasy. They also developed a website with a chat room monitored by peer counselors.[14]

Stepping Stone, in San Diego, California, is a residential drug treatment facility for gay men and lesbians. Most of their clients are poly drug users and most are dually diagnosed with psychiatric disorders. They address sexual behaviors and mental health issues in the context of drug abuse treatment. Stepping Stone sponsors a harm reduction social marketing campaign to increase awareness of the dangers of club drugs and alcohol.[15]

What needs to be done?

Several organizations are currently addressing the negative effects of club drugs at raves and parties across the country. More education is needed about the toxicity of club drugs, poly drug use, and the connection between drug use and unsafe sex. Referrals for mental health counseling should also be made available at these venues.

The gay community needs to address the very real pressures in some sub-communities to party and be highly sexually active, and ask the question "is drug use worth the risks men are taking?"[3] It is not enough to attempt to reduce drug use and abuse at circuit parties without also addressing the powerful sexual motivations to using drugs.[3,9]

When prescribing Viagra, physicians should counsel men on safer sex and the harmful effects of combining Viagra with methamphetamines, poppers, and ecstasy. Physicians should inquire about club drug use among their HIV-positive patients and counsel them on the danger of combining them with HIV treatment drugs.[16] Physicians should be aware that club drug use can affect adherence to HIV drugs.

Says who?

1. Freese TE, Miotto K et al. The effects and consequences of selected club drugs. *Journal of Substance Abuse Treatment.* 2002;23:151–56.

2. Swanson J, Cooper A. Dangerous liaison: club drug use and HIV/AIDS. *IAPAC Monthly.* 2002;8:1–15.

3. Halkitis PN, Parsons JT, Stirratt MJ. A double epidemic: crystal methamphetamine drug use in relation to HIV transmission among gay men. *Journal of Homosexuality*. 2001;41:17–35.

4. Stall R, Paul JP, Greenwood G et al. Alcohol use, drug use and alcohol-related problems among men who have sex with men: the Urban Men's Health Study. *Addiction*. 2001;96:1589–1601.

5. Colfax GN, Mansergh G, et al. Drug use and sexual risk behavior among gay and bisexual men who attend circuit parties: a venue-based comparison. *Journal of Acquired Immune Deficiency Syndromes*. 2001;28:373–79.

6. Fendrich M, Wislar JS, Johnson TP et al. A contextual profile of club drug use among adults in Chicago. *Addiction*. 2003;98:1693–1703.

7. Semple SJ, Patterson TL, Grant I. The context of sexual risk behavior among heterosexual methamphetamine users. *Addictive Behavior*. 2004;29:807–10.

8. Klitzman RL, Pope HG, Hudson JI. MDMA ("ecstasy") abuse and high-risk sexual behaviors among 169 gay and bisexual men. *American Journal of Psychiatry*. 2000;157:1162–64.

9. Task Force on Crystal, Syphilis and HIV. Confronting crystal methamphetamine use in New York City. Public policy recommendations. Gay Men's Health Crisis, New York, NY. July 2004. http://www.gmhc.org/policy/nyc/crystaltaskforce04.php

10. Adlaf EM, Smart RG. Party subculture or dens of doom? An epidemiological study of rave attendance and drug use patterns among adolescent students. *Journal of Psychoactive Drugs*. 1997;29:193–98.

11. Shoptaw S, Reback CJ. Drug and sex risk behavior reductions with behavioral treatments for methamphetamine dependence among gay/bisexual men. Presented at the National HIV Prevention Conference, Atlanta, GA. 2003. Abstract #T3-D1004.

12. www.dancesafe.org

13. www.crystalmeth.org, www.na.org, www.aa.org

14. Rothaus S. Workshop targets young gays with a penchant for club drugs. *Miami Herald*. July 16, 2003.

15. Johnson SB. Stepping Stone: a catalyst for change. Presented at Methamphetamine Use and Gay Men Meeting. Sacramento, CA. April 24, 2003.

16. Romanelli F, Smith KS, Pomeroy C. Use of club drugs by HIV-seropositive and HIV-seronegative gay and bisexual men. *Topics in HIV Medicine*. 2003;11:25–32.

Section 6.3

Injection Drug Use and HIV Risk

Reprinted from "Substance Abuse," AIDS.gov, October 2010.

In 2007, people infected with human immunodeficiency virus (HIV) through injection drug use (IDU) accounted for 9 percent of all HIV diagnoses (5,694 persons). Sharing needles and other equipment for drug injection is a well-known way to transmit HIV. People who have sex with an injection drug user are also at risk for infection through the sexual transmission of HIV.

Why Does Injecting Drugs Put You at Risk for HIV?

Sharing drug equipment (or "works") is a major risk factor for spreading HIV. Infected blood can be introduced into drug solutions by the following means:

- Using blood-contaminated syringes to prepare drugs

- Reusing bottle caps, spoons, or other containers ("spoons" and "cookers") used to dissolve drugs in water and to heat drug solutions

- Reusing small pieces of cotton or cigarette filters ("cottons") used to filter out particles that could block the needle

- Reusing water used to dissolve drugs or clean syringes

How Can Injection Drug Users Reduce Their Risk for HIV Infection?

The best way to reduce your risk of HIV is to stop injecting drugs— but here are some other things that will reduce your risk of getting HIV or transmitting it to others:

- Never reuse or "share" syringes, water, or drug preparation equipment.

- Only use syringes obtained from a reliable source (such as pharmacies or needle-exchange programs).

- Use a new, sterile syringe each time to prepare and inject drugs.

- If possible, use sterile water to prepare drugs—otherwise, use clean water from a reliable source (such as fresh tap water).

- Use a new or disinfected container ("cooker") and a new filter ("cotton") each time you prepare drugs.

- Clean the injection site with a new alcohol swab before you inject.

- Safely dispose of syringes after one use.

In recent years, new cases of IDU-related HIV infection have decreased, thanks to prevention programs aimed at substance users. Prevention measures work!

Other Drug-Related Risks for HIV

Methamphetamine ("meth") is a highly addictive stimulant drug that can increase sexual arousal while reducing inhibitions. It can also be injected. These factors put meth users at an increased risk of getting or transmitting HIV infection, through both sexual transmission and injection drug use.

Although meth use is an HIV risk factor for anyone who uses it, research suggests that there is a particularly strong link between meth use and HIV transmission for men who have sex with men (MSM). Studies show that MSM who use meth may increase their sexual *and* drug-use risk factors. They may do the following:

- Use condoms less often

- Have more sex partners

- Engage in unprotected anal sex

- Inject meth instead of smoking or snorting it

Alcohol and Other Drugs

The risk for HIV associated with substance abuse involves more than simply the sharing of drug injecting equipment. Use of drugs and alcohol can interfere with judgment about sexual and other behavior. As a result, substance users may be more likely to have unplanned and unprotected sex.

Section 6.4

Sexual Risk Factors and HIV Transmission

Reprinted from AIDS.gov, October 2010

Risky Business

There is evidence to show that some sexual behaviors are riskier than others. All sexual practices can be made "safer" (meaning less risk of transmitting/contracting sexually transmitted diseases [STDs] and human immunodeficiency virus [HIV]), but some activities are regarded as much safer than others.

Receptive Anal Intercourse (Bottoming)

- The odds of contracting HIV from "bottoming" without a condom are higher than any other sexual behavior.

- Do not douche before sex. If you are concerned about cleanliness, clean the rectum gently, with a soapy finger and water.

- Always use large quantities of water-based lubricant with a polyurethane or latex condom when bottoming to minimize trauma to the rectum and prevent the transmission of STDs and HIV.

- HIV has been found in pre-ejaculatory fluid, so having your partner pull out before he ejaculates may not decrease your risk.

Insertive Anal Sex (Topping)

- "Topping" without a condom is considered a high-risk behavior for transmission of HIV and other STDs.

- Your partner may have sores or other signs of infection in his/ her rectum that are not noticeable because they are not outside the body.

- Transmission can occur if you have tears or cuts on the shaft of your penis.

- There is a potential for blood and other fluids containing HIV to infect the cells in the urethra of the penis.

Receptive Vaginal Intercourse

- During sex, HIV is transmitted from men to women much more easily than from women to men.

- Unprotected vaginal sex without a condom is considered a high-risk behavior for HIV infection.

- The risk for transmission is increased if you currently have another STD or vaginal infection. Many STDs or infections may be "silent"—meaning you may not be aware that you are infected because you have no symptoms.

- Many barrier methods that are used to prevent pregnancy (diaphragm, cervical cap, etc.) *do not* protect against STDs or HIV infection because they still allow infected semen to contact your vaginal membranes.

- Oral or hormonal contraceptives (i.e., birth control pills) *do not* protect against STDs or HIV infection.

- Female condoms *do* prevent against HIV infection, if used correctly and consistently.

Insertive Vaginal Intercourse

- Unprotected vaginal sex is less risky for the male partner than the female partner—but there is still a risk that you could contract HIV and other STDs.

- Some STDs are "silent," meaning that a woman may have an STD but not have any symptoms. Your partner may not know she has an infection, so it is important to use a condom.

- Use a latex or polyurethane condom with a water-based lubricant each and every time you have insertive vaginal sex to prevent infection by HIV or other STDs.

Performing Oral Sex on a Man (Receptive Oral Sex)

- HIV transmission is a risk, though not as great as with anal or vaginal sex.

- There is a risk of contracting other STDs, like chlamydia and gonorrhea.

- Your risk of contracting HIV is reduced if the person does not ejaculate (cum) in your mouth.

- Your risk of HIV is reduced if you do not have open sores or cuts in your mouth.

- Using condoms for oral sex reduces the risk of HIV and other STD transmission.

Receiving Oral Sex If You Are a Man (Insertive Oral Sex)

- There is less associated risk for HIV infection with this sexual activity.

- There is a risk of contracting other STDs, similar to the risks associated with receptive oral sex.

- There is a theoretical risk of contracting HIV in this way.

Receiving Oral Sex If You Are a Woman (Receptive Oral Sex)

- The risk for contracting HIV this way is significantly lower than for unprotected vaginal intercourse.

- There is still a theoretical risk for HIV.

- There is still a risk of contracting other STDs (e.g., herpes) and bacterial infections.

- There are effective barriers you can use for receptive oral sex. You can cut open an unlubricated latex condom and lay it over your vulva. This will protect your partner from contact with your vaginal fluids. Dental dams or nonmicrowaveable plastic wrap are also effective means of preventing transmission by providing a barrier to infection. (Plastic wrap that can be microwaved will not protect you—viruses are small enough to pass through that type of wrap.)

Performing Oral Sex on a Women (Insertive Oral Sex)

- HIV has been found in vaginal secretions, so there is a risk of contracting HIV through this activity.

- It may be possible to contract other STDs through this activity.

- A barrier method (cut-open unlubricated condom, dental dam, or nonmicrowaveable plastic wrap) should be used to prevent against transmission of both HIV and most STDs. These barriers will protect you from contact with your partner's vaginal fluid.

Digital Stimulation

- There is risk of contracting HIV from digital stimulation if there are cuts or sores present on the fingers or in the rectum or vagina.

- Use latex or non-latex medical grade gloves, and lots of water-based lubricant to prevent this risk.

Sex Toys

- Using sex toys can be a safe practice but be sure to follow cleaning instructions on the packaging that comes with the toy.

- Clean your toys with soap and water, or a stronger disinfectant if indicated on the cleaning instructions. It is important to do this *after each use*!

- If possible, use a condom over the toy.

- Don't share your sex toys. It is best to have your own personal toy. If you do choose to share your toy with your partner, use a condom on the toy if possible and change the condom before your partner uses it.

Safer Sex Activities

These activities carry no risk of HIV transmission. There are still possibilities of contracting other STDs, like genital ulcer diseases (e.g., herpes) or parasites (e.g., "crabs" or pubic lice) with masturbation or frottage:

- Nonsexual massage

- Casual or dry kissing

- Masturbation (without your partner's body fluids)

- Frottage—also known as "dry humping" or body-to-body rubbing

There are still possibilities of contracting other STDs, like genital ulcer diseases (e.g., herpes) or parasites (e.g., "crabs" or pubic lice) with masturbation or frottage.

Section 6.5

Sexually Transmitted Diseases and HIV Risk

Reprinted from "The Role of STD Detection and Treatment in HIV Prevention," Centers for Disease Control and Prevention, April 10, 2008.

Testing and treatment of sexually transmitted diseases (STDs) can be an effective tool in preventing the spread of human immunodeficiency virus (HIV), the virus that causes acquired immunodeficiency syndrome (AIDS). An understanding of the relationship between STDs and HIV infection can help in the development of effective HIV prevention programs for persons with high-risk sexual behaviors.

Individuals who are infected with STDs are at least two to five times more likely than uninfected individuals to acquire HIV infection if they are exposed to the virus through sexual contact. In addition, if an HIV-infected individual is also infected with another STD, that person is more likely to transmit HIV through sexual contact than other HIV-infected persons (Wasserheit, 1992).

There is substantial biological evidence demonstrating that the presence of other STDs increases the likelihood of both transmitting and acquiring HIV:

- **Increased susceptibility:** STDs appear to increase susceptibility to HIV infection by two mechanisms. Genital ulcers (e.g., syphilis, herpes, or chancroid) result in breaks in the genital tract lining or skin. These breaks create a portal of entry for

HIV. Additionally, inflammation resulting from genital ulcers or non-ulcerative STDs (e.g., chlamydia, gonorrhea, and trichomoniasis) increases the concentration of cells in genital secretions that can serve as targets for HIV (e.g., CD4+ cells).

- **Increased infectiousness:** STDs also appear to increase the risk of an HIV-infected person transmitting the virus to his or her sex partners. Studies have shown that HIV-infected individuals who are also infected with other STDs are particularly likely to shed HIV in their genital secretions. For example, men who are infected with both gonorrhea and HIV are more than twice as likely to have HIV in their genital secretions than are those who are infected only with HIV. Moreover, the median concentration of HIV in semen is as much as ten times higher in men who are infected with both gonorrhea and HIV than in men infected only with HIV. The higher the concentration of HIV in semen or genital fluids, the more likely it is that HIV will be transmitted to a sex partner.

How can STD treatment slow the spread of HIV infection?

Evidence from intervention studies indicates that detecting and treating STDs may reduce HIV transmission:

- STD treatment reduces an individual's ability to transmit HIV. Studies have shown that treating STDs in HIV-infected individuals decreases both the amount of HIV in genital secretions and how frequently HIV is found in those secretions (Fleming, Wasserheit, 1999).

- Herpes can make people more susceptible to HIV infection, and it can make HIV-infected individuals more infectious. It is critical that all individuals, especially those with herpes, know whether they are infected with HIV and, if uninfected with HIV, take measures to protect themselves from infection with HIV.

- Among individuals with both herpes and HIV, trials are underway studying if treatment of the genital herpes helps prevent HIV transmission to partners.

What are the implications for HIV prevention?

Strong STD prevention, testing, and treatment can play a vital role in comprehensive programs to prevent sexual transmission of HIV.

Furthermore, STD trends can offer important insights into where the HIV epidemic may grow, making STD surveillance data helpful in forecasting where HIV rates are likely to increase. Better linkages are needed between HIV and STD prevention efforts nationwide in order to control both epidemics.

In the context of persistently high prevalence of STDs in many parts of the United States and with emerging evidence that the U.S. HIV epidemic increasingly is affecting populations with the highest rates of curable STDs, the Centers for Disease Control and Prevention (CDC)/ Health Resources and Services Administration (HRSA) Advisory Committee on HIV/AIDS and STD Prevention (CHAC) recommended the following:

- Early detection and treatment of curable STDs should become a major, explicit component of comprehensive HIV prevention programs at national, state, and local levels.

- In areas where STDs that facilitate HIV transmission are prevalent, screening and treatment programs should be expanded.

- HIV testing should always be recommended for individuals who are diagnosed with or suspected to have an STD.

- HIV and STD prevention programs in the United States, together with private and public sector partners, should take joint responsibility for implementing these strategies.

CHAC also notes that early detection and treatment of STDs should be only one component of a comprehensive HIV prevention program, which also must include a range of social, behavioral, and biomedical interventions.

Section 6.6

Tattoos and Piercings and HIV Risk

"Body Art and HIV Risk" is excerpted from "HIV Transmission: Questions and Answers," Centers for Disease Control and Prevention, March 25, 2010. "Safety Procedures" is excerpted from "Body Art: Tattoos and Piercings," Centers for Disease Control and Prevention, January 21, 2008.

Body Art and HIV Risk

A risk of human immunodeficiency virus (HIV) transmission during tattooing or body piercing does exist if instruments contaminated with blood are either not sterilized or disinfected or are used inappropriately between clients. The Centers for Disease Control and Prevention (CDC) recommends that single-use instruments intended to penetrate the skin be used once, then disposed of. Reusable instruments or devices that penetrate the skin and/or contact a client's blood should be thoroughly cleaned and sterilized between clients.

Personal service workers who do tattooing or body piercing should be educated about how HIV is transmitted and take precautions to prevent transmission of HIV and other blood-borne infections in their settings.

Safety Procedures

Health and safety procedures for body artists may be regulated by city, county, or state agencies. Reputable shops and tattoo parlors govern themselves and follow strict safety procedures to protect their clients—and their body artists.

If you decide to get a tattoo or body piercing, make sure you go to a licensed facility and take time to discuss the safety procedures with the artists working at the shop or tattoo parlor. They should explain the process and clarify what they do to keep everyone safe and healthy by using sterile needles and razors, washing hands, wearing gloves, and keeping surfaces clean.

Body piercers and tattoo artists protect themselves and their clients when following safe and healthy practices, such as the following:

- Use single-use, disposable needles and razors. Disposable piercing needles, tattoo needles, and razors are used on one person and then thrown away. Reusing needles or razors is not safe.

- Safely dispose of needles and razors. Used needles and razors should be thrown away in a biohazard-labeled, disposable container to protect both the client and the person changing or handling the trash bag from getting cut.

- Wash hands before and after putting on disposable gloves. Gloves are always worn while working with equipment and clients, changed when necessary, and are not reused.

- Clean and sterilize reusable tools and equipment. Some tools and equipment can be reused when creating body art. Reusable tools and equipment should be cleaned and then sterilized to remove viruses and bacteria.

- Frequently clean surfaces and work areas. Chairs, tables, workspaces, and counters should be disinfected between procedures to protect the health of both the client and the artist. Cross-contamination (spreading bacteria and viruses from one surface to another) can occur if surfaces are not disinfected frequently and between clients. Any disinfectant that claims to be able to eliminate the tuberculosis germ can also kill HIV, hepatitis B, and hepatitis C viruses. Use a commercial disinfectant, following the manufacturer's instructions, or a mixture of bleach and water (one part bleach to nine parts water).

By following safety procedures, tattoo artists and body piercers protect themselves and their clients against exposure risks.

Chapter 7

HIV Risk in the Healthcare Setting

Chapter Contents

Section 7.1

Occupational Exposure

How can HIV be transmitted?

Blood, semen, vaginal secretions, vomitus, breast milk, or pus from a person who is infected with HIV (human immunodeficiency virus) may contain HIV and may cause infection. The risk of acquiring HIV from a needle-stick injury is less than 1 percent, and the risk of infection from exposure not involving a puncture or a cut (such as a splash of body fluid onto the skin or the mucous membrane) is less than 0.1 percent. The risk of HIV infection from a human bite is between 0.1 percent and 1 percent.

"Clear" body fluids such as tears, saliva, sweat, and urine contain little or no virus and do not transmit HIV unless they are contaminated with blood.

What should I do if I think I have been exposed?

If a skin puncture has occurred, induce bleeding at the puncture site by applying gentle pressure as you wash the area with soap and water. If skin or mucous membranes have been splashed by body fluid, immediately rinse the area thoroughly with water.

Get the name, address, and phone number of the source person (patient) and the name, address, and phone number of the source person's attending physician. If you do not know the patient's HIV status, ask the attending physician to help. If you are at work, notify your supervisor. Do not spend time now on details of how or why the exposure happened. There will be time for this later.

When do I first need to get medical care?

Seek immediate assessment and treatment from your employee health unit, your private physician, or the emergency department. If anti-HIV medication is indicated, it should be taken as soon as possible. If you have a skin puncture or cut, you might need a tetanus toxoid booster, depending on the nature of the injury. Your physician will need to ask questions about the incident and other details in order to determine what treatment, if any, is necessary.

What details will I need to give my physician?

For a puncture injury. Is it a deep or surface puncture? If the puncture was caused by a needle, what gauge was the needle? Was the needle solid (suturing) or hollow? Could you see blood or bloody material on the surface of the needle or scalpel? Was the device previously in contact with patient's body fluids? If blood was injected into you, how much? Were you wearing protective gloves?

For a skin or mucous membrane splash. Were you exposed to blood or other body fluid? How much? On what part of the body were you exposed? What size was the area of contact? What was the length of contact time? Was there a break in the skin? A rash? A bite? Were you wearing protection (e.g., gloves, eyeglasses)?

What will my physician need to know about the source person?

The HIV status of the source person. If the source person is HIV-negative, he or she could be infected but may not yet have positive HIV tests (he or she may be in the "window" period). Will he or she agree to be tested or retested for HIV infection?

If the source person is HIV-positive, does he or she have AIDS? Has the source person taken anti-HIV therapy? If so, what medications is he or she taking? Is he or she at the end stage of the disease (with a high quantity of virus in his or her blood and body fluids)?

If the source person will not agree to HIV testing, whether he or she is in a high-risk HIV group. Is the person an intravenous drug user or the sexual partner of an intravenous drug user, a bisexual or homosexual male, and/or a person with multiple partners? Did he or she receive a blood transfusion between 1980 and 1985? Has he or she received a blood transfusion recently?

What will I need to tell my physician about myself?

Information about any medical conditions, medications, and allergies. Have you been exposed to HIV before? If so, when? How? Are you pregnant? Are you breast-feeding? Are you sexually active?

131

Whether you will agree to testing. Will you agree to confidential testing in order to document seroconversion (in the rare event of HIV transmission by occupational exposure)?

Should I receive post-exposure HIV prophylaxis?

Based on answers to the questions above, your physician may advise you to take medication to reduce your risk of developing HIV. Your doctor may also give medicine to protect you against hepatitis and syphilis. You will need baseline blood work, especially for evaluation of bone marrow, liver, and kidney function. These tests will be repeated during the course of therapy.

Does prophylactic treatment work?

Early post-exposure prophylaxis can reduce the risk of HIV infection tenfold. Even if infection occurs despite prophylaxis, early suppression of the virus can lower the "set point" for viral load and slow the course of HIV disease substantially.

Does the treatment have side effects?

Some of the medicines used can cause side effects. For example, zidovudine may cause headache, fatigue, insomnia, and gastrointestinal symptoms (nausea, diarrhea, abdominal discomfort). In rare instances, lamivudine may cause pancreatitis and gastrointestinal symptoms. Indinavir and saquinavir may cause gastrointestinal upset and diarrhea. Indinavir has also been associated with kidney stones. Two quarts of fluid should be taken daily to reduce this risk.

How can I protect others from possible exposure to HIV?

Until HIV infection is ruled out, you should avoid the exchange of body fluids during sex, postpone pregnancy, and refrain from blood or organ donation. If you are breast-feeding, your baby's doctor may ask you to switch to formula feeding.

When should I be retested for HIV?

HIV testing may be repeated at six weeks, three months, and six months. Nearly all people found to be negative at three months are confirmed to be uninfected. However, the Centers for Disease Control and Prevention recommend retesting up to six months following the last possible exposure. If you have not formed antibodies to HIV by six months, then infection did not occur. Until then, you should report and seek medical evaluation if you have any acute illness. An acute illness, especially if accompanied by fever, rash, or swollen lymph nodes, may be a sign of HIV infection or another medical condition.

How can I cope with my feelings?

It is natural to feel anger, self-recrimination, fear, and depression after occupational exposure to HIV. During the difficult time of prevention therapy and waiting, you may want to seek support from employee-assistance programs or local mental health professionals.

Section 7.2

Patient Exposure

Excerpted from "HIV Transmission: Questions and Answers,"
Centers for Disease Control and Prevention, March 25, 2010.

Are patients in a healthcare setting at risk of getting HIV?

Although human immunodeficiency virus (HIV) transmission is possible in healthcare settings, it is extremely rare. Medical experts emphasize that the careful practice of infection control procedures, including universal precautions (i.e., using protective practices and personal protective equipment to prevent HIV and other blood-borne infections), protects patients as well as healthcare providers from possible HIV transmission in medical and dental offices and hospitals.

In 1990, the Centers for Disease Control and Prevention (CDC) reported on an HIV-infected dentist in Florida who apparently infected some of his patients while doing dental work. Studies of viral deoxyribonucleic acid (DNA) sequences linked the dentist to six of his patients who were also HIV-infected. The CDC has not yet been able to establish how the transmission took place. No additional studies have found any evidence of transmission from provider to patient in healthcare settings.

CDC has documented rare cases of patients contracting HIV in healthcare settings from infected donor tissue. Most of these cases occurred due to failures in following universal precautions and infection control guidelines. Most also occurred early in the HIV epidemic, before established screening procedures were in place.

Section 7.3

Blood Transfusion and Organ Donation Recipients

Excerpted from "Blood Transfusions and Organ Donation," AIDS.gov, October 2010.

Our Nation's Blood Supply

In the early years of the human immunodeficiency virus (HIV) epidemic, blood transfusions and blood products were a prime source of HIV infection. In 1985, however, an HIV test became available, and screening of all blood donations became mandatory. Of those who contracted HIV through blood transfusions or products, nearly all did so before 1985.

The U.S. blood supply is now among the safest in the world:

- All blood donors are prescreened for HIV risk factors.

- Three different HIV screening tests, including the p24 antigen test, are performed on all donated blood.

- Blood and blood products that test positive for HIV are safely discarded and are not used for transfusions. Donors whose blood tests positive for HIV are notified by the collecting agency.

It is important to know that you cannot get HIV from donating blood. Blood collection procedures are highly regulated and safe.

If you know in advance that you are going to need blood for surgery, you can choose to donate and store your own blood with a blood banking service. This is called an autologous donation.

Using Blood Donation to Learn Your HIV Status

Some people think that donating blood is a more private way to learn their HIV status than asking their doctor for an HIV test or visiting a clinic. You should not donate blood to find out if you are HIV-positive.

Why? Because the HIV tests used to screen donor blood are highly accurate—but they aren't perfect. If you have been infected with HIV recently, even the most sensitive test may not show it, but you could still infect others who receive your blood.

If you have engaged in high-risk sexual or drug-taking behaviors, you should not donate blood. To learn your HIV status, find an HIV testing center. By taking an HIV test, you can protect your own health, as well as the health of people who need blood!

The U.S. Food and Drug Administration (FDA) regulates the U.S. blood supply and safeguards over 3.5 million blood transfusion recipients each year. The FDA also certifies all assay test kits used to detect diseases in donated blood. Each unit of donated blood is tested for the following:

- Hepatitis B and C (HBV and HCV)

- Human immunodeficiency virus (HIV 1 and HIV 2)

- Human T-lymphotropic virus (types I and II)

- Syphilis

Organ/Tissue Transplants

The risks of transplant-related HIV infection are low. All donor organs are screened for infectious diseases, including HIV.

But HIV tests do not always detect the virus in people with very recent infection. In 2007, there were four documented cases of HIV spread through organ transplants. These were the first cases in twenty years, and they were linked to a single donor, who tested negative for HIV in pre-transplant testing.

Patients awaiting organ transplant need to be aware of the very small risk of HIV infection—and to balance that risk against their particular health needs and the limited availability of donor organs.

The Centers for Disease Control and Prevention (CDC) has issued criteria designed to identify "high-risk" organ donors and to exclude them from donating organs or tissue in most circumstances. Because of the very limited number of organs available for transplant, however, the CDC's guidelines state that high-risk donors are acceptable if "the risk to the recipient of not performing the transplant is deemed to be greater than the risk of HIV transmission and disease."

Chapter 8

Other HIV Transmission Rumors and Risks

Chapter Contents

Section 8.1

Insect Bites

Excerpted from "HIV Transmission: Questions and Answers," Centers
for Disease Control and Prevention, March 25, 2010.

Can I get human immunodeficiency virus (HIV) from mosquitoes?

No. From the start of the HIV epidemic there has been concern
about HIV transmission from biting and bloodsucking insects, such
as mosquitoes. However, studies conducted by the Centers for Disease
Control and Prevention (CDC) and elsewhere have shown no evidence
of HIV transmission from mosquitoes or any other insects—even in areas where there are many cases of AIDS and large populations of mosquitoes. Lack of such outbreaks, despite intense efforts to detect them,
supports the conclusion that HIV is not transmitted by insects.

The results of experiments and observations of insect biting behavior indicate that when an insect bites a person, it does not inject
its own or a previously bitten person's or animal's blood into the next
person bitten. Rather, it injects saliva, which acts as a lubricant so the
insect can feed efficiently. Diseases such as yellow fever and malaria
are transmitted through the saliva of specific species of mosquitoes.
However, HIV lives for only a short time inside an insect and, unlike
organisms that are transmitted via insect bites, HIV does not reproduce (and does not survive) in insects. Thus, even if the virus enters
a mosquito or another insect, the insect does not become infected and
cannot transmit HIV to the next human it bites.

There also is no reason to fear that a mosquito or other insect could
transmit HIV from one person to another through HIV-infected blood
left on its mouth parts. Several reasons help explain why this is so.
First, infected people do not have constantly high levels of HIV in
their bloodstreams. Second, insect mouth parts retain only very small
amounts of blood on their surfaces. Finally, scientists who study insects
have determined that biting insects normally do not travel from one
person to the next immediately after ingesting blood. Rather, they fly
to a resting place to digest the blood meal.

Section 8.2

Kissing, Biting, Scratching, or Spitting

Excerpted from "HIV Transmission: Questions and Answers," Centers for Disease Control and Prevention, March 25, 2010.

Can human immunodeficiency virus (HIV) be transmitted by kissing?

It depends on the type of kissing. There is no risk from closed-mouth kissing.

There are extremely rare cases of HIV being transmitted via deep "French" kissing but in each case, infected blood was exchanged due to bleeding gums or sores in the mouth. Because of this remote risk, it is recommended that individuals who are HIV-infected avoid deep, open-mouth "French" kissing with a non-infected partner, as there is a potential risk of transferring infected blood.

Summary: There is no risk of transmission closed-mouth kissing. There is a remote risk from deep, open-mouth kissing if there are sores or bleeding gums and blood is exchanged. Therefore, persons living with HIV should avoid this behavior with a non-infected partner.

Can HIV be transmitted by human bite?

It is very rare, but in specific circumstances HIV can be transmitted by a human bite. In 1997, the Centers for Disease Control and Prevention (CDC) published findings from a state health department investigation of an incident that suggested blood-to-blood transmission of HIV by a human bite. There have been other rare reports in the medical literature in which HIV appeared to have been transmitted by a human bite. Biting is not a common way of transmitting HIV, in fact, there are numerous reports of bites that did not result in HIV infection. Severe trauma with extensive tissue damage and the presence of blood were reported in each of the instances where transmission was documented or suspected. Bites that do not involve broken skin have no risk for HIV transmission, as intact skin acts as a barrier to HIV transmission.

Summary: There is no risk from a bite where the skin is not broken. There is a remote risk of transmission by human bite. All documented cases where transmission did occur included severe trauma with extensive tissue damage and the presence of blood.

Can HIV be transmitted by being scratched?

No. There is no risk of transmission from scratching because there is no transfer of body fluids between individuals. Any person with open wounds should have them treated as soon as possible.

Can HIV be transmitted by being spit on by an HIV-infected person?

No. In some persons living with HIV, the virus has been detected in saliva, but in extremely low quantities. Contact with saliva alone has never been shown to result in transmission of HIV, and there is no documented case of transmission from an HIV-infected person spitting on another person.

Section 8.3

Needle-Stick Injuries in a Non-Healthcare Setting

Excerpted from "HIV Transmission: Questions and Answers," Centers for Disease Control and Prevention, March 25, 2010.

Have people been infected with human immunodeficiency virus (HIV) from being stuck by needles in non-healthcare settings?

No. While it is possible to get infected with HIV if you are stuck with a needle that is contaminated with HIV, there are no documented cases of transmission outside of a healthcare setting.

The Centers for Disease Control and Prevention (CDC) have received inquiries about used needles left by HIV-infected injection drug users in coin return slots of pay phones, the underside of gas pump handles, and on movie theater seats. Some reports have falsely indicated that CDC "confirmed" the presence of HIV in the needles. CDC has not tested such needles nor has CDC confirmed the presence or absence of HIV in any sample related to these rumors. The majority of these reports and warnings appear to be rumors/myths.

CDC was informed of one incident in Virginia of a needle stick from a small-gauge needle (believed to be an insulin needle) in a coin return slot of a pay phone and a needle found in a vending machine that did not cause a needle-stick injury. There was an investigation by the local police and health department and there was no report of anyone contracting an infectious disease from these needles.

Discarded needles are sometimes found in the community. These needles are believed to have been discarded by persons who use insulin or inject illicit drugs. Occasionally the public and certain workers (e.g., sanitation workers or housekeeping staff) may sustain needle-stick injuries involving inappropriately discarded needles. Needle-stick injuries can transfer blood and blood-borne pathogens (e.g., hepatitis B, hepatitis C, and HIV), but the risk of transmission is extremely low and there are no documented cases of transmission outside of a healthcare setting.

CDC does not recommend routinely testing discarded needles to assess the presence or absence of infectious agents in the needles. Management of exposed persons should be done on a case-by-case basis to determine the risk of a blood-borne pathogen infection in the source and the nature of the injury. Anyone who is injured from a needle-stick in a community setting should contact their healthcare provider or go to an emergency room as soon as possible. Antiretroviral medications given shortly after being stuck by a needle infected with HIV can reduce the risk of HIV infection. The healthcare provider should then report the injury to the local or state health department.

Section 8.4

Sports

Excerpted from "HIV Transmission: Questions and Answers," Centers for Disease Control and Prevention, March 25, 2010.

Can I get human immunodeficiency virus (HIV) while playing sports?

There are no documented cases of HIV being transmitted during participation in sports. The very low risk of transmission during sports participation would involve sports with direct body contact in which bleeding might be expected to occur.

If someone is bleeding, their participation in the sport should be interrupted until the wound stops bleeding and is both antiseptically cleaned and securely bandaged. There is no risk of HIV transmission through sports activities where bleeding does not occur.

Chapter 9

HIV/AIDS Risks and Prevention Strategies in Targeted Populations

Chapter Contents

Section 9.1

Youth

Excerpted from "HIV/AIDS among Youth,"
Centers for Disease Control and Prevention, August 3, 2008.

Young people in the United States are at persistent risk for human immunodeficiency virus (HIV) infection. This risk is especially notable for youth of minority races and ethnicities. Continual HIV prevention outreach and education efforts, including programs on abstinence and on delaying the initiation of sex, are required as new generations replace the generations that benefited from earlier prevention strategies. Unless otherwise noted, this section defines youth, or young people, as persons who are thirteen to twenty-four years of age.

Statistics

HIV/AIDS in 2004

The following are based on data from the 35 areas with long-term, confidential name-based HIV reporting:

- An estimated 4,883 young people received a diagnosis of HIV infection or acquired immunodeficiency syndrome (AIDS), representing about 13 percent of the persons given a diagnosis during that year.[1]

- HIV infection progressed to AIDS more slowly among young people than among all persons with a diagnosis of HIV infection. The following are the proportions of persons in whom HIV infection did not progress to AIDS within twelve months after diagnosis of HIV infection: 81 percent of persons aged fifteen to twenty-four; 70 percent of persons aged thirteen to fourteen; 61 percent of all persons.

- African Americans were disproportionately affected by HIV infection, accounting for 55 percent of all HIV infections reported among persons aged thirteen to twenty-four.[2]

- Young men who have sex with men (MSM), especially those of minority races or ethnicities, were at high risk for HIV infection. In the seven cities that participated in the Centers for Disease Control and Prevention's (CDC's) Young Men's Survey during 1994 to 1998, 14 percent of African American MSM and 7 percent of Hispanic MSM aged fifteen to twenty-two were infected with HIV.[3]

- During 2001–2004, in the thirty-three states with long-term, confidential name-based HIV reporting, 62 percent of the 17,824 persons thirteen to twenty-four years of age given a diagnoses of HIV/AIDS were males, and 38 percent were females.

AIDS in 2004

An estimated 2,174 young people received a diagnosis of AIDS (5.1 percent of the estimated total of 42,514 AIDS diagnoses), and 232 young people with AIDS died.[1]

An estimated 7,761 young people were living with AIDS, a 42 percent increase since 2000, when 5,457 young people were living with AIDS.[1]

Young people for whom AIDS was diagnosed during 1996–2004 lived longer than persons with AIDS in any other age group except those younger than thirteen years. Nine years after receiving a diagnosis of AIDS, 76 percent of those aged thirteen to twenty-four were alive, compared with 81 percent of those younger than age thirteen, 74 percent of those aged twenty-five to thirty-four, 70 percent of those aged thirty-five to forty-four, 63 percent of those aged forty-five to fifty-four, and 53 percent of those aged fifty-five and older.[1]

Since the beginning of the epidemic, an estimated 40,059 young people in the United States had received a diagnosis of AIDS, and an estimated 10,129 young people with AIDS had died. They accounted for about 4 percent of the estimated total of 944,306 AIDS diagnoses and 2 percent of the 529,113 deaths of people with AIDS.[1]

Risk Factors and Barriers to Prevention

Sexual Risk Factors

Early age at sexual initiation. According to CDC's Youth Risk Behavioral Survey (YRBS), many young people begin having sexual intercourse at early ages: 47 percent of high school students have had sexual intercourse, and 7.4 percent of them reported first sexual intercourse before age thirteen.[4] HIV/AIDS education needs to take place at correspondingly young ages, before young people engage in sexual behaviors that put them at risk for HIV infection.

Heterosexual transmission. Young women, especially those of minority races or ethnicities, are increasingly at risk for HIV infection through heterosexual contact. According to data from a CDC study of HIV prevalence among disadvantaged youth during the early to mid-1990s, the rate of HIV prevalence among young women aged sixteen to twenty-one was 50 percent higher than the rate among young men in that age group.[5] African American women in this study were seven times as likely as white women and eight times as likely as Hispanic women to be HIV-positive. Young women are at risk for sexually transmitted HIV for several reasons, including biologic vulnerability, lack of recognition of their partners' risk factors, inequality in relationships, and having sex with older men who are more likely to be infected with HIV.

MSM. Young MSM are at high risk for HIV infection, but their risk factors and the prevention barriers they face differ from those of persons who become infected through heterosexual contact. According to a CDC study of 5,589 MSM, 55 percent of young men (aged fifteen to twenty-two) did not let other people know they were sexually attracted to men.[6] MSM who do not disclose their sexual orientation are less likely to seek HIV testing, so if they become infected, they are less likely to know it. Further, because MSM who do not disclose their sexual orientation are likely to have one or more female sex partners, MSM who become infected may transmit the virus to women as well as to men. In a small study of African American MSM college students and nonstudents in North Carolina, the participants had sexual risk factors for HIV infection, and 20 percent had a female sex partner during the preceding twelve months.[7]

Sexually transmitted diseases (STDs). The presence of an STD greatly increases a person's likelihood of acquiring or transmitting HIV.[8] Some of the highest STD rates in the country are those among young people, especially young people of minority races and ethnicities.[9]

Substance Abuse

Young people in the United States use alcohol, tobacco, and other drugs at high rates.[10] Both casual and chronic substance users are more likely to engage in high-risk behaviors, such as unprotected sex, when they are under the influence of drugs or alcohol.[11] Runaways and other homeless young people are at high risk for HIV infection if they are exchanging sex for drugs or money.

Lack of Awareness

Research has shown that a large proportion of young people are not concerned about becoming infected with HIV.[12] Adolescents need accurate, age-appropriate information about HIV infection and AIDS, including how to talk with their parents or other trusted adults about HIV and AIDS, how to reduce or eliminate risk factors, how to talk with a potential partner about risk factors, where to get tested for HIV, and how to use a condom correctly. Information should also include the concept that abstinence is the only 100 percent effective way to avoid infection.

Poverty and Out-of-School Youth

Nearly one in four African Americans and one in five Hispanics live in poverty.[13] The socioeconomic problems associated with poverty, including lack of access to high-quality healthcare, can directly or indirectly increase the risk for HIV infection.[14] Young people who have dropped out of school are more likely to become sexually active at younger ages and to fail to use contraception.[15]

The Coming of Age of HIV-Positive Children

Many young people who contracted HIV through perinatal transmission are facing decisions about becoming sexually active. They will require ongoing counseling and prevention education to ensure that they do not transmit HIV.

Prevention

CDC estimates that 56,300 new HIV infections occurred in the United States in 2006.[16] Populations of minority races or ethnicities are disproportionately affected by the HIV epidemic. To reduce further the incidence of HIV, CDC announced a new initiative, Advancing HIV Prevention, in 2003. This initiative comprises four strategies: making HIV testing a routine part of medical care, implementing new models for diagnosing HIV infections outside medical settings, preventing new infections by working with HIV-infected persons and their partners, and further decreasing perinatal HIV transmission.

Through the Minority AIDS Initiative, CDC explores ways to reduce health disparities in communities made up of persons of minority races or ethnicities who are at high risk for HIV. These funds are used to address the high-priority HIV prevention needs in such communities.

CDC provides nine awards to community-based organizations (CBOs) that focus primarily on youth and provides indirect funding through state, territorial, and local health departments to organizations serving youth. Of these nine awards, five are focused on African Americans, three on Hispanics, one on Asians and Pacific Islanders, and one on whites. The following are some CDC-tested prevention programs that state and local health departments and CBOs can provide for youth:

- Teens Linked to Care is focused on young people aged thirteen to twenty-nine who are living with HIV.

- Street Smart is an HIV/AIDS and STD prevention program for runaway and homeless youth.

- PROMISE (Peers Reaching Out and Modeling Intervention Strategies for HIV/AIDS Risk Reduction in their Community) is a community-level HIV prevention intervention that relies on role-model stories and peers from the community.

- Adult Identity Mentoring project, which encourages students to articulate personal goals and then teaches them the skills required to achieve those goals, can be effective in helping at-risk youth delay the initiation of sex.[17]

CDC research has shown that early, clear parent-child communication regarding values and expectations about sex is an important step in helping adolescents delay sexual initiation and make responsible decisions about sexual behaviors later in life. Parents are in a unique position to engage their children in conversations about HIV, STD, and teen pregnancy prevention because the conversations can be ongoing and timely.[18]

Schools also can be important partners for reaching youth before high-risk behaviors are established, as evidenced by the YRBS finding that 88 percent of high school students in the United States reported having been taught about AIDS or HIV infection in school.

Overall, a multifaceted approach to HIV/AIDS prevention, which includes individual, peer, familial, school, church, and community programs, is necessary to reduce the incidence of HIV/AIDS in young people.

References

1. CDC *HIV / AIDS Surveillance Report, 2004.* Vol. 16. Atlanta: US Department of Health and Human Services, CDC: 2005:1–46.

2. CDC. *HIV Prevention in the Third Decade.* Atlanta: US Department of Health and Human Services, CDC; 2005.

3. CDC. HIV incidence among young men who have sex with men—seven US cities, 1994–2000. *MMWR* 2001;50:440–44.

4. CDC. Youth Risk Behavior Surveillance United States, 2003. *MMWR* 2004;53(SS-2):1–29.

5. Valleroy LA, MacKellar DA, Karon JM, Janssen RS, Hayman DR. HIV infection in disadvantaged out-of-school youth: prevalence for U.S. Job Corps entrants, 1990 through 1996. *Journal of Acquired Immune Deficiency Syndromes* 1998;19:67–73.

6. CDC. HIV/STD risks in young men who have sex with men who do not disclose their sexual orientation—six US cities, 1994–2000. *MMWR* 2003;52:81–85.

7. CDC. HIV transmission among black college student and non-student men who have sex with men—North Carolina, 2003. *MMWR* 2004;53:731–34.

8. Fleming DT, Wasserheit JN. From epidemiological synergy to public health policy and practice: the contribution of other sexually transmitted diseases to sexual transmission of HIV infection. *Sexually Transmitted Infections* 1999;75:3–17.

9. CDC. *Sexually Transmitted Disease Surveillance, 2004.* Atlanta: US Department of Health and Human Services, CDC; 2005.

10. Substance Abuse and Mental Health Services Administration. 2004 National Survey on Drug Use & Health.

11. Leigh BC, Stall R. Substance use and risky sexual behavior for exposure to HIV: issues in methodology, interpretation, and prevention. *American Psychologist* 1993;48:1035–45.

12. The Kaiser Family Foundation. National Survey of Teens on HIV/AIDS, 2000.

13. U.S. Census Bureau. Poverty: 1999. Census 2000 Brief. May 2003.

14. Diaz T, Chu SY, Buehler JW, et al. Socioeconomic differences among people with AIDS: results from a multistate surveillance project. *American Journal of Preventive Medicine* 1994;10:217–22.

15. Office of the Surgeon General. The Surgeon General's call to action to promote sexual health and responsible sexual behavior, July 9, 2001.

16. Hall HI, Ruiguang S, Rhodes P, et al. Estimation of HIV incidence in the United States. *JAMA*. 2008;300:520–29.

17. Clark LF, Miller KS, Nagy SS, et al. Adult identity mentoring: reducing sexual risk for African-American seventh grade students. *Journal of Adolescent Health* 2005;37:337.e1–337.e10.

18. Dittus P, Miller KS, Kotchick BA, Forehand R. Why Parents Matter!: the conceptual basis for a community-based HIV prevention program for the parents of African American youth. *Journal of Child and Family Studies* 2004;13(1):5–20.

Section 9.2

Women

Human Immunodeficiency Virus (HIV) in Women

Women who are HIV-positive may experience the following symptoms:

- Persistent yeast infections

- Persistent vaginal infections

- Menstrual irregularities

- Severe herpes simplex virus

- Chronic pelvic inflammatory disease (PID)

- Human papilloma virus (HPV), which can cause genital warts or cervical cancer

Biology and Body Fluids

Men and women have a different anatomy so women's bodies often respond differently to the same illnesses or infections. For example, during vaginal sex, with all other factors being equal, a woman can be at a higher risk for contracting HIV than a man. Here are some reasons why:

- The thin lining of the vagina and cervix provides a larger surface area for HIV transmission. In men, the equivalent surface area (the entrance to the urethra, or the delicate skin under the foreskin) is smaller.

- Semen contains a higher concentration of HIV than vaginal fluids.

151

- Semen stays in the vaginal canal so unlike men, women can't wash away bodily fluids after having sex. Young women have less vaginal fluid than mature women. This makes vaginal intercourse "drier" and delicate tissue more likely to tear. HIV can easily enter the body through these tiny tears.

- Normal aging changes, particularly experienced by postmenopausal women, such as a decrease in vaginal lubrication and thinning vaginal walls, can increase HIV risk. This makes vaginal intercourse "drier" and delicate tissue more likely to tear.

Women's HIV Risk Factors

There are various economic, social, and cultural factors that increase a woman's risk for HIV. Unequal gender relations, discrimination, sexual violence, poverty, low self-esteem, and substance abuse may lead to behaviors or situations associated with high rates of HIV among women. Also, the lack of focus on women in research programs can increase a woman's risk for contracting HIV.

Access to Resources

Many women lack access to resources especially Aboriginal women, female injection drug users, and female prisoners. These women often receive inadequate education, treatment, and support services.

If you are a woman living in a remote or rural area, you may not have the same access to preventive and clinical services that urban women do.

If you are a woman who is street-involved or work in the sex trade you may choose to have sex at a young age or have multiple partners in order to access income, housing, food, or to meet other basic needs.

HIV disproportionately affects women living in poverty; the struggle for daily survival can lead to activities that place them at high risk for HIV.

Sociocultural Issues

For some women, their social status is linked to pregnancy and motherhood. As such, safer sex practices and/or using contraception are not always options chosen by women.

For some men, having multiple sex partners is an essential part of their status. Thus, women's risk for HIV and other sexually transmitted infections (STIs) may increase because of their partner's sexual decisions.

Some men in monogamous male-female relationships choose to have sex with other men while still in the relationship. This can put their primary partner at risk for HIV and other STIs if their partner is not aware of the male partner's additional sexual activity.

Female genital cutting can increase a woman's risk for HIV. Any open wounds provide an easy entry point for the virus. Women who promote condom use are sometimes seen as promiscuous; some women may be hesitant to suggest condom use because of this stigma.

Some lesbians and women who have sex with women assume that they are not at risk for contracting HIV or other sexually transmitted infections; however, lesbians and women who have sex with women can contract HIV from other women who have HIV.

Despite common myths and stereotypes, older women and seniors are sexually active and some use injection drugs. Some seniors may be less likely to consistently use condoms during sex because of a generational mindset, unfamiliarity with STI/HIV prevention methods, and, for postmenopausal women, preventing pregnancy is no longer an issue.

What Are U.S. Women's HIV Prevention Needs?

Are Women at Risk?

Yes. HIV is taking an increasing toll on women and girls in the United States. In 1985, women comprised 8 percent of all acquired immunodeficiency syndrome (AIDS) cases in the United States, while by 2005, women made up 27 percent of all AIDS cases.[1]

In 2005, women accounted for 30 percent of all new HIV infections. Of these, 60 percent occurred among African Americans, 19 percent among whites, 19 percent among Hispanics, and 1 percent each among Asian/Pacific Islanders and American Indian/Alaska Natives.[2]

Who Are Women Most Affected by HIV?

African American and Hispanic women in particular are disproportionately affected by HIV/AIDS. Although African American and Hispanic women comprise only 23 percent of the total female population in the United States, in 2005 they accounted for 79 percent of all new HIV infections (African American women: 60 percent, Hispanic women: 19 percent).[2,3] Accordingly, in 2004 HIV infection was the leading cause of death for black women (including African American women) aged twenty-five to thirty-four years.[3]

Younger women are also affected by HIV/AIDS. In recent years, the largest number of HIV/AIDS diagnoses among women occurred in women fifteen to thirty-nine years old.[3] In 2005, young women represented 28 percent of AIDS cases among young men and women aged twenty to twenty-four.[1]

What Places Women at Risk?

Most women are infected with HIV through heterosexual contact, especially women with injection drug using partners. In 2005, 80 percent of all new infections in women were from heterosexual contact.[3] Women are more likely than men to acquire HIV via sexual intercourse, due to greater exposed surface area in the female genital tract.[4]

Injection and non-injection drug use places women at an increased risk for HIV and is strongly linked to unsafe sexual practices. Approximately 20 percent of new HIV cases in women are related to injection drug use.[3] Women who use crack cocaine may also be at high risk of sexual transmission of HIV, particularly if they sell or trade sex for drugs.[5]

Sexually transmitted infections (STIs) other than HIV can increase the likelihood of getting or transmitting HIV.[6] In the United States, Chlamydia and gonorrhea (both asymptomatic) are the most commonly reported STIs, with highest rates in women of color and young women and adolescents.[7]

Sexual abuse (both childhood and adult) and domestic violence play a substantial role in placing women at risk for HIV infection. In the United States, annually 2.1 million women are raped and 4 million become victims of domestic violence; of these women, more than 10,000 rape victims and 79,000 violence victims require hospitalization.[8] Women who report early and chronic sexual abuse are seven times more likely to engage in HIV-related risk behaviors compared to women without trauma history.[9]

Women disproportionately suffer from poverty, in particular women of color who are affected by HIV. Because of this, women are less likely than men to have health insurance and access to quality healthcare or prevention services. Approximately two-thirds of women with HIV in the United States have an annual income of less than $10,000.[10] Poverty can increase HIV risks such as exchanging sex for money, shelter, or drugs. In a survey of young and low-income women in California, women who reported sex work were more likely to have syphilis, herpes, hepatitis C, and a history of sexual abuse.[11]

Abuse, violence, and poverty can all lessen a woman's power to negotiate condom use or choose safer partners. They also can lead to psychological distress, such as depression, anxiety, and post-traumatic stress disorder (PTSD).[9]

Having relationships that overlap in time (concurrent partners) can increase women's risk of HIV transmission. Concurrency is more likely to occur among women who are not married, are young adults, and are poor.[12]

What Can Help?

Involving male partners. For women to protect themselves from HIV, they must not only rely on their own skills, attitudes, and behaviors regarding condom use, but also on those of their male partner. Often, men and women in relationships may find intimacy to be more important than protection against HIV. Involving women's partners in HIV prevention programs can help strengthen intimacy and trust and improve sexual communication and negotiation, including asking about past and current partners.

Support from other women. Many prevention programs for women offer groups to reduce women's isolation and allow women to support each other and normalize safer behaviors. Greater social support can increase self-esteem and allow women to make healthier choices. A program in Washington, DC, helped build support and empowerment for HIV-positive African American women by holding educational groups during shared meals and providing small gifts (along with condoms) as incentives or thank-yous.[13]

Help with non-HIV factors. Women at risk for HIV face many behavioral and structural challenges beyond HIV: poverty and economic strain, unemployment, violence and unhealthy gender relations, migration, STIs, drug use, and caring for children and family members.[14] HIV prevention programs for women should provide transportation, child care, nutritious food, and compensation such as money, phone or store cards, or gift packs. Programs should provide up-to-date referrals for employment, housing, medical care, and mental health services for trauma, abuse, and depression.

What Is Being Done?

Currently seventeen women-specific interventions exist that have been approved by the Centers for Disease Control and Prevention (CDC) as best evidence or promising evidence or are part of the Diffusion of Effective Behavioral Interventions (DEBI) project: CHOICES, Communal Effectance-AIDS Prevention, Female and Culturally

Specific Negotiation, Project FIO (the Future Is Ours), Project SAFE, Real AIDS Prevention Project (RAPP), Sisters Informing Healing Living and Empowering (SIHLE), Sisters Informing Sisters on Topics about AIDS (SISTA), Sisters Saving Sisters, Sister to Sister, Women's Health Promotion (WHP), Women Involved in Life Learning from Other Women (WILLOW), Women's Co-op, Condom Promotion, Insights, Safer Sex, and Salud, Educacion, Prevencion y Autocuidado (SEPA).[15]

The Women's Leadership and Community Planning project in San Francisco offers a two-day training for women with HIV in California who want to take greater leadership roles in state planning councils. At the training, women network with each other, as well as learn skills in public speaking, decision-making, and conflict management. Women stay in touch through monthly conference calls. After the first training, six of thirteen women moved into leadership positions on their local or state councils.[16]

Respeto/Proteger: Respecting and Protecting our Relationships is an HIV prevention program for Latino teen mothers and fathers in Los Angeles, California. Developed and tested with a community agency and academic researchers, the program recognizes risks young women face, including poverty, drug and alcohol use, history of STIs, and physical or sexual abuse. The six-session intervention focuses on healing the wounded spirit and builds on feelings of maternal and paternal protectiveness using cultural and traditional teachings.[17]

What Needs to Be Done?

Because women are more likely to get HIV from their male partners, programs that target men (especially IDUs) will have a beneficial impact on women. Needle exchange and drug treatment strategies are critical. Public health agencies need to raise awareness about sexual abuse and domestic violence to not only help men and women develop the skills to prevent it, but also to curb its effect on the HIV epidemic. HIV testing campaigns that target women and women-friendly testing sites are also needed.

Behavioral and structural HIV prevention interventions for women continue to be necessary, given the lack of evidence from biomedical interventions (microbicides, vaccines).[18] However, research needs to continue on how women can protect themselves with an accessible, affordable, comfortable, and discrete tool for safer sex.

Although research has highlighted the subpopulations of women most affected by HIV/AIDS, it is even more important to translate and materialize study findings into tangible public health programs and effective policies. Interventions that address sexuality, family, culture, empowerment, self-esteem, and negotiating skills, as well as interventions located in varying community settings are especially valuable.

Says Who?

1. Kaiser Family Foundation. Women and HIV/AIDS in the United States. Policy Fact Sheet. July 2007.

2. Centers for Disease Control and Prevention. Cases of HIV infection and AIDS in the United States and Dependent Areas, 2005. HIV/AIDS Surveillance Report. 2007;17.

3. Centers for Disease Control and Prevention. HIV/AIDS fact sheet: HIV/AIDS among women. June 2007.

4. National Institute of Allergy and Infectious Diseases at National Institutes of Health. Research on HIV infection in women. 2006.

5. Theall KP, Sterk CE, Elifson KW, et al. Factors associated with positive HIV serostatus among women who use drugs: continued evidence for expanding factors of influence. *Public Health Reports*. 2003;118:415–24.

6. Sangani P, Rutherford G, Wilkinson D. Population-based interventions for reducing sexually transmitted infections, including HIV infection. *Cochrane Database of Systematic Reviews*. 2004; 2:CD001220.

7. Weinstock H, Berman S, Cates W. Sexually transmitted diseases among American youth: incidence and prevalence estimates, 2000. *Perspectives in Sexual and Reproductive Health*. 2004;36:6–10.

8. Koenig LJ, Moore J. Women, violence, and HIV: A critical evaluation with implications for HIV services. *Maternal and Child Health Journal*. 2000;4:103–9.

9. Wyatt GE, Myers HF, Loeb TB. Women, trauma, and HIV: an overview. *AIDS and Behavior*. 2004;8:401–3.

10. Bozzette SA, Berry SH, Duan N, et al. The care of HIV-infected adults in the United States. HIV Cost and Services Utilization Study Consortium. *New England Journal of Medicine*. 1998;339:1897–1904.

11. Cohan DL, Kim A, Ruiz J, et al. Health indicators among low income women who report a history of sex work: the

population based Northern California Young Women's Survey. *Sexually Transmitted Infections*. 2005;81:428–33.

12. Adimora AA, Schoenbach VJ, Bonas DM, et al. Concurrent sexual partnerships among women in the United States. *Epidemiology*. 2002;13:320–27.

13. Prosper! The Women's Collective, Washington DC.

14. Dworkin SL, Ehrhardt AA. Going beyond "ABC" to include "GEM": critical reflections on progress in the HIV/AIDS epidemic. *American Journal of Public Health*. 2007;97:13–18.

15. Centers for Disease Control and Prevention. Updated Compendium of Evidence-Based Interventions, 2007.

16. Women's Leadership and Community Planning project, CompassPoint, San Francisco, CA.

17. Lesser J, Koniak-Griffin D, Gonzalez-Figueroa E, et al. Childhood abuse history and risk behaviors among teen parents in a culturally rooted, couple-focused HIV prevention program. *Journal of the Association of Nurses in AIDS Care*. 2007;18:18–27.

18. Landovitz RJ. Recent efforts in biomedical prevention of HIV. *Topics in HIV Medicine*. 2007;15:99–103.

Section 9.3

Men Who Have Sex with Men

Reprinted from "HIV and AIDS among Gay and Bisexual Men,"
Centers for Disease Control and Prevention, March 2010.

Gay and bisexual men—referred to in Centers for Disease Control and Prevention (CDC) surveillance systems as men who have sex with men (MSM)[1]—of all races continue to be the risk group most severely affected by human immunodeficiency virus (HIV). Additionally, this is the only risk group in the United States in which the annual number of new HIV infections is increasing. There is an urgent need to expand access to proven HIV prevention interventions for gay and bisexual men, as well as to develop new approaches to fight HIV in this population.

A Snapshot

MSM account for nearly half of the more than one million people living with HIV in the United States (48 percent, or an estimated 532,000 total persons).

MSM account for more than half of all new HIV infections in the United States each year (53 percent, or an estimated 28,700 infections).

While CDC estimates that MSM account for just 4 percent of the U.S. male population aged thirteen and older, the rate of new HIV diagnoses among MSM in the United States is more than forty-four times that of other men (range: 522–989 per 100,000 MSM vs. 12 per 100,000 other men).

MSM is the only risk group in the United States in which new HIV infections are increasing. While new infections have declined among both heterosexuals and injection drug users, the annual number of new HIV infections among MSM has been steadily increasing since the early 1990s.

According to the latest estimates, white MSM represent a greater number of new HIV infections than any other population, followed closely by black MSM—who are one of the most disproportionately affected subgroups in the United States.

The primary ages at which MSM become infected differ by race:

- **Young black MSM:** Most new infections among black MSM occur among young black MSM. In fact, there are more new HIV infections among young black MSM (aged thirteen to twenty-nine) than among any other age and racial group of MSM. The number of new infections among black MSM in this age group is roughly twice that of their white and Hispanic counterparts (5,220 infections in blacks vs. 3,330 among whites and 2,300 among Hispanics).

- **White MSM in their thirties and forties:** Most new infections among white MSM occur among those aged thirty to thirty-nine (4,670), followed by those aged forty to forty-nine (3,740).

- **Young Hispanic MSM:** Among Hispanic MSM, most new infections occur in the youngest (thirteen to twenty-nine) age group (2,300), though a substantial number of new HIV infections also occur among those aged thirty to thirty-nine (1,870).

A study of MSM in five U.S. cities found extremely high levels of infection among MSM, and many of those infected did not know it:

- Overall, one in four MSM participating in the study was infected. Black MSM were twice as likely to be infected with HIV than other MSM.

- Among all of those who were infected, about half were unaware of their HIV status. Results were particularly alarming for black MSM and young MSM, with more than two-thirds of infected black MSM, and nearly 80 percent of infected young MSM (aged eighteen to twenty-four) unaware that they were infected.

Acquired immunodeficiency syndrome (AIDS) continues to claim the lives of too many MSM. Since the beginning of the epidemic, more than 274,000 MSM with AIDS have died.

Complex Factors Increase Risk

High prevalence of HIV: The high prevalence of HIV among gay and bisexual men means MSM face a greater risk of being exposed to infection with each sexual encounter, especially as they get older. For young black MSM, partnering with older black men (among whom HIV prevalence is high) may also lead to increased risk.

Lack of knowledge of HIV status: Studies show that individuals who know they are infected take steps to protect their partners. Yet many MSM are unaware of their status and may unknowingly be transmitting the virus to others. Additionally, some MSM may make false assumptions or have inaccurate information about their partner's HIV status. It is critical to ensure that sexually active MSM get tested for HIV at least annually, or more frequently as needed.

Complacency about risk: Among young MSM in particular, complacency about HIV may play a key role in HIV risk, since these men did not personally experience the severity of the early AIDS epidemic. Additional challenges for many MSM include maintaining consistently safe behaviors over time, underestimating personal risk, and the false belief that because of treatment advances, HIV is no longer a serious health threat. We must reach each generation of MSM and develop programs that can help MSM remain uninfected throughout the course of their lives.

Social discrimination and cultural issues: For some MSM, social and economic factors, including homophobia, stigma, and lack of access to healthcare may increase risk behaviors or be a barrier to receiving HIV prevention services.

Substance abuse: Some MSM use alcohol and illegal drugs, contributing to increased risk for HIV infection and other sexually transmitted diseases (STDs). Substance use can increase the risk for HIV transmission through risky sexual behaviors while under the influence and through sharing needles or other injection equipment.

HIV: Protect Yourself

Be smart about HIV. Here's what you can do to reduce your risk of infection:

- **Get the facts:** Arm yourself with basic information. Are you at risk? How is HIV spread? How can you protect yourself?

- **Take control:** You have the facts; now protect yourself and your loved ones. There are three essential ways to reduce your risk: Don't have sex (anal, vaginal, or oral); only have sex (anal, vaginal, or oral) if you're in a mutually monogamous relationship with a partner you know is not infected; and use a condom every time you have anal, vaginal, or oral sex. Correct and consistent use of the male latex condom is highly effective in reducing HIV transmission.

- **Put yourself to the test:** Knowing your HIV status is a critical step toward stopping HIV transmission, because if you know you are infected, you can take steps to protect your partners. Also, if you are infected, the sooner you find out, the sooner you can receive life-extending treatment. In fact, CDC recommends that everyone between the ages of thirteen and sixty-four be tested for HIV. Because other STDs can play a role in the acquisition of HIV, knowing whether you are infected with either is critical in reducing your risk for infection.

- **Start talking:** Talk to everyone you know about HIV—friends and family, co- workers and neighbors, at work and at places of worship. Have ongoing and open discussions with your partners about HIV testing and risk behaviors. Talking openly about HIV can reduce the stigma that keeps too many from seeking the testing, prevention and treatment services, and support they need.

HIV doesn't have to become part of your life. Each of us can and must be part of the solution.

Section 9.4

Older Adults

Reprinted from "HIV/AIDS among Persons Aged Fifty and Older,"
Centers for Disease Control and Prevention, February 28, 2008.

The number of persons aged fifty years and older living with human immunodeficiency virus (HIV) and acquired immunodeficiency syndrome (AIDS) has been increasing in recent years. This increase is partly due to highly active antiretroviral therapy (HAART), which has made it possible for many HIV-infected persons to live longer, and partly due to newly diagnosed infections in persons over the age of fifty. As the U.S. population continues to age, it is important to be aware of specific challenges faced by older Americans and to ensure that they get information and services to help protect them from infection.

The Numbers

In 2005, persons aged fifty and older accounted for the following:

- 15 percent of new HIV/AIDS diagnoses[1]
- 24 percent of persons living with HIV/AIDS (increased from 17 percent in 2001)[1]
- 19 percent of all AIDS diagnoses[1]
- 29 percent of persons living with AIDS[1]
- 35 percent of all deaths of persons with AIDS[1]

The rates of HIV/AIDS among persons fifty and older were twelve times as high among blacks (51.7/100,000) and five times as high among Hispanics (21.4/100,000) compared with whites (4.2/100,000).[2]

Prevention Challenges

Persons over the age of fifty may have many of the same risk factors for HIV infection that younger persons have.

163

Many older persons are sexually active but may not be practicing safer sex to reduce their risk for HIV infection.[3] Older women may be especially at risk because age-related vaginal thinning and dryness can cause tears in the vaginal area.[4]

Some older persons inject drugs or smoke crack cocaine, which can put them at risk for HIV infection. HIV transmission through injection drug use accounts for more than 16 percent of AIDS cases among persons aged fifty and older.[5]

Some older persons, compared with those who are younger, may be less knowledgeable about HIV/AIDS and therefore less likely to protect themselves. Many do not perceive themselves as at risk for HIV, do not use condoms, and do not get tested for HIV.[6,7]

Older persons of minority races/ethnicities may face discrimination and stigma that can lead to later testing, diagnosis, and reluctance to seek services.[8]

Healthcare professionals may underestimate their older patients' risk for HIV/AIDS and thus may miss opportunities to deliver prevention messages, offer HIV testing, or make an early diagnosis that could help their patients get early care.[3]

Physicians may miss a diagnosis of AIDS because some symptoms can mimic those of normal aging, for example, fatigue, weight loss, and mental confusion. Early diagnosis, which typically leads to the prescription of HAART and to other medical and social services, can improve a person's chances of living a longer and healthier life.

The stigma of HIV/AIDS may be more severe among older persons, leading them to hide their diagnosis from family and friends. Failure to disclose HIV infection may limit or preclude potential emotional and practical support.

What the Centers for Disease Control and Prevention (CDC) Is Doing

CDC recommends routine HIV screening for adults and adolescents, including pregnant women, in healthcare settings in the United States and recommends reducing barriers to HIV testing.[9] The recommendations specify routine testing for persons up to age sixty-four. (Persons aged sixty-four and over should be counseled to receive HIV testing if they have risk factors for HIV infection.) Routine testing is intended not only to identify persons who are unaware that they are HIV infected but also to remove the stigma of being tested. Making testing routine for older persons can help open a discussion about risk behavior between a physician and an older person.

Prevention strategies should be developed for older persons who are potentially at risk for HIV infection: education to increase awareness and knowledge, skills training to help them negotiate risk-reduction behaviors, and messages that are age-appropriate and culturally sensitive. Intervention strategies to help older women negotiate safer sexual behavior are especially important.

A recent review of HIV/AIDS behavioral interventions for persons fifty and older recommended simultaneous multilevel approaches, including building on our current understanding of behavior change and HIV prevention successes with younger populations while considering important intervention principles gathered from work with older populations in other health areas.

References

1. CDC. *HIV/AIDS Surveillance Report, 2005*. Vol. 17. Rev ed. Atlanta: U.S. Department of Health and Human Services, CDC; 2007:1–54.

2. Linley L, Hall HI, An Q, et al. HIV/AIDS diagnoses among persons fifty years and older in 33 states, 2001–2005. National HIV Prevention Conference, December 2007; Atlanta. Abstract B08-1.

3. Lindau ST, Schumm MA, Laumann EO, et al. A study of sexuality and health among older adults in the United States. *N Eng J Med* 2007;357:762–74.

4. Center for AIDS Prevention Studies. What are HIV prevention needs of adults over 50 [fact sheet 29E]? September 1997.

5. Linsk NL. HIV among older adults. *AIDS Reader* 2000;10(7):430–40.

6. Lindau ST et al. Older women's attitudes, behavior, and communication about sex and HIV: a community-based study. *J Womens Health* 2006;6:747–53.

7. Henderson SJ et al. Older women and HIV: how much do they know and where are they getting their information? *J Am Geriatr Soc* 2004;52:1549–53.

8. Zingmond DS et al. Circumstances at HIV diagnosis and progression of disease in older HIV-infected Americans. *Am J Public Health* 2001;91:1117–20.

9. CDC. Revised recommendations for HIV testing of adults, adolescents, and pregnant women in health-care settings. *MMWR* 2006;55(RR-14):1–17.

Section 9.5

Homeless Populations

"What Are Homeless Persons' HIV Prevention Needs?" reprinted with permission from the Center for AIDS Prevention Studies (CAPS), University of California at San Francisco (www.caps.ucsf.edu). © 2005 Regents of the University of California. Reviewed by David A. Cooke, MD, FACP, November 2010.

Who are the homeless?

Homelessness is a growing problem in the United States. It is estimated that on any given day there are more than 800,000 homeless individuals in the United States, while over the course of a year there are 2.3 to 3.5 million individuals who experience a period of homelessness.[1] In the 2004 mayors' report on homelessness 70 percent of cities surveyed registered an increase in the number of requests for emergency shelter during the preceding year.[2]

The U.S. homeless population is typically divided into three major groups: single adults, members of homeless families, and youth. It is estimated that single adults make up 54 percent of the population, families 40 percent, and unaccompanied youth 5 percent.[2]

Do homeless populations have a high prevalence of human immunodeficiency virus (HIV) infection?

People who are homeless have poorer health and higher mortality than the general population.[3] The prevalence of HIV/AIDS (acquired immunodeficiency syndrome) varies widely among homeless subgroups, but generally exceeds that of the non-homeless population. The elevated prevalence of infection combined with limited access to treatment and poor living conditions have contributed to HIV/AIDS becoming a leading cause of death in this population.[4]

A study in San Francisco, California, reported an overall HIV prevalence of 10.5 percent for currently homeless and marginally housed adults, which is five times higher than that of the general San Francisco population. The same study reported an HIV prevalence of 30 percent among homeless men who have sex with men (MSM) and 8 percent among homeless injection drug users (IDUs).[5]

The association between homelessness and HIV appears to be a two-way street. HIV-positive persons are at greater risk of homelessness due to discrimination and the high costs of housing and medical care. At the same time, homeless people have an elevated risk of contracting HIV.

What puts a homeless person at risk?

Homeless persons are in transient living situations, typically in impoverished communities with high HIV prevalence. Thus, risky behaviors they may engage in are more likely to result in infection.

Homeless persons are also more likely to evidence drug, alcohol, and mental disorders than the general population. By one estimate in 2000, 88 percent of homeless single men and 69 percent of homeless single women had one of these three disorders.[6] Overall, almost one-fourth of the single adult homeless population suffers from severe and persistent mental illness.[1] The impulsivity and impaired judgment often associated with severe mental illness or substance abuse contribute to risky behaviors such as unprotected sex, multiple partners, sharing needles, or exchanging sex for drugs.

The conditions of homelessness and extreme poverty also contribute to risky behaviors. For example, most homeless shelters provide communal sleeping and bathing, are single sex, and offer limited privacy. Under these restrictions, it is more difficult to have stable sexual relationships.

Other characteristics that are common among homeless persons and associated with HIV risk behaviors include: adverse childhood experiences such as physical and sexual abuse,[1,7] sexual assault, partner violence and other traumatic histories, and poor social support.[8]

What are barriers to prevention?

A common misconception is that the greatest barrier to delivering prevention services to homeless persons is finding them. The reality, however, is that homeless people are often visible by living or working in the streets or readily accessible in shelters. Forming trusting relationships, making consistent contact over time, and working through already existing social networks can help find and retain homeless persons for follow-up and services. In one HIV testing program for homeless persons with severe mental illness, 90 percent of those tested returned to receive their results.[9]

Institutional barriers and settings can restrict HIV prevention activities. Staffing at shelters is often only adequate to provide basic needs, and shelters may be reluctant to allow outside HIV prevention programs to talk explicitly about sex and drugs or to distribute condoms because those activities are forbidden in most shelters. A lack of private space for counseling and education around sensitive topics can also be a barrier.

What's being done?

The quantity and quality of services available to homeless individuals varies greatly across the nation. Historically, services have concentrated on serving single male clients and few have formed coordinated networks of care to facilitate comprehensive ongoing services.[1] Here we provide just a few examples of effective interventions designed specifically to serve homeless individuals at risk for or living with HIV.

Sex, Games and Videotapes is a program for homeless mentally ill men in a New York City, New York, shelter that is built around activities central to shelter life: competitive games, storytelling, and watching videos. For many men sex is conducted in public spaces, revolves around drug use, and must be done quickly. The program allows for sex issues to be brought up in a nonjudgmental way. One component is a competition to see who can put a condom (without tearing it) on a banana fastest—this teaches important skills for using a condom quickly. The program reduced sexual risk behavior threefold.[10]

Boston HAPPENS provides health education, case management, basic medical care, HIV testing, counseling, and mental health care for HIV-positive, at-risk youth, many of whom are homeless. Boston HAPPENS' collaborators run drop-in services and storefront clinics in places where young people hang out. Through persistent outreach and individualized case management, HAPPENS retains homeless at-risk youth in care.[11]

Providing homeless individuals with housing and cash benefits has been shown to reduce risk-taking behaviors such as unprotected sex, drug use, and needle sharing.[12,13]

Housing Works is an AIDS service organization that specializes in providing comprehensive care to HIV-positive homeless persons in New York City. Their services include housing, healthcare, job training and placement, as well as a variety of other advocacy services for homeless HIV-positive persons.[14]

What needs to be done?

There is an ongoing need to deliver effective prevention activities in culturally appropriate service settings that homeless persons use, such as soup kitchens, shelters, residential hotels, and clinics. Staff of these organizations should be trained in HIV prevention education methods that recognize specific risk factors related to homelessness, employ realistic expectations for change, and give homeless people concrete goals that they can accomplish.

Coordinated care networks need to be developed so that staff can link individuals quickly and easily to the services they need.[15] Group interventions that have worked in certain settings need to be broadly disseminated and adapted for use in other locations.

Efforts to prevent HIV transmission among homeless persons will flounder without a concerted effort to better address their survival needs including long-term housing, jobs, income, adequate nutrition, substance abuse treatment, and regular medical and mental health services. Unfortunately, despite the announcement of new initiatives to help the homeless, recent trends in government support in these areas are discouraging and the growing federal budget deficit does not bode well for increases in the near future. As one of the most vulnerable populations in our society, homeless persons need support, respect, protection, and continued prevention efforts.

Says who?

1. Burt M, Laudan Y, Lee E, et al. *Helping America's homeless: emergency shelter or affordable housing?* Washington, D.C.: Urban Institute Press. 2001.

2. U.S. Conference of Mayors. A status report on hunger and homelessness in America's cities: 2004. www.usmayors.org/uscm/hungersurvey/2004/onlinereport/HungerAnd HomelessnessReport2004.pdf (accessed 4/20/06).

3. Burt, MR, Laudan, AY, Douglas T, et. al. 1999 Homelessness: Programs and the People They Serve—Summary Report. Washington, DC: DHUD/DHHS. http://www.huduser.org/publications/homeless/homelessness/contents.php (accessed 4/20/06).

4. Cheung AM, Hwang SW. Risk of death among homeless women: a cohort study and review of the literature. *Canadian Medical Association Journal*. 2004;170:1243.

5. Robertson MJ, Clark RA, Charlebois ED, et al. HIV seroprevalence among homeless and marginally housed adults in San Francisco. *American Journal of Public Health*. 2004;94:1207–17.

6. North CS, Eyrich KM, Pollio DE, et al. Are rates of psychiatric disorders in the homeless population changing? *American Journal of Public Health*. 2004;94:103–8.

7. Herman DB, Susser ES, Struening EL, et al. Adverse childhood experiences: are they risk factors for adult homelessness? *American Journal of Public Health*. 1997;87:249–55.

8. Zlotnick C, Tam T, Robertson MJ. Adverse childhood events, substance abuse, and measures of affiliation. *Addiction and Behavior*. 2004;29:1177–81.

9. Desai MM, Rosenheck RA. HIV testing and receipt of test results among homeless persons with severe mental illness. *American Journal of Psychiatry*. 2004;161:2287–94.

10. Susser E, Valencia E, Berkman A, et al. Human immunodeficiency virus sexual risk reduction in homeless men with mental illness. *Archives of General Psychiatry*. 1998;55:266–72.

11. Harris SK, Samples CL, Keenan PM, et al. Outreach, mental health, and case management services: can they help to retain HIV-positive and at-risk youth and young adults in care? *Maternal and Child Health Journal*. 2003;7:205–18.

12. Aidala A, Cross JE, Stall R, Harre D, et. al. Housing status and HIV risk behaviors: implications for prevention and policy. *AIDS and Behavior*. 2005;9:1–15.

13. Riley ED, Moss AR, Clark RA, et. al. Cash benefits are associated with lower risk behavior among the homeless and marginally housed in San Francisco. *Journal of Urban Health*. 2005;82:142–50.

14. Housing Works, www.housingworks.org (accessed 4/20/06).

15. Woods ER, Samples CL, Melchiono MW, et. al. Initiation of services in the Boston HAPPENS Program: human immunodeficiency virus-positive, homeless, and at-risk youth can access services. *AIDS Patient Care STDs*. 2002;16:497–510.

Section 9.6

Prison Populations

"What Is the Role of Prisons and Jails in HIV Prevention?" reprinted with permission from the Center for AIDS Prevention Studies (CAPS), University of California at San Francisco (www.caps.ucsf.edu). © 2009 Regents of the University of California.

Is prevention in prisons and jails important?

Absolutely. The United States has the highest incarceration rate in the world, and the numbers keep growing.[1] In 2007, the United States had over 2.4 million people in state, federal, and local correctional facilities.[2] For the first time, more than one in every one hundred adults in the United States is confined in a jail or prison.[1]

Persons in prison and jail have higher rates of many diseases and health problems than the general population. Human immunodeficiency virus (HIV) rates among incarcerated persons are two and a half times higher than in the general population.[3] In any given year, about 25 percent of all HIV-positive persons in the United States pass through a correctional facility.[4] Persons in prison and jail also have higher rates of sexually transmitted infections (STIs), tuberculosis, and viral hepatitis, as well as substance abuse and mental illness.[5]

These high infection rates in prisons and jails in the United States reflect the fact that the majority of persons who are incarcerated come from impoverished and disenfranchised communities with limited access to prevention, screening, and treatment services.[6] These are the same neighborhoods with high rates of HIV, STIs, and other infectious diseases.

Criminal justice and public health systems can work together to provide comprehensive prevention and treatment inside and outside facilities. Incarceration presents a window of opportunity for primary prevention, screening, treatment, and establishing comprehensive, proactive transitional linkages for persons approaching release and follow-up.

171

What is the HIV connection between prisons, jails, and the community?

At least 95 percent of persons in prison are released into the community at some point.[7] The impact of incarceration and disease is not limited to the men and women being locked up, but extends to their families, partners, and communities.

There is a mistaken belief that men and women acquire HIV inside, when in fact, the vast majority of HIV-positive persons in prison and jail enter the criminal justice system HIV-positive.[8,9]

Persons with a history of mental illness, trauma, or physical and sexual abuse, who do not have access to mental health services, may self-medicate with substance use. This combination puts them at increased risk for behaviors that may both lead to HIV and land them in jail or prison. Rates of mental health diagnoses for persons in jail and prison are 45 to 65 percent, while rates of substance abuse are as high as 75 percent.[10]

How does incarceration impact HIV risk?

Persons in prison and jail may engage in risk behaviors before, during, and after incarceration. However, behavior during incarceration may be riskier for those who do not have access to condoms, clean syringes, and other prevention tools. Sexual activity (both consensual and coerced), substance use, injecting, and tattooing can all put individuals at risk for HIV/STIs and viral hepatitis.[11] In one study of incarcerated young men, 50 percent had used substances and 17 percent had consensual sex with men or women while confined.[12]

Release from correctional settings and re-entry into the community can be a stressful time and often carries higher risks than being incarcerated. Persons released from prison and jail may celebrate their release with HIV risk-related behaviors such as drinking, drug use, and sex. Persons released with few resources often return to the same precarious environments where they were arrested. A study of persons formerly incarcerated in Washington found a high risk of drug overdose within the first two weeks of release.[13]

There is a misperception that incarcerated men are responsible for increasing rates of HIV/STIs. Imprisonment does affect HIV/STI rates in the community, but not from men getting infected on the inside and bringing it out to their female sexual partners once they are released. Instead, incarceration decreases the number of men in the community, which disrupts stable partnerships, changes the male-to-female ratio, and promotes higher-risk concurrent, or overlapping, partnerships.[14]

What can be done inside?

Across the United States, many HIV prevention agencies and public health departments are working with the criminal justice system to improve the health of persons who are incarcerated and their communities. Agencies can provide: peer-based prevention programs, including prevention with positives; harm reduction programs; quality healthcare; treatment for HIV/STIs; treatment for substance abuse and mental illness; links to community services pre-release; help with community reintegration post-release.[10,15]

Counseling, testing, and treatment for HIV/STI/hepatitis/ tuberculosis (TB). Incarceration can be an opportunity for screening and treating a group of individuals with high-risk behaviors. This should include comprehensive pre-test counseling with a consent process describing the implications of testing positive or negative, as these can have consequences within correctional facilities, such as limiting housing and work assignments, and restricting visiting privileges. It should also include providing treatment for those who test positive and prevention education to those who test positive and negative.

Mental health treatment. Persons in prison and jail have high rates of mental illness. Conditions in correctional settings such as overcrowding, violence, and isolation have negative effects on mental health. Prisons and jails can help by providing assessment and effective treatment. Persons with mental illness who have committed minor offenses should be diverted to mental health services before or instead of prison or jail.[16]

Comprehensive substance abuse treatment. While many jails and prisons in the United States offer detoxification, professional and peer counseling, self-help groups, and drug and alcohol education, very few offer methadone maintenance. The capacity of effective substance abuse treatment programs falls far short of the need. The Key Extended Entry Program (KEEP), based in New York, New York, provides jail-based methadone treatment and dedicated treatment slots to released individuals in the community.[17]

What are transitional interventions?

Effective transitional interventions ensure that prevention and treatment services provided on the inside are continued on the outside. Many communities will have an increasing role in transitional planning with enactment of the Second Chance Act.[18]

Project START is the only intervention for incarcerated populations in the Center for Disease Control and Prevention's (CDC's) Compendium of Evidence-Based Interventions. Project START is a client-centered, six-session HIV, STI, and hepatitis risk reduction intervention for persons being released from a correctional setting. Based in harm reduction, it uses a prevention case management model and motivational enhancement to encourage risk reduction. The first two sessions are pre-release and the last four are post-release. All sessions include facilitated referrals for housing, employment, substance abuse and mental health treatment, legal issues, and avoiding reincarceration. Research demonstrated that Project START was effective in reducing unprotected sex among young men after their release from prison.[19]

Project Bridge in Providence, Rhode Island, provides intensive case management for HIV-positive persons being released from state prison. Enrollees receive eighteen months of case management by a social worker and an outreach worker. Participants meet weekly for twelve weeks, then once a month, at a minimum. Project Bridge is effective in helping HIV-positive persons obtain and maintain much needed post-release services. Research showed that despite high levels of addiction (97 percent) and mental illness (34 percent), participants received post-release medical care (95 percent), secured housing (46 percent), linked to mental health care (71 percent), and linked to addiction services (51 percent).[20]

What are next steps?

Effectively addressing HIV in prisons, jails, and communities requires both effective prevention strategies (such as peer education, access to condoms, HIV counseling and testing) and effective structural and medical strategies. Some of the proven effective strategies and policies that can help reduce HIV/STIs in prisons and jails include: harm reduction programs (providing clean syringes);[21] substance abuse treatment;[17] mental health treatment;[16] STI/HIV treatment;[5] transitional discharge planning;[19,20] housing;[5] alternatives to incarceration;[15] and sentencing and parole reform.[1]

Collaboration between the criminal justice system (prison, jail, parole, and probation) and the community public health system (social services, medical/health clinics, treatment programs, etc.) is essential, and there are several effective models. Building partnerships can help tackle public health issues while understanding the challenges of public safety and custody priorities. If we truly want to decrease rates of HIV, STIs, and hepatitis in our communities, we have to work together to create a seamless continuum that will improve prevention, care, and treatment both inside prisons and jails as well as in disproportionately affected communities.

Says who?

1. PEW Center on the States. One in 31: The long reach of American corrections. March 2009.

2. West HC, Sabol WJ. Prisoners in 2007. *Bureau of Justice Statistics Bulletin.* 2008.

3. Maruschak L. HIV in Prisons, 2006. *Bureau of Justice Statistics Bulletin.* 2008.

4. Hammett TM, Harmon MP, Rhodes W. The burden of infectious disease among inmates of and releasees from US correctional facilities, 1997. *American Journal of Public Health.* 2002;92:1789–94.

5. The Foundation for AIDS Research. HIV in correctional settings: implications for prevention and treatment policy. Issue Brief No 5, March 2008.

6. Golembeski C, Fullilove R. Criminal (in)justice in the city and its associated health consequences. *American Journal of Public Health.* 2005;95:1701–6.

7. Hughes T, James Wilson D. Reentry trends in the United States. Bureau of Justice Statistics.

8. Vlahov D, Putnam S. From corrections to communities as an HIV priority. *Journal of Urban Health.* 2006;83:339–48.

9. Zack B, Kramer K. HIV prevention education in correctional settings. Project UNSHACKLE discussion paper. May 2008.

10. James DJ, Glaze LE. Mental health problems of prison and jail inmates. Bureau of Justice Statistics Special Report. September 2006.

11. HIV transmission among male inmates in a state prison system—Georgia, 1992–2005. *Morbidity and Mortality Weekly Report.* 2006;55:421–26.

12. Seal DW, Margolis AD, Morrow KM, et al. Substance use and sexual behavior during incarceration among 18- to 29-year-old men: prevalence and correlates. *AIDS and Behavior.* 2008;12:27–40.

13. Binswanger IA, Stern MF, Deyo RA, et al. Release from prison—a high risk of death for former inmates. *New England Journal of Medicine.* 2007;356:157–65.

14. Aral SO, Adimora AA, Fenton KA. Understanding and responding to disparities in HIV and other sexually transmitted infections in African Americans. *Lancet.* 2008;372:337–40.

15. Freudenberg N. Jails, prisons, and the health of urban populations: a review of the impact of the correctional system on community health. *Journal of Urban Health.* 2001;78:214–35.

16. World Health Organization. Mental health and prisons. 2005.

17. Tomasino V, Swanson AJ, Nolan J, et al. The Key Extended Entry Program (KEEP): A methadone treatment program for opiate-dependent inmates. *The Mount Sinai Journal of Medicine.* 2001;68:14–20.

18. Second Chance Act.

19. Wolitski RJ, The Project START study group. Relative efficacy of a multi-session sexual risk-reduction intervention for young men released from prison in 4 states. *American Journal of Public Health.* 2006;96:1845–61.

20. Zaller ND, Holmes L, Dyl AC, et al. Linkage to treatment and supportive services among HIV-positive ex-offenders in Project Bridge. *Journal of Health Care for the Poor and Underserved.* 2008;19:522–31.

21. Jürgens R, Ball A, Verster A. Interventions to reduce HIV transmission related to injecting drug use in prison. *Lancet Infectious Diseases.* 2009;9:57–66.

Chapter 10

HIV/AIDS Prevention

Chapter Contents

Section 10.1

Safer Sex

"Reducing Your Sexual Risk" is reprinted from "Sexual Risk Factors," AIDS.gov, October 2010. "Tips for Using Condoms and Dental Dams" is reprinted from U.S. Department of Veterans Affairs, December 10, 2009.

Reducing Your Sexual Risk

Human immunodeficiency virus (HIV) can be spread by having unprotected sexual contact (sex without barrier protection, like a condom) with an HIV-positive person.

Some of the ways to reduce your risk of getting HIV through sexual contact include the following:

- **Abstinence:** Abstaining from sexual behavior (vaginal, anal, or oral sex) of any kind is the only 100 percent sure way to prevent HIV infection.

- **Be faithful:** Being faithful means you are in a sexual relationship with only one person, both of you are having sex only with each other, and you have both been tested and know each other's HIV status.

- **Get tested and know your partner's status:** Knowing your own status is important for both your health and the health of your partner. You also need to ask your sexual partner(s) if they have been tested for HIV, when they were last tested, and what the results were. Talking about your HIV status can be a difficult or uncomfortable—but it's important to start the discussion early and *before* you have sex. If you and your partner decide to have sexual partners outside of your relationship, this is a conversation you need to be having continuously with your partner. In addition you both should continue to be tested for HIV and other sexually transmitted diseases (STDs) every three to six months.

- **Correct and consistent use of the male latex or polyurethane condom:** If you use a condom incorrectly, it can slip or break, which lessens the chance it will protect you. And if you use a condom inconsistently (i.e., you don't use a fresh condom with every act of oral, anal, or vaginal intercourse), you can get STDs, including HIV, because transmission can occur with a single act of intercourse. It is important to note that female polyurethane condoms are also effective in preventing HIV and certain STDs. You should always use a water-based lubricant when you use a condom for vaginal or anal sex. Lubricants reduce friction and help prevent condom breakage. Do *not* use an oil-based lubricant (like petroleum jelly, hand lotion, or cooking oil). Oil-based lubricants can damage condoms and make them less effective.

Condoms do not provide 100 percent protection against all sexually transmitted diseases. Protection against genital ulcer diseases (e.g., herpes, human papilloma virus [HPV]) depends on the site of the sore/ulcer or infection. Latex condoms can protect against transmission only when the ulcers or infections are in genital areas that are covered or protected by the condom. Thus, consistent and correct use of latex condoms would be expected to protect against transmission of genital ulcer diseases and HPV in some, but not all, instances.

Condoms with the spermicide Nonoxynol-9 are *not* recommended for STD/HIV prevention. Nonoxynol-9 (N9) has been found to irritate rectal and vaginal walls, thus increasing the chance of HIV infection in the event that semen does come in contact with them.

Tips for Using Condoms and Dental Dams

Some people think that using a condom makes sex less fun. Other people have become creative and find condoms sexy. Not having to worry about infecting someone will definitely make sex much more enjoyable!

If you are not used to using condoms: practice, practice, practice.

Condom Do's and Don'ts

Shop around. Use lubricated latex condoms. Always use latex, because lambskin condoms don't block HIV and STDs, and polyurethane condoms break more often than latex. Shop around and find your favorite brand. Try different sizes and shapes. (Yes, they come in different sizes and shapes!) There are a lot of choices—one will work for you.

Keep it fresh. Store condoms loosely in a cool, dry place (not your wallet). Make sure your condoms are fresh—check the expiration date. Throw away condoms that have expired, been very hot, or been washed in the washer. If you think the condom might not be good, get a new one. You and your partner are worth it.

Take it easy. Open the package carefully, so that you don't rip the condom. Be careful if you use your teeth. Make sure that the condom package has not been punctured (there should be a pocket of air). Check the condom for damaged packaging and signs of aging such as brittleness, stickiness, and discoloration.

Keep it hard. Put on the condom after the penis is erect and before it touches any part of a partner's body. If a penis is uncircumcised (uncut), the foreskin must be pulled back before putting on the condom.

Heads up. Make sure the condom is right-side out. It's like a sock—there's a right side and a wrong side. Before you put it on the penis, unroll the condom about half an inch to see which direction it is unrolling. Then put it on the head of the penis and hold the tip of the condom between your fingers as you roll it all the way down the shaft of the penis from head to base. This keeps out air bubbles that can cause the condom to break. It also leaves a space for semen to collect after ejaculation.

Slippery when wet. If you use a lubricant (lube), it should be a water-soluble lubricant (for example, ID Glide, K-Y Jelly, Slippery Stuff, Foreplay, Wet, Astroglide) in order to prevent breakdown of the condom. Products such as petroleum jelly, massage oils, butter, Crisco, Vaseline, and hand creams are not considered water-soluble lubricants and should not be used. Put lubricant on after you put on the condom, not before—it could slip off. Add more lube often. Dry condoms break more easily.

Come and go. Withdraw the penis immediately after ejaculation, while the penis is still erect; grasp the rim of the condom between your fingers and slowly withdraw the penis (with the condom still on) so that no semen is spilled.

Clean up. Throw out the used condom right away. Tie it off to prevent spillage or wrap it in bathroom tissue and put it in the garbage. Condoms can clog toilets. Use a condom only once. Never use the same condom for vaginal and anal intercourse. Never use a condom that has been used by someone else.

Do You Have to Use a Condom for Oral Sex?

It is possible for oral sex to transmit HIV, whether the infected part-ner is performing or receiving oral sex. But the risk is low compared with unprotected vaginal or anal sex.

If you choose to perform oral sex, and your partner is male, use a latex condom on the penis, or if you or your partner is allergic to latex, plastic (polyurethane) condoms can be used.

If you choose to have oral sex, and your partner is female, use a latex barrier (such as a natural rubber latex sheet, a dental dam, or a cut-open condom that makes a square) between your mouth and the vagina. A latex barrier such as a dental dam reduces the risk of blood or vaginal fluids entering your mouth. Plastic food wrap also can be used as a barrier.

If you choose to perform oral sex with either a male or female partner and this sex includes oral contact with your partner's anus (anilingus or rimming), use a latex barrier (such as a natural rubber latex sheet, a dental dam, or a cut-open condom that makes a square) between your mouth and the anus. Plastic food wrap also can be used as a barrier. This barrier is to prevent getting another sexually trans-mitted disease or parasites, not HIV.

If you choose to share sex toys, such as dildos or vibrators, with your partner, each partner should use a new condom on the sex toy; and be sure to clean sex toys between each use.

Female Condom

Most people have never heard of these, but they may be helpful for you. The female condom is a large condom made of polyurethane fit-ted with larger and smaller rings at each end that help keep it inside the vagina. They may seem a little awkward at first, but can be an alternative to the male condom. They are made of polyurethane, so any lubricant can be used without damaging them. Female condoms generally cost more than male condoms, and if you aren't used to them, you'll definitely need to practice. Here are some tips:

- Store the condom in a cool dry place, not in direct heat or sunlight.

- Throw away any condoms that have expired—the date is printed on individual condom wrappers.

- Check the package for damage and check the condom for signs of aging such as brittleness, stickiness, and discoloration. The female condom is lubricated, so it will be somewhat wet.

- Before inserting the condom, you can squeeze lubricant into the condom pouch and rub the sides together to spread it around.

- Put the condom in before sex play because pre-ejaculatory fluid, which comes from the penis, may contain HIV. The condom can be inserted up to eight hours before sex.

- The female condom has a firm ring at each end of it. To insert the condom, squeeze the ring at the closed end between the fingers (like a diaphragm), and push it up into the back of the vagina. The open ring must stay outside the vagina at all times, and it will partly cover the lip area.

- Do not use a male condom with the female condom.

- Do not use a female condom with a diaphragm.

- If the penis is inserted outside the condom pouch or if the outer ring (open ring) slips into the vagina, stop and take the condom out. Use a new condom before you start sex again.

- Don't tear the condom with fingernails or jewelry.

- Use a female condom only once and properly dispose of it in the trash (not the toilet).

Dental Dams and Plastic Wrap

Even though oral sex is a low-risk sexual practice, you may want to use protection when performing oral sex on someone who has HIV.

Dental dams are small squares of latex that were made originally for use in dental procedures. They are now commonly used as barriers when performing oral sex on women, to keep in vaginal fluids or menstrual blood that could transmit HIV or other STDs.

Some people use plastic wrap instead of a dental dam. It's thinner. Here are some things to remember:

- Before using a dental dam, first check it visually for any holes.

- If the dental dam has cornstarch on it, rinse that off with water (starch in the vagina can lead to an infection).

- Cover the woman's genital area with the dental dam.

- For oral-anal sex, cover the opening of the anus with a new dental dam.

- A new dental dam should be used for each act of oral sex; it should never be reused.

Section 10.2

Circumcision

"Male Circumcision and Risk for HIV Transmission and Other Health
Conditions: Implications for the United States," Centers for Disease
Control and Prevention, February 7, 2008.

What Is Male Circumcision?

Male circumcision is the surgical removal of some or all of the foreskin (or prepuce) from the penis.[1]

Male Circumcision and Risk for HIV Transmission

Several types of research have documented that male circumcision
significantly reduces the risk of human immunodeficiency virus (HIV)
acquisition by men during penile-vaginal sex.

Biologic Plausibility

Compared with the dry external skin surface, the inner mucosa
of the foreskin has less keratinization (deposition of fibrous protein),
a higher density of target cells for HIV infection (Langerhans cells),
and is more susceptible to HIV infection than other penile tissue in
laboratory studies.[2] The foreskin may also have greater susceptibility
to traumatic epithelial disruptions (tears) during intercourse, providing a portal of entry for pathogens, including HIV.[3] In addition, the
microenvironment in the preputial sac between the unretracted foreskin and the glans penis may be conducive to viral survival.[1] Finally,
the higher rates of sexually transmitted genital ulcerative disease,
such as syphilis, observed in uncircumcised men may also increase
susceptibility to HIV infection.[4]

International Observational Studies

A systematic review and meta-analysis that focused on male circumcision and heterosexual transmission of HIV in Africa was published
in 2000.[5] It included nineteen cross-sectional studies, five case-control

studies, three cohort studies, and one partner study. A substantial protective effect of male circumcision on risk for HIV infection was noted, along with a reduced risk for genital ulcer disease. After adjustment for confounding factors in the population-based studies, the relative risk for HIV infection was 44 percent lower in circumcised men. The strongest association was seen in men at high risk, such as patients at sexually transmitted disease (STD) clinics, for whom the adjusted relative risk was 71 percent lower for circumcised men.

Another review that included stringent assessment of ten potential confounding factors and was stratified by study type or study population was published in 2003.[6] Most of the studies were from Africa. Of the thirty-five observational studies in the review, the sixteen in the general population had inconsistent results. The one large prospective cohort study in this group showed a significant protective effect: the odds of infection were 42 percent lower for circumcised men.[7] The remaining nineteen studies were conducted in populations at high risk. These studies found a consistent, substantial protective effect, which increased with adjustment for confounding. Four of these were cohort studies: all demonstrated a protective effect, with two being statistically significant.

Ecologic studies also indicate a strong association between lack of male circumcision and HIV infection at the population level. Although links between circumcision, culture, religion, and risk behavior may account for some of the differences in HIV infection prevalence, the countries in Africa and Asia with prevalence of male circumcision of less than 20 percent have HIV infection prevalences several times higher than those in countries in these regions where more than 80 percent of men are circumcised.[8]

International Clinical Trials

Three randomized controlled clinical trials were conducted in Africa to determine whether circumcision of adult males will reduce their risk for HIV infection. The study conducted in South Africa[9] was stopped in 2005, and those in Kenya[10] and Uganda[11] were stopped in 2006 after interim analyses found a statistically significant reduction in male participants' risk for HIV infection from medical circumcision.

In these studies, men who had been randomly assigned to the circumcision group had a 60 percent (South Africa), 53 percent (Kenya), and 51 percent (Uganda) lower incidence of HIV infection compared with men assigned to the wait-list group to be circumcised at the end of the study. In all three studies, a few men who had been assigned to be circumcised did not undergo the procedure, and vice versa. When the data were reanalyzed to account for these occurrences, men who had been circumcised had a 76 percent (South Africa), 60 percent (Kenya), and 55 percent (Uganda) reduction in risk for HIV infection compared with those who were not circumcised. The Uganda study investigators are also examining the following in an ongoing study: safety and acceptability of male circumcision in HIV-infected men and men of unknown HIV infection status, safety and acceptability of male circumcision in the men's female sex partners, and effect of male circumcision on male-to-female transmission of HIV and other STDs.

Male Circumcision and Male-to-Female Transmission of HIV

In an earlier study of couples in Uganda in which the male partner was HIV infected and the female partner was initially HIV-seronegative, the infection rates of the female partners differed by the circumcision status and viral load of the male partners. If the male's HIV viral load was less than 50,000 copies/mL, there was no HIV transmission if the man was circumcised, compared with a transmission rate of 9.6 per 100 person-years if the man was uncircumcised.[7] When viral load was not controlled for, there was a nonsignificant trend toward a reduction in the male-to-female transmission rate from circumcised men compared with uncircumcised men. Such an effect may be due to decreased viral shedding from circumcised men or to a reduction in ulcerative STDs acquired by female partners of circumcised men.[12] A clinical trial in Uganda to assess the impact of circumcision on male-to-female transmission reported that its first interim safety analysis showed a nonsignificant trend toward a higher rate of HIV acquisition in women partners of HIV-seropositive men in couples who had resumed sex prior to certified postsurgical wound healing and did not detect a reduction in HIV acquisition by female partners engaging in sex after wound healing was complete.[13]

Male Circumcision and Other Health Conditions

Lack of male circumcision has also been associated with sexually transmitted genital ulcer disease and Chlamydia, infant urinary tract infections, penile cancer, and cervical cancer in female partners of uncircumcised men.[1] The latter two conditions are related to human papillomavirus (HPV) infection. Transmission of this virus is also associated with lack of male circumcision. A recent meta-analysis included twenty-six studies that assessed the association between male circumcision and risk for genital ulcer disease. The analysis concluded that there was a significantly lower risk for syphilis and chancroid among circumcised men, whereas the reduced risk of herpes simplex virus type 2 infection had a borderline statistical significance.[4]

Risks Associated with Male Circumcision

Reported complication rates depend on the type of study (e.g., chart review vs. prospective study), setting (medical vs. nonmedical facility), person operating (traditional vs. medical practitioner), patient age (infant vs. adult), and surgical technique or instrument used. In large studies of infant circumcision in the United States, reported inpatient complication rates range from 0.2 percent to 2.0 percent.[1,14,15] The most common complications in the United States are minor bleeding and local infection. In the recently completed African trials of adult circumcision, the rates of adverse events possibly, probably, or definitely attributable to circumcision ranged from 2 percent to 8 percent. The most commonly reported complications were pain or mild bleeding. There were no reported deaths or long-term sequelae documented.[9,10,11,16] A recent case-control study of two outbreaks of methicillin-resistant *Staphylococcus aureus* (MRSA) in otherwise healthy male infants at one hospital identified circumcision as a potential risk factor. However, in no case did MRSA infections involve the circumcision site, anesthesia injection site, or the penis, and MRSA was not found on any of the circumcision equipment or anesthesia vials tested.[17]

Effects of Male Circumcision on Penile Sensation and Sexual Function

Well-designed studies of sexual sensation and function in relation to male circumcision are few, and the results present a mixed picture. Taken as a whole, the studies suggest that some decrease in sensitivity of the glans to fine touch can occur following circumcision.[18] However, several studies conducted among men after adult circumcision suggest that few men report their sexual functioning is worse after circumcision; most report either improvement or no change.[19–22] The three African trials found high levels of satisfaction among the men after circumcision;[9,10,11,16] however, cultural differences limit extrapolation of their findings to U.S. men.

HIV Infection and Male Circumcision in the United States

In 2005, men who have sex with men (MSM) (48 percent), MSM who also inject drugs (4 percent), and men (11 percent) and women

(21 percent) exposed through high-risk heterosexual contact accounted for an estimated 84 percent of all HIV/AIDS cases diagnosed in U.S. areas with confidential name-based HIV infection reporting. Blacks accounted for 49 percent of cases and Hispanics for 18 percent. Infection rates for both groups were several-fold higher than the rate for whites. An overall prevalence of 0.5 percent was estimated for the general population.[23] Although data on HIV infection rates since the beginning of the epidemic are available, data on circumcision and risk for HIV infection in the United States are limited. In one cross-sectional survey of MSM, lack of circumcision was associated with a twofold increase in the odds of prevalent HIV infection.[24] In another, prospective study of MSM, lack of circumcision was also associated with a twofold increase in risk for HIV seroconversion.[25] In both studies, the results were statistically significant, and the data had been controlled statistically for other possible risk factors. However, in another prospective cohort study of MSM, there was no association between circumcision status and incident HIV infection, even among men who reported no unprotected anal receptive intercourse.[26] And in a recent cross-sectional study of African American and Latino MSM, male circumcision was not associated with previously known or newly diagnosed HIV infection.[27] In one prospective study of heterosexual men attending an urban STD clinic, when other risk factors were controlled, uncircumcised men had a 3.5-fold higher risk for HIV infection than men who were circumcised. However, this association was not statistically significant.[28] And in an analysis of clinic records for African American men attending an STD clinic, circumcision was not associated with HIV status overall, but among men with known HIV exposure, circumcision was associated with a statistically significant 58 percent reduction in risk for HIV infection.[29]

Status of Male Circumcision in the United States

In national probability samples of adults surveyed during 1999 to 2004, the National Health and Nutrition Examination Surveys (NHANES) found that 79 percent of men reported being circumcised, including 88 percent of non-Hispanic white men, 73 percent of non-Hispanic black men, 42 percent of Mexican American men, and 50 percent of men of other races/ethnicities.[30] It is important to note that reported circumcision status may be subject to misclassification. In a study of adolescents, only 69 percent of circumcised and 65 percent of uncircumcised young men correctly identified their circumcision status as verified by physical exam.[31]

According to the National Hospital Discharge Survey (NHDS), 65 percent of newborns were circumcised in 1999, and the overall proportion of newborns circumcised was stable from 1979 through 1999.[32] Notably, the proportion of black newborns circumcised increased during this reporting period (from 58 percent to 64 percent); the proportion of white newborns circumcised remained stable (66 percent). In addition, the proportion of newborns who were circumcised in the Midwest increased during the twenty-year period—from 74 percent in 1979 to 81 percent in 1999; the proportion of infants born in the West who were circumcised decreased from 64 percent in 1979 to 37 percent in 1999. In another survey, the National Inpatient Sample (NIS), circumcision rates increased from 48 percent during 1988–1991 to 61 percent during 1997–2000. Circumcision was more common among newborns who were born to families of higher socioeconomic status, who were born in the Northeast or Midwest, and who were black.[33]

In 1999, the American Academy of Pediatrics (AAP) changed from a neutral stance on circumcision to a position that the data then available were insufficient to recommend routine neonatal male circumcision. The Academy also stated, "It is legitimate for the parents to take into account cultural, religious, and ethnic traditions, in addition to medical factors, when making this choice."[34] This position was reaffirmed by the Academy in 2005. This change in policy may have influenced reimbursement for, and the practice of, neonatal circumcision. In a 1995 review, 61 percent of circumcisions were paid for by private insurance, 36 percent were paid for by Medicaid, and 3 percent were self-paid by the parents of the infant. Compared with infants of self-pay parents, those covered by private insurance were 2.5 times as likely to be circumcised.[35] Since 1999, sixteen states have eliminated Medicaid payments for circumcisions that were not deemed medically necessary.[36] However, AAP has recently (2007) convened a panel to reconsider its circumcision policy in light of additional data now available.

Cost-Benefits and Ethical Issues for Neonatal Circumcision in the United States

A large retrospective study of circumcision in nearly fifteen thousand infants found neonatal circumcision to be highly cost-effective, considering the estimated number of averted cases of infant urinary tract infection and lifetime incidence of HIV infection, penile cancer, balanoposthitis, and phimosis. The cost of postneonatal circumcision was tenfold the cost of neonatal circumcision.[37] Many parents now make decisions about infant circumcision based on cultural, religious, or parental desires rather than health concerns.[38]

Some persons have raised ethical objections to asking parents to make decisions about elective surgery during infancy, particularly when it is done primarily to protect against risks of HIV and STDs that don't occur until young adulthood, but other ethicists have found it an appropriate parental proxy decision.[39]

Considerations for the United States

A number of important differences from sub-Saharan African settings where the three male circumcision trials were conducted must be considered in determining the possible role for male circumcision in HIV prevention in the United States. Notably, the overall risk of HIV infection is considerably lower in the United States, changing risk-benefit and cost-effectiveness considerations. Also, studies to date have demonstrated efficacy only for penile-vaginal sex, the predominant mode of HIV transmission in Africa, whereas the predominant mode of sexual HIV transmission in the United States is by penile-anal sex among MSM. There are as yet no convincing data to help determine whether male circumcision will have any effect on HIV risk for men who engage in anal sex with either a female or male partner, as either the insertive or receptive partner. Receptive anal sex is associated with a substantially greater risk of HIV acquisition than is insertive anal sex. It is more biologically plausible that male circumcision would reduce HIV acquisition risk for the insertive partner rather than for the receptive partner, but few MSM engage solely in insertive anal sex.[40]

In addition, although the prevalence of circumcision may be somewhat lower in U.S. racial and ethnic groups with higher rates of HIV infection, most American men are already circumcised, and it is not known whether men at higher risk for HIV infection would be willing to be circumcised or whether parents would be willing to have their infants circumcised to reduce possible future HIV infection risk. Lastly, whether the effect of male circumcision differs by HIV-1 subtype, predominately subtype B in the United States and subtypes A, C, and D in circulation at the three clinical trial sites in Africa, is also unknown.

Summary

Male circumcision has been associated with a lower risk for HIV infection in international observational studies and in three randomized controlled clinical trials. It is possible, but not yet adequately assessed, that male circumcision could reduce male-to-female transmission of HIV, although probably to a lesser extent than female-to-male transmission.

Male circumcision has also been associated with a number of other health benefits. Although there are risks to male circumcision, serious complications are rare. Accordingly, male circumcision, together with other prevention interventions, could play an important role in HIV prevention in settings similar to those of the clinical trials.[41,42]

Male circumcision may also have a role in the prevention of HIV transmission in the United States. The Centers for Disease Control and Prevention (CDC) consulted with external experts in April 2007 to receive input on the potential value, risks, and feasibility of circumcision as an HIV prevention intervention in the United States and to discuss considerations for the possible development of guidelines.

As CDC proceeds with the development of public health recommendations for the United States, individual men may wish to consider circumcision as an additional HIV prevention measure, but they must recognize that circumcision does carry risks and costs that must be considered in addition to potential benefits; has only proven effective in reducing the risk of infection through insertive vaginal sex; and confers only partial protection and should be considered only in conjunction with other proven prevention measures (abstinence, mutual monogamy, reduced number of sex partners, and correct and consistent condom use).

References

1. Alanis MC, Lucidi RS. Neonatal circumcision: a review of the world's oldest and most controversial operation. *Obstet Gynecol Surv*. 2004 May;59(5):379–95.

2. Patterson BK, Landay A, Siegel JN, et al. Susceptibility to human immunodeficiency virus-1 infection of human foreskin and cervical tissue grown in explant culture. *Am J Pathol*. 2002 Sep;161(3):867–73.

3. Szabo R, Short RV. How does male circumcision protect against HIV infection? *BMJ*. 2000 Jun 10;320(7249):1592–94.

4. Weiss HA, Thomas SL, Munabi SK, Hayes RJ. Male circumcision and risk of syphilis, chancroid, and genital herpes: a systematic review and meta-analysis. *Sex Transm Infect*. 2006 Apr;82(2):101–9; discussion 10.

5. Weiss HA, Quigley MA, Hayes RJ. Male circumcision and risk of HIV infection in sub-Saharan Africa: a systematic review and meta-analysis. *AIDS*. 2000 Oct 20;14(15):2361–70.

6. Siegfried N, Muller M, Volmink J, et al. Male circumcision for prevention of heterosexual acquisition of HIV in men. *Cochrane Database Syst Rev*. 2003;(3):CD003362.

7. Gray RH, Kiwanuka N, Quinn TC, et al. Male circumcision and HIV acquisition and transmission: cohort studies in Rakai, Uganda. *AIDS*. 2000 Oct 20;14(15):2371–81.

8. Halperin DT, Bailey RC. Male circumcision and HIV infection: 10 years and counting. *Lancet*. 1999 Nov 20;354(9192):1813–15.

9. Auvert B, Taljaard D, Lagarde E, Sobngwi- Tambekou J, Sitta R, Puren A. Randomized, controlled intervention trial of male circumcision for reduction of HIV infection risk: the ANRS 1265 Trial. *PLoS Med*. 2005 Nov;2(11):e298. Erratum in: *PLoS Med*. 2006 May;3(5):e298.

10. Bailey RC, Moses S, Parker CB, et al. Male circumcision for HIV prevention in young men in Kisumu, Kenya: a randomised controlled trial. *Lancet*. 2007 Feb 24;369(9562):643–56.

11. Gray RH, Kigozi G, Serwadda D, et al. Male circumcision for HIV prevention in men in Rakai, Uganda: a randomised trial. *Lancet*. 2007 Feb 24;369(9562):657–66.

12. Gray R, Wawer MJ, Thoma M, et al. Male circumcision and the risks of female HIV and sexually transmitted infections acquisition in Rakai, Uganda [Abstract 128]. Presented at: 13th Conference on Retroviruses and Opportunistic Infections. Feb 5–9, 2006; Denver, CO. Accessed Jan 24, 2008.

13. Wawer MJ. Trial of male circumcision: HIV, sexually transmitted disease (STD) and behavioral effects in men, women and the community. Accessed Jan 23, 2008.

14. Wiswell TE, Geschke DW. Risks from circumcision during the first month of life compared with those for uncircumcised boys. *Pediatrics*. 1989;83(6):1011–15.

15. Christakis DA, Harvey E, Zerr DM, Feudtner C, Wright JA, Connell FA. A trade-off analysis of routine newborn circumcision. *Pediatrics*. 2000 Jan;105(1 Pt 3):246–49.

16. Kigozi G, Watya S, Polis CB, et al. The effect of male circumcision on sexual satisfaction and function, results from a randomized trial of male circumcision for human immunodeficiency virus prevention, Rakai, Uganda. *BJU Int*. 2008 Jan;101(1):65–70.

17. Nguyen DM, Bancroft E, Mascola L, et al. Risk factors for neonatal methicillin resistant Staphylococcus aureus infection in a well-infant nursery. *Infect Control Hosp Epidemiol.* 2007;28:406-11.

18. Sorrells ML, Snyder JL, Reiss MD, et al. Fine-touch pressure thresholds in the adult penis. *BJU Int.* 2007 Apr;99(4):864–69. Erratum in: *BJU Int.* 2007 Aug;100(2):481.

19. Krieger JN, Bailey RC, Opeya JC, et al. Adult male circumcision outcomes: experience in a developing country setting. *Urol Int.* 2007;78(3):235–40.

20. Collins S, Upshaw J, Rutchik S, et al. Effects of circumcision on male sexual function: debunking a myth? *J Urol.* 2002;167:2111–12.

21. Senkul T, Iseri C, Sen B, et al. Circumcision in adults: effect on sexual function. *Urology.* 2004;63:155–58.

22. Masood S, Patel HRH, Himpson RC, et al. Penile sensitivity and sexual satisfaction after circumcision: are we informing men correctly? *Urol Int.* 2004;75:62–66.

23. Centers for Disease Control and Prevention. *HIV/AIDS Surveillance Report, 2005. Vol. 17. Rev. ed.* Atlanta: U.S. Department of Health and Human Services, Centers for Disease Control and Prevention; June 2007:1–54.

24. Kreiss JK, Hopkins SG. The association between circumcision status and human immunodeficiency virus infection among homosexual men. *J Infect Dis.* 1993 Dec;168(6):1404–8.

25. Buchbinder SP, Vittinghoff E, Heagerty PJ, et al. Sexual risk, nitrite inhalant use, and lack of circumcision associated with HIV seroconversion in men who have sex with men in the United States. *J Acquir Immune Defic Syndr.* 2005 May 1;39(1):82–89.

26. Templeton DJ, Jin F, Prestage GP, et al. Circumcision status and risk of HIV seroconversion in the HIM cohort of homosexual men in Sydney [Abstract WEAC103]. Presented at: 4th IAS Conference on HIV Pathogenesis, Treatment, and Prevention; Jul 22–25, 2007; Sydney, Australia. Accessed Jan 23, 2008.

27. Millett GA, Ding H, Lauby J, et al. Circumcision status and HIV infection among black and Latino men who have sex

with men in 3 US cities. *J Acquir Immune Defic Syndr*. 2007 Dec;46(5):643–50.

28. Telzak EE, Chiasson MA, Bevier PJ, Stoneburner RL, Castro KG, Jaffe HW. HIV-1 seroconversion in patients with and without genital ulcer disease: a prospective study. *Ann Intern Med*. 1993 Dec 15;119(12):1181–86.

29. Warner L, Ghanem KG, Newman D, et al. Male circumcision and risk of HIV infection among heterosexual men attending Baltimore STD clinics: an evaluation of clinic-based data [Abstract 326]. Presented at: National STD Prevention Conference; May 8–11, 2006; Jacksonville, FL. Accessed Jan 23, 2008.

30. Xu F, Markowitz LE, Sternberg MR, Aral SO. Prevalence of circumcision and herpes simplex virus type 2 infection in men in the United States: the National Health and Nutrition Examination Survey (NHANES), 1999–2004. *Sex Transm Dis*. 2007 July; 34(7):479–84.

31. Risser JM, Risser WL, Eissa MA, Cromwell PF, Barratt MS, Bortot A. Self-assessment of circumcision status by adolescents. *Am J Epidemiol*. 2004 Jun 1;159(11):1095–97.

32. Centers for Disease Control and Prevention. Trends in circumcisions among newborns. Accessed Jan 24, 2008.

33. Nelson CP, Dunn R, Wan J, Wei JT. The increasing incidence of newborn circumcision: data from the nationwide inpatient sample. *J Urol*. 2005 Mar;173(3):978–81.

34. American Academy of Pediatrics, Task Force on Circumcision. Circumcision policy statement. *Pediatrics*. 1999 Mar;103(3):686–93.

35. Mansfield CJ, Hueston WJ, Rudy M. Neonatal circumcision: associated factors and length of hospital stay. *J Fam Pract*. 1995 Oct;41(4):370–76.

36. National Conference of State Legislatures. State Health Notes: Circumcision and infection. Accessed Jan 23, 2008.

37. Schoen EJ, Oehrli M, Colby CJ, Machin G. The highly protective effect of newborn circumcision against invasive penile cancer. *Pediatrics*. 2000 Mar;105(3):e36. Accessed Jan 24, 2008.

38. Adler R, Ottaway S, Gould S. Circumcision: we have heard from the experts; now let's hear from the parents. *Pediatrics.* 2001:107:e20. Accessed Jan 24, 2008.

39. Benatar M, Benatar D. Between prophylaxis and child abuse: the ethics of neonatal male circumcision. *Am J Bioeth.* 2003 Spring;3(2):35–48.

40. Koblin BA, Chesney MA, Husnik MJ, et al. High-risk behaviors among men who have sex with men in 6 US cities: baseline data from the EXPLORE study. *Am J Public Health.* 2003 Jun;93(6):926–32. Erratum in: *Am J Public Health* 2003 Aug;93(8):1203.

41. World Health Organization and UNAIDS. New data on male circumcision and HIV prevention: policy and programme implications. 2007 Mar. Accessed Jan 24, 2008.

42. Williams BG, Lloyd-Smith JO, Gouws E, et al. The potential impact of male circumcision on HIV in sub-Saharan Africa. *PLoS Med.* 2006;3(7):e262. Accessed Jan 24, 2008.

Section 10.3

Protecting Our Blood Supply

"Blood Safety" is reprinted from Centers for Disease Control and Prevention, October 20, 2006. Reviewed by David A. Cooke, MD, FACP, November 2010. "Transfusion Safety" is reprinted from the National Institutes of Health, September 2007.

Blood Safety

How Safe Is the Blood Supply in the United States?

The U.S. blood supply is among the safest in the world. Nearly all people infected with human immunodeficiency virus (HIV) through blood transfusions received those transfusions before 1985, the year HIV testing began for all donated blood.

The Public Health Service has recommended an approach to blood safety in the United States that includes stringent donor selection practices and the use of screening tests. U.S. blood donations have been screened for antibodies to HIV-1 since March 1985 and HIV-2 since June 1992. The p24 antigen test was added in 1996. Blood and blood products that test positive for HIV are safely discarded and are not used for transfusions.

The improvement of processing methods for blood products also has reduced the number of infections resulting from the use of these products.

Currently, the risk of infection with HIV in the United States through receiving a blood transfusion or blood products is extremely low and has become progressively lower, even in geographic areas with high HIV prevalence rates.

Transfusion Safety

Yesterday

The earliest attempts to transfuse blood, which sometimes entailed giving animal blood to humans, were often unsuccessful due to poor understanding of the fundamental immunologic principles of transfusion. It was not until the early 1800s that attempts to perform cross-species blood transfusions were finally abandoned.

Table 10.1. Tests Performed on Each Unit of Donated Blood

Disease	Test	Year Implemented
HIV/AIDS	HIV/AIDS HIV- 1 antibody test	1985
	HIV-1/2 antibody test	1992
	HIV-1 p24 antigen test	1996
HIV/AIDS and Hepatitis C	Nucleic acid test (NAT)	1999
Hepatitis C	Hepatitis C anti-HCV	1990
Hepatitis B	Hepatitis B surface antigen test	1971
	Hepatitis B core antibody	1987
Hepatitis	Hepatitis alanine aminotransferase (ALT)	1986
Syphilis	Syphilis serologic test	1948
Human T-cell Lymphotropic Virus (HTLV)	HTLV-I antibody	1989
	HTLV-I/II antibody	1998

Note: This list is subject to change as new blood safety opportunities and requirements emerge. Additional tests may be performed to meet special patient needs.
Source: American Red Cross

Improved understanding of the immunological components of transfusion, such as the discovery of the ABO blood group antigens by Karl Landsteiner in 1901, led to improved transfusion results. However, the extent of problems arising from transmission of infectious agents was just beginning to be appreciated.

In the early 1980s, the acquired immunodeficiency syndrome (AIDS) epidemic emerged and a significant number of people were infected by receiving blood or blood products tainted with human immunodeficiency virus type 1 (HIV-1), the retrovirus that causes AIDS.

The National Institutes of Health (NIH) funded the Retrovirus Epidemiology Donor Study (REDS) to determine the prevalence and incidence of HIV among blood donors and the risks of transmitting HIV and other viruses via transfusions. Since 1989, REDS has conducted these studies at selected blood centers throughout the country.

A new technology, called nucleic acid amplification testing (NAT) greatly improved detection of HIV in donated blood. Previous HIV screening tests relied on detecting circulating antibodies. However, the time between viral infection and development of antibodies is often three weeks or more. During this "window period" the older tests could yield negative results for infected blood. NAT reduced the window period for HIV to as few as eleven days. Similarly, NAT reduced the window period for hepatitis C virus (HCV) from seventy to ten days.

In 2003, with the emergence of the West Nile virus (WNV), the NAT procedure was rapidly modified to detect WNV. In just nine months, a test for WNV was developed and approved by the Food and Drug Administration. As a result, nearly one thousand blood donors with WNV infection were identified before their donations entered the blood supply.

Today

REDS-II is now under way to improve the safety and availability of the U.S. blood supply. Its primary objectives are to monitor the appearance of newly discovered infectious agents in the blood supply, evaluate the characteristics and behaviors of voluntary blood donors, determine the causes of transfusion reactions of unknown etiology, assess the results of new donor screening methods, assess the effects of new blood bank technologies on blood safety and availability, and evaluate the donation process to improve the adequacy of the blood supply.

Current REDS-II protocols are evaluating the risks of transfusion-transmitted infectious agents; the transmissibility of parvovirus B19 by blood transfusion; the prevalence of influenza virus in blood of otherwise healthy donors; the frequency and characteristics of HIV, HCV, and hepatitis B virus (HBV) in infected, permanently-deferred donors; and depletion of iron in blood donors.

An international component of REDS-II is conducting epidemiological, laboratory, and survey research on blood donors in selected countries seriously affected by AIDS to ensure the safety and availability of blood for transfusion. The World Health Organization estimates that 5 to 10 percent of AIDS cases continue to be acquired from blood transfusions.

Investigators are working to develop tests to detect transmissible spongiform encephalopathies, such as Creutzfeldt-Jakob disease (CJD) and new variant CJD, and to develop methods to inactivate or remove abnormal prion proteins from blood and blood components.

NAT is now used to screen virtually all whole blood and plasma donations collected in the United States for HIV, HCV, and WNV, thereby reducing the risk of infection associated with blood transfusion to about 1 in 2,000,000 blood units. Before NAT screening, the risk of acquiring HIV was about 1 in 500,000 and the risk of HCV about 1 in 100,000.

Ongoing research efforts continue to improve our understanding of the incidence, epidemiology, and mechanisms of transfusion-related acute lung injury (TRALI), a potentially life-threatening syndrome with an incidence of approximately 1 in every 5,000 units of blood and blood components transfused.

Research is under way to address concerns regarding emerging threats, such as CJD and severe acute respiratory syndrome (SARS), and to respond to recent isolated human outbreaks of chikungunya virus and avian influenza virus.

Tomorrow

Newly developed technologies will routinely be used to provide rapid and accurate detection of infectious agents transmissible in blood, such as HIV, HCV, HBV, Chagas disease, and malaria. Tests will also detect emerging agents that pose a threat to transfusion safety.

New tests will allow blood collection services to discern between individuals who have circulating HIV antibodies due to HIV infection and those who have antibodies due to previous immunization with an HIV vaccine.

A wide range of safe and effective oxygen-carrying blood substitutes may become available that would be extremely useful when blood is not immediately available or in short supply, such as in the case of a rare blood type or a major disaster. The substitutes would be free of infectious agents and would pose no major risks of toxicity to recipients.

Section 10.4

Syringe Exchange Programs

"Syringe Exchange Programs," Centers for Disease Control and Prevention, December 2005. Reviewed by David A. Cooke, MD, FACP, November 2010.

In 1997, a report to Congress concluded that needle exchange programs can be an effective component of a comprehensive strategy to prevent human immunodeficiency virus (HIV) and other blood-borne infectious diseases in communities that choose to include them.[1] Federal funding to carry out any program of distributing sterile needles or syringes to injection drug users (IDUs) has been prohibited by Congress since 1988. In addition, several states have restricted the funding or operation of syringe exchange programs (SEPs).

As of 2004, injection drug use accounted for about one-fifth of all HIV infections and most hepatitis C infections in the United States.[2,3] Injection drug users (IDUs) become infected and transmit the viruses to others through sharing contaminated syringes and other drug injection equipment and through high-risk sexual behaviors. Women who become infected with HIV through sharing needles or having sex with an infected IDU can also transmit the virus to their babies before or during birth or through breastfeeding.

To succeed in effectively reducing the transmission of HIV and other blood-borne infections, programs must consider a comprehensive approach to working with IDUs. Such an approach incorporates a range of pragmatic strategies that address both drug use and sexual risk behaviors. One of the most important of these strategies is ensuring that IDUs who cannot or will not stop injecting drugs have access to sterile syringes. This strategy supports the "one-time-only use of sterile syringes" recommendation of several institutions and governmental bodies, including the U.S. Public Health Service.[4]

What Are Syringe Exchange Programs?

It is estimated that an individual IDU injects about one thousand times a year.[5] This adds up to millions of injections, creating an enormous need for reliable sources of sterile syringes. Syringe exchange programs (SEPs) provide a way for those IDUs who continue to inject to safely dispose of used syringes and to obtain sterile syringes at no cost.

The first organized SEPs in the United States were established in the late 1980s in Tacoma, Washington; Portland, Oregon; San Francisco; and New York City. By 2002, there were 184 programs in more than 36 states, Indian lands, and Puerto Rico. These programs exchanged more than twenty-four million syringes.[6]

In addition to exchanging syringes, many SEPs provide a range of related prevention and care services that are vital to helping IDUs reduce their risks of acquiring and transmitting blood-borne viruses as well as maintain and improve their overall health.

These services may include the following:

- HIV/AIDS (acquired immunodeficiency syndrome) education and counseling

- Condom distribution to prevent sexual transmission of HIV and other sexually transmitted diseases (STDs)

- Referrals to substance abuse treatment and other medical and social services

- Distribution of alcohol swabs to help prevent abscesses and other bacterial infections

- On-site HIV testing and counseling and crisis intervention

- Screening for tuberculosis (TB), hepatitis B, hepatitis C, and other infections

- Primary medical services

SEPs operate in a variety of settings, including storefronts, vans, sidewalk tables, health clinics, and places where IDUs gather. They vary in their hours of operation, with some open for two-hour street-based sessions several times a week, and others open continuously. They also vary in the number of syringes allowed for exchange. Many also conduct outreach efforts in the neighborhoods where IDUs live.[7]

What Is the Public Health Impact of SEPs?

SEPs have been shown to be an effective way to link some hard-to-reach IDUs with important public health services, including TB and STD screening and treatment. Through their referrals to substance abuse treatment, SEPs can help IDUs stop using drugs.[8] Studies also show that SEPs do not encourage drug use among SEP participants or the recruitment of first-time drug users. In addition, a number of studies have shown that IDUs will use sterile syringes if they can obtain them.[9] SEPs provide IDUs with an opportunity to use sterile syringes and share less often.[10]

The results of this research, and the clear dangers of syringe sharing, led the National Institutes of Health Consensus Panel on HIV Prevention to state that: "An impressive body of evidence suggests powerful effects from needle exchange programs. . . . Studies show reduction in risk behavior as high as 80 percent, with estimates of a 30 percent or greater reduction of HIV in IDUs."[11]

Economic studies have concluded that SEPs are also cost effective. At an average cost of $0.97 per syringe distributed, SEPs can save money in all IDU populations where the annual HIV seroincidence exceeds 2.1 per 100 person years.[12] The cost per HIV infection prevented by SEPs has been calculated at $4,000 to $12,000, considerably less than the estimated $190,000 medical costs of treating a person infected with HIV.[13]

What Issues Do SEPs Face?

SEPs face a variety of issues in their operation. One of the most substantial is coverage. For example, Montreal—a city that has active and well-supported SEPs, allows sales of syringes without prescription, and encourages pharmacy sales—was able to meet less than 5 percent of the need for sterile syringes in 1994.[14] Of the 126 SEPs participating in a 2002 survey, the eleven largest exchanged almost half of the 24.8 million syringes exchanged. Most of the remaining SEPs exchanged much smaller numbers (the twenty-two smallest-volume SEPs exchanged fewer than 5,000 syringes each).[6]

SEPs also face significant legal and regulatory restrictions. For example, forty-seven states have drug paraphernalia laws that establish criminal penalties for the distribution and possession of syringes. Eight states and one territory have laws that prohibit dispensing or possessing syringes without a valid medical prescription. Public health authorities in communities have employed a number of strategies to ensure the legal provision of SEP services, including declaring public health emergencies.[15]

Local community opposition also can be an issue. Residents may be concerned that the programs will encourage drug use and drug traffic and increase the number of used discarded syringes in their neighborhoods. Studies have found no evidence of increases in discarded syringes around SEPs.[16] Finally, some IDUs avoid SEPs because they fear that using a program that serves IDUs will identify them as IDUs. For others, the fear of arrest, fines, and possible incarceration if caught carrying syringes to or from the SEP is a potent deterrent.[17]

What Have Communities Done?

Activities have included the following:

- Supporting community-based discussions of the role that SEPs can play in comprehensive HIV and viral hepatitis prevention and care programs, in particular in getting SEP users into substance abuse treatment programs

- Educating policy makers about the facts of injection-related transmission of blood-borne pathogens and the public health benefits of providing access to sterile syringes as part of a comprehensive public health approach

- Encouraging collaborative review of the public health impact of repealing drug paraphernalia laws that penalize the possession or carrying of syringes

Sources

1. Shalala, DE. *Needle Exchange Programs in America: Review of Published Studies and Ongoing Research.* Report to the Committee on Appropriations for the Departments of Labor, Health and Human Services, Educations and Related Agencies. February 18, 1997.

2. Glynn M, Rhodes P. Estimated HIV prevalence in the United States at the end of 2003. 2005 National HIV Prevention Conference; June 12–15, 2005. Atlanta, GA. Abstract T1-B1101.

3. Centers for Disease Control and Prevention (CDC). Hepatitis C fact sheet. Accessed December 22, 2005 from http://www.cdc.gov/ncidod/diseases/hepatitis/c/fact.htm.

4. Centers for Disease Control and Prevention, Health Resources and Services Administration, National Institute on Drug Abuse and Substance Abuse and Mental Health Services Administration. *HIV prevention bulletin: Medical advice for persons who inject illicit drugs.* May 9, 1997.

5. Lurie P, Jones TS, Foley J. A sterile syringe for every drug user injection: how many injections take place annually, and how might pharmacists contribute to syringe distribution? *Journal of Acquired Immune Deficiency Syndromes and Human Retrovirology* 1998;18(Suppl 1):S45–S51.

6. Centers for Disease Control and Prevention (CDC). Update: syringe exchange programs—United States, 2002. *Morbidity and Mortality Weekly Report* 2005; 54(27);673–76.

7. Centers for Disease Control and Prevention (CDC). Update: syringe exchange programs—United States, 1997. *Morbidity and Mortality Weekly Report* 1998;47(31):652–55.

8. Vlahov D, Junge B. The role of needle exchange programs in HIV prevention. *Public Health Reports* 1998;113(Suppl 1):75–80.

9. Des Jarlais DC, Friedman SR, Sotheran JL, Wenston J, Marmor M, Yancovitz SR, Frank B, Beatrice S, Mildvan D. Continuity and change within an HIV epidemic: injecting drug users in New York City, 1984–1992. *JAMA* 1994;271:121–27.

10. Heimer R, Khoshnood K, Bigg D, Guydish J, Junge B. Syringe use and reuse: effects of needle exchange programs in three cities. *Journal of Acquired Immune Deficiency Syndromes and Human Retrovirology* 1998;18(Suppl 1):S37–S44.

11. National Institutes of Health. *Consensus Development Statement. Interventions to prevent HIV risk behaviors*, February 11–13, 1997:7–8.

12. Lurie P, Gorsky R, Jones TS, Shomphe L. An economic analysis of needle exchange and pharmacy-based programs to increase sterile syringe availability for injection drug users. *Journal of Acquired Immune Deficiency Syndromes and Human Retrovirology* 1998;18(Suppl 1):S126–32.

13. Holtgrave DR, Pinkerton SD. Updates of cost of illness and quality of life estimates for use in economic evaluations of HIV prevention programs. *Journal of Acquired Immune Deficiency Syndromes and Human Retrovirology* 1997; 16:54–62.

14. Remis RS, Bruneau J, Hankins CA. Enough sterile syringes to prevent HIV transmission among injection drug users in Montreal? *Journal of Acquired Immune Deficiency Syndromes and Human Retrovirology* 1998;18(Suppl 1):S57–S59.

15. Burris S, Finucane D, Gallagher H, Grace J. The legal strategies used in operating syringe exchange programs in the United States. *American Journal of Public Health* 1996;86(8 Pt 1): 1161–66.

16. Doherty MC, Garfein RS, Vlahov D, Junge B, Rathouz PJ, Galai N, Anthony JC, Beilenson P. Discarded needles do not increase soon after the opening of a needle exchange program. *American Journal of Epidemiology* 1997;145(8):730–37.

17. Springer KW, Sterk CE, Jones TS, Friedman L. Syringe disposal options for injection drug users: a community-based perspective. *Substance Use and Misuse* 1999;34(13):1917–34.

Section 10.5

Universal Precautions for Healthcare Workers

Excerpted from "Universal Precautions for Prevention of Transmission of HIV and Other Bloodborne Infections," Centers for Disease Control and Prevention, February 5, 1999. Reviewed by David A. Cooke, MD, FACP, November 2010.

"Universal precautions," as defined by the Centers for Disease Control and Prevention (CDC), are a set of precautions designed to prevent transmission of human immunodeficiency virus (HIV), hepatitis B virus (HBV), and other blood-borne pathogens when providing first aid or healthcare. Under universal precautions, blood and certain body fluids of all patients are considered potentially infectious for HIV, HBV, and other blood-borne pathogens.

Universal precautions apply to blood, other body fluids containing visible blood, semen, and vaginal secretions. Universal precautions also apply to tissues and to the following fluids: cerebrospinal, synovial, pleural, peritoneal, pericardial, and amniotic fluids. Universal precautions do not apply to feces, nasal secretions, sputum, sweat, tears, urine, and vomitus unless they contain visible blood. Universal precautions do not apply to saliva except when visibly contaminated with blood or in the dental setting where blood contamination of saliva is predictable.

Universal precautions involve the use of protective barriers such as gloves, gowns, aprons, masks, or protective eyewear, which can reduce the risk of exposure of the healthcare worker's skin or mucous membranes to potentially infective materials. In addition, under universal precautions, it is recommended that all healthcare workers take precautions to prevent injuries caused by needles, scalpels, and other sharp instruments or devices.

Pregnant healthcare workers are not known to be at greater risk of contracting HIV infection than are healthcare workers who are not pregnant; however, if a healthcare worker develops HIV infection during pregnancy, the infant is at risk of infection resulting from perinatal transmission. Because of this risk, pregnant healthcare workers should be especially familiar with, and strictly adhere to, precautions to minimize the risk of HIV transmission.

Gloving, Gowning, Masking, and Other Protective Barriers as Part of Universal Precautions

All healthcare workers should routinely use appropriate barrier precautions to prevent skin and mucous membrane exposure during contact with any patient's blood or body fluids that require universal precautions.

Gloves should be worn:

- for touching blood and body fluids requiring universal precautions, mucous membranes, or nonintact skin of all patients, and

- for handling items or surfaces soiled with blood or body fluids to which universal precautions apply.

Gloves should be changed after contact with each patient. Hands and other skin surfaces should be washed immediately or as soon as patient safety permits if contaminated with blood or body fluids requiring universal precautions. Hands should be washed immediately after gloves are removed. Gloves should reduce the incidence of blood contamination of hands during phlebotomy, but they cannot prevent penetrating injuries caused by needles or other sharp instruments. Institutions that judge routine gloving for all phlebotomies is not necessary should periodically reevaluate their policy. Gloves should always be available to healthcare workers who wish to use them for phlebotomy. In addition, the following general guidelines apply:

- Use gloves for performing phlebotomy when the healthcare worker has cuts, scratches, or other breaks in his/her skin.

- Use gloves in situations where the healthcare worker judges that hand contamination with blood may occur, e.g., when performing phlebotomy on an uncooperative patient.

- Use gloves for performing finger and/or heel sticks on infants and children.

- Use gloves when persons are receiving training in phlebotomy.

Masks and protective eyewear or face shields should be worn by healthcare workers to prevent exposure of mucous membranes of the mouth, nose, and eyes during procedures that are likely to generate droplets of blood or body fluids requiring universal precautions. Gowns or aprons should be worn during procedures that are likely to generate splashes of blood or body fluids requiring universal precautions.

All healthcare workers should take precautions to prevent injuries caused by needles, scalpels, and other sharp instruments or devices during procedures; when cleaning used instruments; during disposal of used needles; and when handling sharp instruments after procedures. To prevent needle stick injuries, needles should not be recapped by hand, purposely bent or broken by hand, removed from disposable syringes, or otherwise manipulated by hand. After they are used, disposable syringes and needles, scalpel blades, and other sharp items should be placed in puncture-resistant containers for disposal. The puncture-resistant containers should be located as close as practical to the use area. All reusable needles should be placed in a puncture-resistant container for transport to the reprocessing area.

General infection control practices should further minimize the already minute risk for salivary transmission of HIV. These infection control practices include the use of gloves for digital examination of mucous membranes and endotracheal suctioning, hand washing after exposure to saliva, and minimizing the need for emergency mouth-to-mouth resuscitation by making mouthpieces and other ventilation devices available for use in areas where the need for resuscitation is predictable.

Although universal precautions do not apply to human breast milk, gloves may be worn by healthcare workers in situations where exposures to breast milk might be frequent, for example, in breast milk banking.

Chapter 11

Preventing Mother-to-Child Transmission of HIV

How Do Babies Get AIDS?

The virus that causes acquired immunodeficiency syndrome (AIDS) can be transmitted from an infected mother to her newborn child. Without antiretroviral treatment, and if mothers breast-feed for eighteen to twenty-four months, up to 35 percent of babies of infected mothers get human immunodeficiency virus (HIV).

Mothers with higher viral loads are more likely to infect their babies. However, no viral load is low enough to be "safe." Infection can occur any time during pregnancy, but usually happens just before or during delivery. The baby is more likely to be infected if the delivery takes a long time. During delivery, the newborn is exposed to the mother's blood.

Drinking breast milk from an infected woman can also infect babies. Mothers who are HIV-infected should generally not breast-feed their babies. To reduce the risk of HIV infection when the father is HIV-positive, some couples have used sperm washing and artificial insemination.

How Can We Prevent Infection of Newborns?

What if the father is infected with HIV? Recent studies have shown that it is possible to "wash" the sperm of an HIV-infected man so that it can be used to fertilize a woman and produce a healthy baby. These procedures are effective but very expensive.

"Pregnancy and HIV," Fact Sheet #611. © 2009 AIDS InfoNet. Reprinted with permission. InfoNet fact sheets are updated frequently. Please visit the website at http://www.aidsinfonet.org for the newest version.

Use antiretroviral medications. The risk of transmitting HIV is extremely low if antiretroviral medications are used. Transmission rates are only 1 percent to 2 percent if the mother takes combination antiretroviral therapy (ART). The rate is also about 2 percent when the mother takes azidothymidine (AZT) during the last two months of her pregnancy, the mother takes a single dose of nevirapine during labor, and the newborn takes a single dose of nevirapine within three days of birth.

However, resistance to nevirapine can develop in up to 40 percent of women who take the single dose. This can reduce the success of later ART for the mother. Resistance to nevirapine can also be transmitted to newborns through breast-feeding. However, the shorter regimens are more affordable for developing countries.

Keep delivery time short. The risk of transmission increases with longer delivery times. If the mother uses AZT and has a viral load under 1,000, the risk is almost zero. Mothers with a high viral load might reduce their risk if they deliver their baby by cesarean (C-) section.

Breast-Feeding

Feeding the Newborn

Up to 15 percent of babies may get HIV infection from infected breast milk. Breast-feeding is controversial, especially in the developing world. Most transmission from breast-feeding occurs within the first two months after birth. However, replacement feeding can increase the risk of infant death. This can be due to loss of disease protection provided by the mother's milk or the use of contaminated water to mix baby formula.

A recent study showed that it is possible for a newborn to become infected by eating food that is chewed for it by an infected mother. This practice should be avoided.

How Do We Know If a Newborn Is Infected?

Most babies born to infected mothers test positive for HIV. Testing positive means you have HIV antibodies in your blood. Babies get HIV antibodies from their mother even if they aren't infected.

Another test, similar to the HIV viral load test, can be used to find out if the baby is infected with HIV. Instead of antibodies, these tests detect HIV in the blood. This is the only reliable way to determine if a newborn is infected with HIV.

If babies are infected with HIV, their own immune systems will start to make antibodies. They will continue to test positive. If they are not infected, the mother's antibodies will eventually disappear. The babies will test negative after about twelve to eighteen months.

What about the Mother's Health?

Recent studies show that HIV-positive women who get pregnant do not get any sicker than those who are not pregnant. Becoming pregnant is not dangerous to the health of an HIV-infected woman. This is true even if the mother breast-feeds her newborn for a full term (two years). In fact, a study in 2007 showed that becoming pregnant was good for a woman's health.

However, "short-course" treatments to prevent infection of a newborn are not the best choice for the mother's health. If a pregnant woman takes ART only during labor and delivery, HIV might develop resistance to them. This can reduce the future treatment options for the mother.

A pregnant woman should consider all of the possible problems with antiretroviral medications:

- Pregnant women should not use both ddI (didanosine; Videx®) and d4T (stavudine; Zerit®) in their ART due to a high rate of a dangerous side effect called lactic acidosis.

- Do not use efavirenz (Sustiva®) during the first three months of pregnancy.

- If your CD4 count is more than 250, do not start using nevirapine (Viramune®).

Some doctors suggest that women interrupt their treatment during the first three months of pregnancy for three reasons:

- The risk of missing doses due to nausea and vomiting during early pregnancy, giving HIV a chance to develop resistance.

- The risk of birth defects, which is highest during the first three months. There is almost no evidence of this, except with efavirenz.

- ART might increase the risk of premature or low birth weight babies.

However, current guidelines do not support treatment interruption for pregnant women.

If you have HIV and you are pregnant, or if you want to become pregnant, talk with your healthcare provider about your options for taking care of yourself and reducing the risk of HIV infection or birth defects for your new child.

The Bottom Line

An HIV-infected woman who becomes pregnant needs to think about her own health and the health of her new child. Pregnancy does not seem to make the mother's HIV disease any worse.

The risk of transmitting HIV to a newborn can be virtually eliminated with "short course" treatments taken only during labor and delivery. But short treatments increase the risk of resistance to the drugs used. This can reduce the success of future treatment for both mother and child.

The risk of birth defects caused by ART is greatest during the first three months of pregnancy. If a mother chooses to stop taking some medications during pregnancy, her HIV disease could get worse. Any woman with HIV who is thinking about getting pregnant should carefully discuss treatment options with her healthcare provider.

Note: HIV transmission statistics in this chapter are from a 2005 publication of the United Nations Joint Programme on HIV/AIDS (UNAIDS).

Chapter 12

HIV Vaccines and Microbicides

Chapter Contents

Section 12.1

Preventive Vaccines

"AIDS Vaccines," Fact Sheet #159, © 2010 AIDS InfoNet. Reprinted with permission. InfoNet fact sheets are updated frequently. Please visit the website at http://www.aidsinfonet.org for the newest version.

What Is a Vaccine?

The body's immune system normally reacts to anything it recognizes as foreign and tries to eliminate it. A vaccine is a substance that helps the immune system respond to a specific germ or virus. A vaccine can prevent an infection. However, no vaccine is 100 percent effective. Most vaccines being used in the United States are between 70 and 95 percent effective.

Vaccines can help individuals by protecting them against a disease or by helping them fight the disease. For a community, vaccines can lower the overall infection rate and help stop the spread of a disease.

How Does a Vaccine Work?

A healthy immune system fights anything it thinks is foreign. It produces proteins called antibodies. These proteins lock onto the invading germs or virus and prevent them from infecting cells.

These antibodies keep the germ or virus from multiplying. Once the threat of infection is over, the immune system produces special memory cells that remember how to fight the specific germ.

Most vaccines are used to prevent infections. However, others help your body fight an infection that you already have. These are called "therapeutic vaccines."

Some vaccines are made up of weakened germs or viruses. These are called "live vaccines." They can give you a mild case of disease, but then your immune system kicks in to protect you against a severe case. Examples include measles, mumps, and rubella. Other "killed" or "inactivated" vaccines, like for influenza or rabies, don't use a living germ. You don't get the disease, but your body can still build up its defenses.

Vaccines can have side effects. With live vaccines, you might get a mild case of the disease you are fighting. With inactivated vaccines, you could have pain, redness, and swelling where you got the shot. You might also briefly feel weakness, fatigue, or nausea.

What's Different about AIDS Vaccines?

All of the proposed acquired immunodeficiency syndrome (AIDS) vaccines use copies of parts of human immunodeficiency virus (HIV) to produce an immune reaction. They cannot cause HIV infection or AIDS. These are different from both types of vaccines mentioned above. They are not weakened live vaccines or inactivated or killed vaccines. They are "engineered" vaccines.

AIDS vaccine trial participants will likely develop antibodies to HIV. So people who take part in a study of a proposed AIDS vaccine might test positive for HIV even if they are not infected. If you are in a vaccine trial, you should only have HIV tests at your trial site.

How Are AIDS Vaccines Tested?

Vaccines start with a researcher's idea about how to fight HIV. This idea is tested in the laboratory and then in animals.

If it is successful in these early studies, a vaccine "candidate" can then be tested in humans. Human testing takes place in three phases:

- Phase 1: Is it safe?

- Phase 2: Does it produce an immune response?

- Phase 3: Is it effective in preventing HIV infection? Does it slow disease progression?

No vaccine provides 100 percent protection against infection. So any vaccine is only partially effective. Although that may sound like a problem, vaccines are actually powerful tools for preventing disease. They bring enormous benefits to individuals and communities. For example, if a vaccine can be given to an entire community and reduce the infection rate by 40 percent, it will have a major impact on the overall number of new infections.

This is a very different situation from measuring the success of an antiretroviral treatment in a group of people already infected. We are used to seeing success rates of 80 percent or more in achieving an undetectable viral load.

Vaccine testing takes many years. For example, Scientists have been working for over 126 years to find a malaria vaccine. It took over 100 years of work to develop a vaccine for typhoid. Polio vaccine took 46 years. The measles vaccine was one of the fastest; it took 9 years to develop.

How Close Are We to an AIDS Vaccine?

There is currently no effective AIDS vaccine. Data from a large trial in Thailand were released in late 2009. The study looked at using standard prevention techniques with or without the vaccine. Participants who got the vaccine regimen were about 30 percent less likely to become infected than those who received the placebo. Researchers are trying to understand this result and to use it to develop a more effective vaccine.

In late 2007, two large trials of an AIDS vaccine were stopped. These were the Step and the Phambili trials. The vaccine failed to prevent HIV infection.

Developing an AIDS vaccine is extremely difficult. Even with the modest effect in the Thai trial, we don't yet know how to measure immune protection against HIV. New ways have to be found to measure the immune response to HIV, and to produce it. There are still many vaccine candidates being developed in the lab, and in human clinical trials.

What about People Who Are Already Infected?

Most vaccines are designed to prevent infection. However, some vaccines might also help people who are already HIV-positive. These are called therapeutic vaccines. A good therapeutic vaccine would strengthen the body's immune response against HIV. We still have to identify ways to measure the immune response against HIV. DermaVir® is a therapeutic vaccine that is currently being studied in humans.

What Else Is Being Studied?

Some researchers believe that taking anti-HIV medications might prevent HIV infection. This approach is called pre-exposure prophylaxis, or PrEP. Prophylaxis means prevention. There are several large studies of PrEP underway now.

Microbicides might be another way to prevent HIV infection. These are substances that could be applied as a cream or gel by women or men to prevent HIV infection during vaginal or anal sex. Several microbicides are currently being tested.

Next Steps

Experts agree that a safe and effective AIDS vaccine would be a vital way to help deal with the global epidemic. It would work along with effective antiretroviral drugs that treat existing HIV infection.

Section 12.2

Microbicides

A microbicide for human immunodeficiency virus (HIV) does not yet exist, but the idea is currently being researched and developed.

What Is a Microbicide?

A microbicide is something designed to destroy microbes (bacteria and viruses) or to reduce their ability to establish an infection. A microbicide for preventing HIV infection would be applied to the vagina or rectum to prevent the virus being passed on during sex.

What Are the Advantages of HIV Microbicides?

A microbicide would share many of the advantages of an acquired immunodeficiency syndrome (AIDS) vaccine. It would be especially useful for women unable to insist on their partner using condoms, who might be able to use a microbicide without their partners knowing. However, a microbicide would not be able to prevent all forms of HIV transmission, and would require regular reapplication. Unlike vaccines, an effective microbicide must be made into a commodity that people will want to use regularly, such as a cream, gel, or vaginal ring.

How Might an HIV Microbicide Work?

A microbicide could work in at least four different ways:

- Kill or inactivate HIV

- Stop the virus entering human cells

- Enhance the body's normal defense mechanisms against HIV

- Inhibit HIV replication

The first microbicide candidates developed were made from barrier gels, among them nonxoynol-9 and cellulose sulfate. More recent trials have been testing antiretroviral-based microbicides, which aim to prevent HIV infection in the same way as pre-exposure prophylaxis might.

What Are the Challenges in Developing HIV Microbicides?

There are many chemicals that kill HIV, including undiluted household bleach. But what is needed for a microbicide is something that works against HIV without causing discomfort or irritation. For example, when researchers investigated using the spermicide nonoxynol-9 as an HIV microbicide they were surprised to find it actually increased the rate of transmission, probably because it caused vaginal lesions and inflammation, which made it easier for HIV to establish an infection, even though nonoxynol-9 killed the virus in lab tests.[1]

For a microbicide to become popular, researchers must develop not only the active ingredient but also a microbicide that is socially acceptable, affordable, and easy to apply. Ideally it would provide protection for several days or even weeks at a time.

Other major issues include how a microbicide might affect sperm and whether it might cause adverse effects for a woman's reproductive health.[2]

How Are the Possible Microbicides Tested?

There are three phases of clinical trials that a potential microbicide must pass through before it is judged effective and safe. Phase I tends to last between twelve and eighteen months, whereas the final phase can take up to three or four years:

- Phase I involves a small number of volunteers to test the safety of various doses.

- Phase II involves hundreds of volunteers to further assess safety and, in some cases, positive responses.

- Phase III involves thousands of volunteers to test safety and effectiveness.

The Phase IIb trial, a recent innovation, is a larger variant of the Phase II trial.

All microbicide trials provide condoms and prevention counseling to all participants, as an ethical obligation. As a result, the overall rate of HIV transmission is lowered, which means more volunteers are needed to produce a significant result. Most volunteers must be HIV-negative at the beginning of the trial, though it is also important to test safety in those who are already infected.

How Many Microbicides Trials Are Under Way?

Several microbicide candidates are currently being studied in over twenty clinical trials.[3] The results of a Phase IIb trial, CAPRISA 004, were presented at the 2010 International AIDS Conference in Vienna. The randomized, controlled trial assessed the safety and effectiveness of tenofovir gel in nine hundred HIV-negative, sexually active women between the ages of eighteen and forty years in South Africa. The results were statistically significant, with the gel reducing the risk of HIV acquisition by 39 percent overall.[4] The protective effect increased to 54 percent among women with high gel adherence. The study is the first to provide proof of concept for microbicides. Although plans for further trials are in place, funding shortfalls are currently restricting progress.[5,6]

A Phase IIb safety and effectiveness study of tenofovir gel, oral tenofovir, and emtricitabine/tenofovir is due to enroll 4,200 women in various sites in Africa.[7] First reports are expected in 2011.

Which Microbicide Trials Have Recently Ended?

In August 2006, Family Health International decided to halt a Phase III trial of a surfactant called SAVVY® after preliminary results showed no evidence of a protective effect. The organization has no plans to further investigate this product.[8]

Two Phase III trials of an entry inhibitor called cellulose sulphate (also known as Ushercell®) were halted in January 2007 after some sites recorded a higher HIV infection rate among women who used the gel, compared to those who were given a version that had no medicinal properties (a placebo). This result led to speculation that the gel may have increased the risk of HIV transmission. Later analysis indicated that the higher infection rate may have been due to chance.[9]

In February 2008, researchers announced the results of a Phase III trial of Carraguard®, an entry inhibitor based on carrageenan, which is derived from seaweed. The product—the first ever to complete Phase

III testing—was shown to be safe, but had no significant effect on HIV transmission.[10]

In 2009 two large-scale trials of the microbicide candidate PRO 2000® ended. PRO 2000, is a type of entry inhibitor that binds to viruses to prevent them from infecting healthy cells.[11]

Results from the smaller trial of the two were released in February 2009. There were 30 percent fewer HIV infections among trial participants who used PRO 2000, compared to women who used the placebo. Although these results seemed promising, they were not statistically significant and therefore could have been down to chance.[12,13]

The results from the second larger trial were released in December 2009. Of the 3,156 women who were given PRO 2000, 130 became infected with HIV, while 123 of the 3,112 women given the placebo gel become infected with the virus. There is therefore no evidence the PRO 2000 gel reduces the risk of HIV infection in women.[14,15]

Who Is Supporting Research and Development?

In 2008 around $244 million was invested in microbicide research and development—up by 8 percent on the previous year. About 85 percent of this money came from the public sector, 14 percent came from the philanthropic sector, and 1 percent was accounted for by commercial companies (only $2.5 million).[16]

At present no major pharmaceutical firm is investing significant amounts of its own money in microbicide research because it is complex and the market is uncertain.[17] As Professor Jonathon Weber has stated: "[Microbicides] are perceived as drugs for Africa, and no one makes money from Africa."[18]

Conclusion

If one of the microbicide candidates were successful in preventing HIV infection, it would be a while before it would become widely available. Any successful product would have to undergo review and licensing by regulatory agencies before becoming available to the public. It would take time to work out the best formulation and dosage, find a suitable delivery method, and distribute the product. Also, if an effective product is produced it may be difficult finding investors, as the microbicide will have to be available to women in low- and middle-income countries and therefore profit margins will be low.[19] In addition, any successful microbicide will only be partially protective and so would have to be complemented with other prevention methods.[20]

While it is important to ensure continued funding and support for microbicide development, it would not be helpful to be overly optimistic about the effectiveness and potential availability of such a product. A microbicide will not be a "silver bullet" for ending the epidemic, but rather another tool to add to existing prevention efforts.

References

1. Global Campaign for Microbicides "Nonoxynol-9" http://www .global-campaign.org/whatsup_with_n9.htm#N-9

2. World Health Organization (2009, September) "Regulatory issues in microbicide development" http://www.who.int/reproductive health/publications/rtis/9789241599436/en/index.html

3. Alliance for Microbicide Development (2010) "Microbicide and PrEP candidates in ongoing clinical trials, summary as of September 2009" http://www.avac.org/ht/d/sp/i/325/pid/325http:// www.avac.org/ht/d/sp/i/325/pid/325http://www.avac.org/ht/d/ http://www.avac.org/ht/d/sp/i/325/pid/325

4. Karim, Q.A. et al (2010) "Effectiveness and safety of tenofovir gel, an antiretroviral microbicide, for the prevention of HIV infection in women," 19 July 2010, Sciencexpress http://www .sciencemag.org/content/329/5996/1168

5. The New York Times (2010, 3 September) "H.I.V. prevention gel hits snag: Money" http://www.nytimes.com/2010/09/04/ world/africa/04safrica.html?_r=1

6. Centre for the AIDS Programme of Research in South Africa "Next steps for tenofovir gel" http://www.caprisa.org/joomla/

7. Microbicides Trial Network (2010) "MTN-003" http://www .mtnstopshiv.org/node/70

8. Family Health International (2006, 28 August) "Phase 3 trial in Nigeria evaluating the effectiveness of SAVVY gel in preventing HIV infection in women will close" http:// www .fhi.org/en/AboutFHI/Media/Releases/pr2006/Phase3 SAVVY082806.htm

9. Van Damme, L. et al (2008) "Lack of effectiveness of Cellulose Sulfate gel for the prevention of vaginal HIV transmission," *NEJM* 359:463–72. http://www.nejm.org/doi/full/10.1056/ NEJMoa0707957

10. Skoler-Karpoff, S. et al (2008) "Efficacy of Carraguard for prevention of HIV infection in women in South Africa: a randomized, double-blind, placebo-controlled trial," *The Lancet*, 372(9654):1977–87. http://www.ncbi.nlm.nih.gov/pubmed/1905904 8?ordinalpos=1&itool=EntrezSystem2.PEntrez.Pubmed.Pubmed_ ResultsPanel.Pubmed_DefaultReportPanel.Pubmed_RVDocSum

11. Global Advocacy for HIV Prevention (AVAC) (2009) "Understanding the results from trials of the PRO 2000 microbicide candidate" http://www.avac.org/ht/d/sp/i/3426/pid/3426

12. National Institute of Allergy and Infectious Diseases (2009, 9 February) "Anti-HIV gel shows promise in large-scale study in women" http://www.niaid.nih.gov/news/newsreleases/2009/ pages/hptn_035_gel.aspx

13. Global Campaign for Microbicides (2009) "Advocates' frequently asked questions about HPTN 035" http://www.global -campaign.org/HPTN-035.htm

14. McCormack, S et al (2010) "PRO2000 vaginal gel for prevention of HIV-1 infection (Microbicides Development Programme 301): a phase 3, randomised, double-blind, parallel-group trial," *The Lancet*, September 20;SO140 http://www.thelancet.com/ journals/lancet/article/PIIS0140-6736%2810%2961086-0/

15. AVAC (2009) "Understanding the results from trials of the PRO 2000 microbicide candidate" http://www.avac.org/ht/d/ sp/i/3426/pid/3426

16. HIV Vaccines and Microbicides Resource Tracking Working Group (2009, July) "Adapting to Realities: Trends in HIV prevention research funding, 2000 to 2008" http://www.unaids.org/ en/KnowledgeCentre/Resources/PressCentre/PressReleases/ 2009/20090720_PR_Funding.asp

17. Global Campaign for Microbicides "Financing" http://www .global-campaign.org/economics.htm

18. *The Guardian* (2004, 22 March) "Taking prevention of Aids beyond ABC" http://www.guardian.co.uk/uk/2004/mar/22/health .aids/print

19. UNAIDS (2008) "Microbicides: challenges to development and distribution (part 2)" http://www.unaids.org/en/Knowledge Centre/Resources/FeatureStories/archive/2008/20080222 -microbicides_Part_2.asp

20. UNAIDS (2008, 20 February) "Microbicides: why are they significant? (Part 1)" http://www.unaids.org/en/KnowledgeCentre/Resources/FeatureStories/archive/2008/20080218_Microbicides_why_are_they_significant_Part1.asp

Chapter 13

HIV Prophylaxis

Chapter Contents

Section 13.1

Pre-Exposure Prophylaxis

"CDC Trials of Pre-Exposure Prophylaxis for HIV Prevention," Centers
for Disease Control and Prevention, February 3, 2010.

New approaches to human immunodeficiency virus (HIV) prevention
are urgently needed to stem the estimated 2.7 million new HIV infections
that occur worldwide each year. While behavior change programs have
contributed to dramatic reductions in the number of annual infections
in the United States and many other nations, far too many individuals
remain at high risk. With an effective vaccine years away, there is mounting evidence that antiretroviral drugs may be able to play an important
role in reducing the risk of HIV infection. As part of its commitment to developing new HIV prevention strategies, the Centers for Disease Control
and Prevention (CDC) is sponsoring three clinical trials of pre-exposure
prophylaxis, or PrEP, for HIV prevention, and is participating in a University of Washington–sponsored trial in Kenya and Uganda. The trials test
the antiretroviral drug tenofovir disoproxil fumarate (or tenofovir, brand
name Viread®) used alone or in combination with emtricitabine (together,
known as the brand name Truvada®) taken as a preventative drug.

The CDC-sponsored trials are designed to answer important questions about the safety and efficacy of a tenofovir or tenofovir plus
emtricitabine pill taken as a daily oral HIV preventative among three
populations at high risk for infection: heterosexuals in Botswana, injection drug users in Thailand, and men who have sex with men (MSM)
in the United States. The trial in Thailand is a safety and efficacy
trial, while the U.S. and Botswana trials are examining clinical and
behavioral safety and adherence. CDC also co-manages two trial sites
in Uganda as part of the University of Washington Partners PrEP
Study, which is examining the safety and efficacy of PrEP among heterosexual couples in which one partner is infected and the other is
not. All of the trials will also assess the effects of taking a daily pill
on HIV risk behaviors, adherence to and acceptability of the regimen,
and in cases where participants become HIV-infected, the resistance
characteristics of the acquired virus. This information will be critical
to guide future studies and HIV prevention programs.

Similar PrEP trials are also being conducted by other agencies. In 2006, Family Health International (FHI), with funding from the Bill and Melinda Gates Foundation, completed a safety trial of tenofovir for HIV prevention among young women in Ghana, Nigeria, and Cameroon. The study provided the first data showing PrEP with tenofovir to be both safe and acceptable for use by HIV-negative individuals. The National Institutes of Health (NIH) is currently evaluating the safety and efficacy of PrEP among MSM in Peru, Ecuador, South Africa, Brazil, Thailand, and the United States, and additional trials investigating PrEP among women have been launched in Africa.

Rationale for Trials of Pre-Exposure Prophylaxis for HIV Prevention

Researchers believe that an antiretroviral drug taken as a daily oral preventative is one of the most important new HIV prevention approaches being investigated today. An effective daily preventative treatment could help address the urgent need for female-controlled prevention methods and, when combined with existing prevention measures, could help reduce new HIV infections among men and women at high risk.

The concept of providing a preventative treatment before exposure to an infectious agent is not new. For example, when individuals travel to an area where malaria is common, they are advised to take medication to fight malaria before and during travel to that region. The medicine to prevent illness will then be in their bloodstream if they are exposed to the infectious agent that causes malaria.

Several sources of data suggest that the use of antiretroviral drugs in this manner may be effective in reducing the risk of HIV infection. Theoretically, if HIV replication can be inhibited from the very first moment the virus enters the body, it may not be able to establish a permanent infection. Providing antiretrovirals (ARVs) to HIV-infected women during labor and delivery and to their newborns immediately following birth has been shown to reduce the risk of mother-to-child transmission by about 50 percent.

Additionally, in observational studies, ARV regimens have been associated with an 80 percent reduction in the risk of HIV infection among healthcare workers following needle sticks and other accidental exposures, when treatment is initiated promptly and continued for several weeks. Finally, animal studies have shown that tenofovir can reduce the transmission of a virus similar to HIV in monkeys when given before and immediately after a single retroviral exposure. Animal studies have also demonstrated that pre-exposure administration of tenofovir plus emtricitabine provided significant protection to monkeys exposed repeatedly to an HIV-like virus. These data, combined with the drugs' favorable resistance and safety profiles as HIV treatments, make tenofovir and tenofovir plus emtricitabine ideal candidates for HIV prevention trials.

Tenofovir was approved by the U.S. Food and Drug Administration in 2001 as a treatment for HIV infection, and the tenofovir plus emtricitabine combination pill was approved for use as an HIV treatment in 2004. Data from Gilead Sciences, Inc. indicate that more than one million HIV-infected people around the world have now used these drugs. As treatments for HIV-infected individuals, tenofovir and tenofovir plus emtricitabine have been shown to be both safe and effective. They have relatively low levels of side effects and slow development of associated drug resistance, compared with other available HIV treatments. Because the therapies are taken orally only once a day, with or without food, they are also among the most convenient-to-use HIV drugs available today. These trials are designed to evaluate the drugs' safety and efficacy among uninfected individuals. Side effects may differ in HIV-negative populations, and it is not yet known if tenofovir or tenofovir plus emtricitabine can prevent HIV infection in humans.

Characteristics of Current PrEP Candidates

- Established safety as HIV treatments
- Potent antiretrovirals
- Long duration of action
- Once-daily dosing
- Low levels of resistance

CDC-Sponsored PrEP Trials

Specific Trial Designs and Objectives

All three of CDC's studies are randomized, double-blind, placebo-controlled trials. All participants receive risk-reduction counseling and other prevention services. In addition, half of the participants are randomly assigned to receive one antiretroviral pill daily (either tenofovir or tenofovir plus emtricitabine, depending on the trial), and the other half are randomly assigned to take one daily placebo pill (a similar tablet without active medication). Neither researchers nor participants know an individual's group assignment. In all, the studies will involve approximately four thousand volunteers. The Thailand and U.S. trials of tenofovir began in 2005 and the Botswana trial of tenofovir plus emtricitabine began in early 2007. The trials are expected to last between three and six years.

To ensure that the studies remain on a solid scientific and ethical foundation, all study procedures and plans are reviewed and approved by scientific and ethical review committees at CDC (called institutional review boards, or IRBs), as well as IRBs established by each host country and research site prior to trial launch. Additionally, data on safety, enrollment, and efficacy will be reviewed regularly by an independent data safety and monitoring board (DSMB) for the Botswana and Thai trials, and by an independent safety review committee for the U.S. trial. These committees review emerging data to ensure that continuing the trial is safe and to determine the point at which the results are conclusive. If scientific questions arise during the course of the research, these committees will meet more frequently.

Thailand

The CDC trial in Thailand is examining the safety and efficacy of tenofovir. The study is being conducted in collaboration with the Bangkok Metropolitan Administration and the Thailand Ministry of Public Health and is enrolling 2,400 HIV-negative intravenous drug users (IDUs)—male and female—at seventeen drug treatment clinics in Bangkok. Participants are recruited at the drug treatment clinics, at community outreach sites, and through a peer referral program.

Botswana and the United States

The Botswana and U.S. trials are assessing the clinical and behavioral safety of once-daily PrEP regimens and adherence to the drugs among key populations at risk. While these trials will not evaluate the drug's efficacy in reducing HIV transmission, they will provide critical information to guide potential implementation of PrEP, should efficacy be demonstrated in other trials.

Botswana. The Botswana study is examining the behavioral and clinical safety of tenofovir plus emtricitabine and adherence to the regimen. This trial began as a safety and efficacy trial, but key challenges—including lower than anticipated HIV incidence and retention rates in the trial population—meant that the trial would be unable to determine efficacy. However, the study will still examine critical questions related to safety and adherence.

227

The trial is being conducted in collaboration with the Botswana government and enrolled 1,200 HIV-negative heterosexual men and women, ages eighteen to thirty-nine, in the nation's two largest cities, Gaborone and Francistown. Participants were recruited through a number of venues, including HIV voluntary counseling and testing centers, sexually transmitted disease (STD) and family planning clinics, youth organizations, and community events.

United States. The U.S. study is being conducted at three sites in collaboration with the San Francisco Department of Public Health, the AIDS Research Consortium of Atlanta, and Fenway Community Health in Boston. The study has enrolled four hundred HIV-negative MSM who reported having had anal intercourse in the prior twelve months. Participants are randomly assigned to one of four study arms. Two arms receive either tenofovir or placebo immediately upon enrollment, while the other two arms receive either tenofovir or placebo after nine months of enrollment. This design will allow researchers to compare risk behaviors among those taking a daily pill and those not taking pills.

Education and Enrollment of Trial Participants

Understanding the potential impact of a daily preventative drug regimen on HIV risk behaviors will be critical, should pre-exposure prophylaxis prove effective in reducing HIV transmission. One of the greatest risks, as efforts progress to identify new biomedical prevention approaches, is that individuals at risk will reduce their use of existing HIV prevention strategies. It will therefore be crucial to reinforce proven behavioral prevention strategies, both within and beyond these trials. All three trials are taking multiple steps to address this issue during the education and enrollment of trial participants and through ongoing participant counseling.

First, it is critical to ensure that participants understand that trial participation may not protect them from HIV infection—either because they may receive a placebo or because they may receive a study drug, the efficacy of which remains unproven. This and other key aspects of the trial, including the potential risks and benefits of participation, are explained to potential volunteers in the language of their choice, prior to their enrollment. To ensure participants fully understand all aspects of their participation, all volunteers are required to pass a comprehension test prior to providing written informed consent. Study participants are also free to withdraw from the trial at any time and for any reason.

Risk-Reduction Counseling and Other Prevention and Treatment Services

To assist participants in eliminating or reducing HIV risk behaviors, extensive counseling is provided at each study visit, and more often if needed. This interactive counseling has proven effective in reducing the risk of HIV and other STDs in multiple populations, including past participants of similar HIV prevention trials. Participants are also offered free condoms and STD testing and treatment to reduce their risk for HIV infection. Additionally, in Thailand, participating IDUs are offered follow-up in a methadone drug treatment program and receive bleach and instructions on how to use it to clean needles. Consistent with Thai government policy, sterile syringes are not provided, but are widely available in Thailand without a prescription and at low cost (one sterile syringe and one needle cost about 5 baht, or about $0.15).

While participants will likely be at lower risk as a result of these prevention services, some individuals will engage in behavior that places them at risk for HIV infection. To ensure that participants who are infected during the trial are quickly referred to the best available medical and psychosocial services, participants receive free rapid HIV testing at every visit. This regular HIV testing will also help guard against the development of drug-resistant virus, as the study drug will be immediately discontinued when infection is detected.

Participants who become infected receive confirmatory testing for infection, post-test risk-reduction and support counseling, and help enrolling in local HIV care programs. Both Thailand and Botswana have antiretroviral treatment and HIV care programs in place at minimal or no cost to patients. In the United States, participants are referred to local healthcare providers or public health programs for needed medical and social services.

Additionally, to help guide treatment decisions and to determine if prior exposure to tenofovir or tenofovir plus emtricitabine has any effect on the course of disease, initial testing will be provided for viral load, CD4 count, and HIV resistance mutations. Participants will also be followed for an additional six months following infection to examine their immune and virologic response. Although study procedures ensure a very low risk of drug-resistant virus emerging, the initial HIV resistance testing will provide important data on the degree to which any resistance does occur.

Monitoring for Side Effects

The health of participants is closely monitored throughout each trial, and participants are linked to any necessary medical care. In addition to scheduled reviews of safety data by the DSMB, both clinical and behavioral safety are closely monitored on an ongoing basis.

Although the drugs being tested have excellent safety profiles, there are potential medical risks. Tenofovir has been associated with minor side effects such as nausea, vomiting, and loss of appetite, as well as rare but more serious effects, such as impaired kidney function or reductions in bone density. Tenofovir plus emtricitabine has similarly been associated with a relatively low level of side effects, including diarrhea, nausea, fatigue, headache, dizziness, and rash, with infrequent reports of more serious side effects, such as impaired kidney function and lactic acidosis (a build-up of lactic acid in the blood). For both drugs, these effects have largely been reversed after use of the drug was discontinued.

Careful monitoring is provided using laboratory testing for any biological abnormalities (such as elevated creatinine or decreased phosphorus), so that the drug being tested can be promptly discontinued if serious concerns are identified. CDC will work with partners in each community to ensure that care is provided if either drug results in any health problems during the trial.

Community Involvement

CDC has and will continue to work closely with community partners at each research site to ensure active community participation during the planning and implementation of these trials.

Botswana. In Botswana, community advisory boards have been established at each site, which include representatives from local governments (elected and traditional), as well as community members and representatives from key stakeholder organizations. Participant advisory boards have also been established. These groups provide input to researchers throughout the trial.

Thailand. In Thailand, a community relations committee, composed of injecting drug users from each of the seventeen drug treatment centers, family members, and representatives of local community organizations, meets regularly and provides advice to study staff on all aspects of study design, implementation, and trial conduct.

United States. In the United States, all three sites have established active community advisory boards that are consulted regularly about study procedures and educational materials for potential participants. Members of these boards provide ongoing advice throughout the trials.

In addition to the regular input received by these established committees, broader outreach and consultations with advocates and community-based organizations representing populations at risk for HIV are held, as needed, to address current and future plans for HIV prevention research and programs.

CDC Participation in Partners PrEP Study

The University of Washington is working with collaborators in Kenya and Uganda to conduct the Partners PrEP Study, which is examining the safety and efficacy of two different PrEP regimens—once-daily tenofovir and once-daily tenofovir plus emtricitabine—among heterosexual couples. CDC co-manages two trial sites in Uganda, in conjunction with The AIDS Support Organization (TASO), the largest indigenous non-governmental organization providing HIV care in Uganda.

This randomized, double-blind, placebo-controlled study operates at nine trial sites in Kenya and Uganda and will include 3,900 serodiscordant couples (couples in which one person is HIV-infected and the other is not). Stable serodiscordant couples are the largest risk group for HIV infection in Africa, and this trial will provide important data on whether PrEP could be used to prevent new HIV infections among this population. HIV-uninfected partners are assigned to one of three groups: tenofovir, tenofovir plus emtricitabine, and placebo. All participants receive ongoing risk reduction counseling and HIV testing, and their safety is monitored by the study's DSMB and local IRBs. HIV-infected members of the discordant couples receive ongoing HIV care.

The trial is the first to test the safety and efficacy of both tenofovir and tenofovir plus emtricitabine in the same population and will allow investigators to simultaneously evaluate the two drugs as candidates for use as PrEP.

Planning for Possible Implementation of PrEP

As we move forward with the search for new HIV prevention strategies, it will be critical to determine how these approaches can best be integrated into existing prevention programs, should they prove effective in reducing risk. Because no strategy is 100 percent effective in preventing HIV infection, the future impact of PrEP on the HIV epidemic will ultimately be determined by how effectively strategies are used in combination to provide the greatest protection to individuals at risk.

CDC has begun to examine potential implementation strategies with a wide range of stakeholders in the United States. CDC's top priority has been preparing for the rapid development of clinical guidelines to ensure the proper use of PrEP in the United States, should it prove effective in clinical trials. The agency has also begun examining how and under what circumstances PrEP could effectively be delivered to populations at highest risk for HIV infection in the United States as part of a comprehensive national HIV prevention strategy.

At the international level, should efficacy be proven, the World Health Organization (WHO) and the Joint United Nations Programme on HIV/AIDS (UNAIDS) would develop normative guidance on global PrEP implementation, and individual countries would develop their own programs and policies for integrating PrEP into prevention efforts. As these plans are developed, CDC will provide technical assistance to its international partners and to countries where CDC trials are being conducted.

Section 13.2

Post-Exposure Prophylaxis

"Post-Exposure Prophylaxis," AIDS.gov, October 2010.

Post-exposure prophylaxis (PEP) is treatment designed to protect you from infection after you have been exposed to a blood-borne pathogen like human immunodeficiency virus (HIV). PEP is generally associated with occupational (workplace) exposure, such as needle sticks for healthcare workers.

PEP is also used to treat accidental exposure outside of the workplace, such as condom breakage or sexual assault. This treatment is classified as non-occupational post-exposure prophylaxis (nPEP).

In order for PEP to be most effective, treatment should begin immediately, but no later than seventy-two hours after exposure.

Types of HIV Exposure in the Workplace

The risk of exposure to infected body fluids and blood is greatest for people who work in a healthcare setting. Exposure to infected blood and body fluids can occur by any of the following means:

- Percutaneous injury (needle sticks or cuts)
- Contact with a mucous membrane (eyes and mouth)
- Contact with non-intact skin (skin that is chapped, scraped, or affected by dermatitis)

The risk of HIV transmission through these routes is extremely low—approximately 0.3 percent after a percutaneous exposure and 0.09 percent after a mucous membrane exposure.

Treatment for HIV Exposure in the Workplace

The sooner you start PEP after you have been exposed to HIV, the lower the risk that you will develop HIV yourself. PEP treatments generally last up to four weeks.

PEP usually consists of a combination of two or three antiretroviral drugs. The choice of medications depends on the type and degree of exposure.

For someone exposed through a shallow puncture wound or by exposure to a small amount of broken skin or mucous membranes, the CDC recommends taking a combination of two antiretrovirals.

For someone exposed through a deep puncture wound, a puncture from a needle with visible blood on it, or contact with a large amount of broken skin or mucous membranes, the CDC recommends taking a combination of three or more antiretrovirals.

Non-Occupational Exposures

These exposures may include sexual assault, a broken condom during sexual activity, or sharing a needle with an HIV-positive individual.

It is best to seek treatment within thirty-six hours of the exposure incident. Some of the places you can go to seek treatment include emergency rooms, urgent care clinics, or a local HIV clinic.

Your healthcare provider will consider whether PEP is right for you based on the type of exposure and the likelihood that the source individual has HIV. You may be asked to return for additional HIV testing for a period of six months.

Part Three

Receiving an
HIV/AIDS Diagnosis

Chapter 14

HIV Testing

Chapter Contents

Section 14.1

HIV Testing Basics

"HIV Testing Basics for Consumers,"
Centers for Disease Control and Prevention, April 9, 2010.

Should I get tested?

The following are behaviors that increase your chances of getting human immunodeficiency virus (HIV). If you answer yes to any of them, you should definitely get an HIV test. If you continue with any of these behaviors, you should be tested every year. Talk to a healthcare provider about an HIV testing schedule that is right for you:

- Have you injected drugs or steroids or shared equipment (such as needles, syringes, works) with others?

- Have you had unprotected vaginal, anal, or oral sex with men who have sex with men, multiple partners, or anonymous partners?

- Have you exchanged sex for drugs or money?

- Have you been diagnosed with or treated for hepatitis, tuberculosis (TB), or a sexually transmitted disease (STD), like syphilis?

- Have you had unprotected sex with someone who could answer yes to any of the above questions?

If you have had sex with someone whose history of sex partners and/or drug use is unknown to you or if you or your partner has had many sex partners, then you have more of a chance of being infected with HIV. Both you and your new partner should get tested for HIV, and learn the results, before having sex for the first time.

For women who plan to become pregnant, testing is even more important. If a woman is infected with HIV, medical care and certain drugs given during pregnancy can lower the chance of passing HIV to her baby. All women who are pregnant should be tested during each pregnancy.

How long after a possible exposure should I wait to get tested for HIV?

Most HIV tests are antibody tests that measure the antibodies your body makes against HIV. It can take some time for the immune system to produce enough antibodies for the antibody test to detect, and this time period can vary from person to person. This time period is commonly referred to as the "window period." Most people will develop detectable antibodies within two to eight weeks (the average is twenty-five days). Even so, there is a chance that some individuals will take longer to develop detectable antibodies. Therefore, if the initial negative HIV test was conducted within the first three months after possible exposure, repeat testing should be considered more than three months after the exposure occurred to account for the possibility of a false-negative result. Ninety-seven percent of persons will develop antibodies in the first three months following the time of their infection. In very rare cases, it can take up to six months to develop antibodies to HIV.

Another type of test is a ribonucleic acid (RNA) test, which detects the HIV virus directly. The time between HIV infection and RNA detection is nine to eleven days. These tests, which are more costly and used less often than antibody tests, are used in some parts of the United States.

For information on HIV testing, you can talk to your healthcare provider or you can find the location of the HIV testing site nearest to you by visiting the National HIV Testing Resources website. Both of these resources are confidential.

How do HIV tests work?

Once HIV enters the body, the immune system starts to produce antibodies (chemicals that are part of the immune system that recognize invaders like bacteria and viruses and mobilize the body's attempt to fight infection). In the case of HIV, these antibodies cannot fight off the infection, but their presence is used to tell whether a person has HIV in his or her body. In other words, most HIV tests look for the HIV antibodies rather than looking for HIV itself. There are tests that look for HIV's genetic material directly, but these are not in widespread use.

The most common HIV tests use blood to detect HIV infection. Tests using saliva or urine are also available. Some tests take a few days for results, but rapid HIV tests can give results in about twenty minutes. All positive HIV tests must be followed up by another test to confirm the positive result. Results of this confirmatory test can take a few days to a few weeks.

239

What are the different HIV screening tests available in the United States?

In most cases the EIA (enzyme immunoassay), used on blood drawn from a vein, is the most common screening test used to look for antibodies to HIV. A positive (reactive) EIA must be used with a follow-up (confirmatory) test such as the Western blot to make a positive diagnosis. There are EIA tests that use other body fluids to look for antibodies to HIV. These include the following:

- Oral fluid tests use oral fluid (not saliva) that is collected from the mouth using a special collection device. This is an EIA antibody test similar to the standard blood EIA test. A follow-up confirmatory Western blot uses the same oral fluid sample.

- Urine tests use urine instead of blood. The sensitivity and specificity (accuracy) are somewhat less than that of the blood and oral fluid tests. This is also an EIA antibody test similar to blood EIA tests and requires a follow-up confirmatory Western blot using the same urine sample.

Rapid tests: A rapid test is a screening test that produces very quick results, in approximately twenty minutes. Rapid tests use blood from a vein or from a finger stick, or oral fluid, to look for the presence of antibodies to HIV. As is true for all screening tests, a reactive rapid HIV test result must be confirmed with a follow-up confirmatory test before a final diagnosis of infection can be made. These tests have similar accuracy rates as traditional EIA screening tests.

Home testing kits: Consumer-controlled test kits (popularly known as "home testing kits") were first licensed in 1997. Although home HIV tests are sometimes advertised through the internet, currently only the Home Access HIV-1 Test System is approved by the Food and Drug Administration. (The accuracy of other home test kits cannot be verified.) The Home Access HIV-1 Test System can be found at most local drugstores. It is not a true home test, but a home collection kit. The testing procedure involves pricking a finger with a special device, placing drops of blood on a specially treated card, and then mailing the card in to be tested at a licensed laboratory. Customers are given an identification number to use when phoning in for the results. Callers may speak to a counselor before taking the test, while waiting for the test result, and when the results are given. All individuals receiving a positive test result are provided referrals for a follow-up confirmatory test, as well as information and resources on treatment and support services.

RNA tests: RNA tests look for genetic material of the virus and can be used in screening the blood supply and for detection of rare very early infection cases when antibody tests are unable to detect antibodies to HIV.

If I test HIV-negative, does that mean that my partner is HIV negative also?

No. Your HIV test result reveals only your HIV status. Your negative test result does not indicate whether or not your partner has HIV. HIV is not necessarily transmitted every time you have sex. Therefore, your taking an HIV test should not be seen as a method to find out if your partner is infected.

Ask your partner if he or she has been tested for HIV and what risk behaviors he or she has engaged in, both currently and in the past. Think about getting tested together.

It is important to take steps to reduce your risk of getting HIV. Not having (abstaining from) sex is the most effective way to avoid HIV. If you choose to be sexually active, having sex with one person who only has sex with you and who is uninfected is also effective. If you are not sure that both you and your partner are HIV-negative, use a latex condom to help protect both you and your partner from HIV and other STDs. Studies have shown that latex condoms are very effective, though not 100 percent, in preventing HIV transmission when used correctly and consistently. If either partner is allergic to latex, plastic (polyurethane) condoms for either the male or female can be used.

What if I test positive for HIV?

If you test positive for HIV, the sooner you take steps to protect your health, the better. Early medical treatment and a healthy lifestyle can help you stay well. Prompt medical care may delay the onset of acquired immunodeficiency syndrome (AIDS) and prevent some life-threatening conditions. There are a number of important steps you can take immediately to protect your health:

- See a licensed healthcare provider, even if you do not feel sick. Try to find a healthcare provider who has experience treating HIV. There are now many medications to treat HIV infection and help you maintain your health. It is never too early to start thinking about treatment possibilities.

- Have a TB (tuberculosis) test. You may be infected with TB and not know it. Undetected TB can cause serious illness, but it can be successfully treated if caught early.

- Smoking cigarettes, drinking too much alcohol, or using illegal drugs (such as methamphetamines) can weaken your immune system. There are programs available that can help you stop or reduce your use of these substances.

- Get screened for other sexually transmitted diseases (STDs). Undetected STDs can cause serious health problems. It is also important to practice safe-sex behaviors so you can avoid getting STDs.

There is much you can do to stay healthy. Learn all that you can about maintaining good health.

Not having (abstaining from) sex is the most effective way to avoid transmitting HIV to others. If you choose to have sex, use a latex condom to help protect your partner from HIV and other STDs. Studies have shown that latex condoms are very effective, though not 100 percent, in preventing HIV transmission when used correctly and consistently. If either partner is allergic to latex, plastic (polyurethane) condoms for either the male or female can be used.

I'm HIV positive. Where can I get information about treatment?

The Centers for Disease Control and Prevention (CDC) recommends that you be in the care of a licensed healthcare provider, preferably one with experience treating people living with HIV. Your healthcare provider can assist you with treatment information and guidance.

Where can I get tested for HIV infection?

Many places provide testing for HIV infection. Common testing locations include local health departments, clinics, offices of private doctors, hospitals, and other sites set up specifically to provide HIV testing. You can also ask your healthcare provider about getting tested, or, for information on HIV testing, you can talk to your healthcare provider or you can find the location of the HIV testing site nearest to you by visiting the National HIV Testing Resources website. Both of these resources are confidential.

Between the time of a possible exposure and the receipt of test results, individuals should consider abstaining from sexual contact with others or use condoms and/or dental dams during all sexual encounters.

If you have questions about HIV or AIDS, it is important to seek testing at a place that also provides counseling about HIV prevention and AIDS. Counselors can answer any questions you might have about risky behaviors and ways you can protect yourself and others in the future. In addition, they can help you understand the meaning of the test results and describe what HIV/AIDS–related resources are available in the local area.

What is CDC doing to get more people tested for HIV?

CDC is the nation's leading source for sharing information on HIV prevention, counseling, and testing. Since the beginning of the epidemic, the agency has provided recommendations and guidelines for HIV counseling and testing, as well as training and education for healthcare providers and the general public.

In September 2006, as part of its continuing efforts to ensure that more people get tested for HIV, CDC released the *Revised Recommendations for HIV Testing of Adults, Adolescents, and Pregnant Women in Health-Care Settings*.

These new recommendations advise routine HIV testing of adults, adolescents, and pregnant women in healthcare settings in the United States. They also recommend reducing barriers to HIV testing.

Why does CDC recommend HIV screening for all pregnant women?

HIV testing during pregnancy is important because antiviral therapy can improve the mother's health and greatly lower the chance that an HIV-infected pregnant woman will pass HIV to her infant before, during, or after birth. The treatment is most effective for babies when started as early as possible during pregnancy. However, there are still great health benefits to beginning treatment even during labor or shortly after the baby is born.

CDC recommends HIV screening for all pregnant women because risk-based testing (when the healthcare provider offers an HIV test based on the provider's assessment of the pregnant woman's risk) misses many women who are infected with HIV. CDC does recommend providing information on HIV (either orally or by pamphlet) and, for women with risk factors, referrals to prevention counseling.

HIV testing provides an opportunity for infected women to find out that they are infected and to gain access to medical treatment that may help improve their own health. It also allows them to make informed choices that can prevent transmission to their infant. For some uninfected women with risks for HIV, the prenatal care period could be an ideal opportunity for HIV prevention and subsequent behavior change to reduce risk for acquiring HIV infection.

Section 14.2

HIV Testing Frequency and Window Period

Excerpted from "HIV Testing Frequency" and "Testing Window Period," AIDS.gov, October 2010.

HIV Testing Frequency

Testing Frequency

How often should you take an human immunodeficiency virus (HIV) test? That depends!

The Centers for Disease Control and Prevention (CDC) recommends that opt-out HIV screening be a part of routine clinical care for all patients aged thirteen to sixty-four. In other words, you should have an HIV test during a medical check-up—just like you have a blood test or a urine test to be sure you are healthy.

In spite of that recommendation, however, most people are tested on the basis of their risk factors for getting HIV. You should get tested for HIV every at least every year if any of the following things apply to you:

- You share needles/syringes or other equipment ("works") for injecting drugs

- You have a history of sexually transmitted diseases (STDs)

- You have had unprotected sex (vaginal, anal, or oral) with multiple or anonymous partners. Or if you have had had unprotected sex with a partner who did not know their own HIV status.

Some healthcare providers may recommend testing every three to six months if you have certain risk factors, including injection drug use and/or unprotected sex with others who engage in high-risk behaviors.

You should consult your healthcare provider to see how often you should be tested.

If you or your partner plan to become pregnant, getting an HIV test is very important. All women who are pregnant should be tested during the first trimester of pregnancy. The CDC also recommends another HIV test in the third trimester of pregnancy for women who live in areas where there are high rates of HIV infection among pregnant women or among women aged fifteen to forty-four.

If you have already been diagnosed with HIV and are pregnant, there are medications and treatment which can lower the chance of passing HIV to your baby. Please contact your doctor or local health department for proper care and information.

Testing Window Period

The Waiting Game: When and How Often?

The timeframe between when you are exposed to HIV and the time you test positive for HIV antibodies can be up to three to six months. This period of time is called a "window period" for HIV testing. On average, you may need to wait two to eight weeks from the time of possible exposure to get a an accurate test result, because it takes at least that long for the immune system to develop enough HIV antibodies to be detectable.

If you took an HIV test within the first three months after possible exposure, you should consider getting another test three months later to confirm your results. Most providers recommend testing at one to three months after your most recent possible exposure.

Section 14.3

Confidential and Anonymous Testing

Excerpted from "Confidential and Anonymous Testing,"
AIDS.gov, October 2010.

HIV Test Results and Privacy Issues

Human immunodeficiency virus (HIV) test results fall under the same privacy rules as all of your medical information. Information about your HIV test cannot be released without your permission. The Health Insurance Portability and Accountability Act of 1996 (HIPAA) ensures that the privacy of individuals' health information is protected while ensuring access to care. However it is important to note that not all HIV testing sites are bound by HIPAA regulations. Before you get tested be sure to inquire about the privacy rules of the HIV test site as well those surrounding your test results.

Available Testing Services

HIV tests can be taken either confidentially or anonymously. Most states offer both anonymous and confidential testing, however some states offer only confidential testing services:

- Confidential testing means that your name and other identifying information will be attached to your test results. The results will go in your medical record and may be shared with your healthcare providers and your insurance company. Otherwise, the results are protected by state and federal privacy laws.

- Anonymous testing means that nothing ties your test results to you. When you take an anonymous HIV test, you get a unique identifier that allows you to get your test results. Not all HIV test sites offer anonymous testing. Contact your local health department to see if there are anonymous test sites in your area.

Names-Based Reporting

Since the beginning of the epidemic, acquired immunodeficiency syndrome (AIDS) cases have been reported to state health departments using name-based reporting. This is now also true for HIV cases. This means, if you test positive for HIV or another STD, the test result and your name will be reported to the state and local health department for the purposes of public health surveillance. Only public health personnel have access to this information at the state level and use this information to get better estimates of the rates of HIV in the state. The state health department will then remove all personal information about you (name, address, etc.) and share the remaining non-identifying information with the Centers for Disease Control and Prevention (CDC) so they can best track national public health trends. The CDC does not share this information with anyone else, including insurance companies.

If you have concerns regarding who can have access to your tests results, it is important to ask your testing center about their privacy policies and to whom they are required to report a positive result.

Section 14.4

Opt-Out Testing

Excerpted from "Opt-Out Testing,"
AIDS.gov, October 2010.

In 2006, the Centers for Disease Control and Prevention (CDC) released its *Revised Recommendations for HIV Testing of Adults, Adolescents, and Pregnant Women in Health-Care Settings*, which advise providers in healthcare settings to do the following things:

- Adopt a policy of routine human immunodeficiency virus (HIV) testing for everyone between the ages of thirteen and sixty-four and all pregnant women

- Use opt-out screening for HIV—meaning that HIV tests will be done routinely unless a patient explicitly refuses to take an HIV test

- Eliminate the requirements for pretest counseling, informed consent, and post-test counseling

"Opt-out testing" does not mean that you *must* take an HIV test. In general, you have the right to refuse an HIV test. (Exceptions include blood and organ donors, military applicants and active duty personnel, federal and state prison inmates under certain circumstances, newborns in some states, and immigrants.)

The CDC believes that opt-out screening for HIV will do the following:

- Help more people find out if they have HIV

- Help those infected with HIV find out earlier, when treatment works best

- Further decrease the number of babies born with HIV

- Reduce stigma associated with HIV testing

- Enable those who are infected to take steps to protect the health of their partners

Section 14.5

Pre- and Post-Test Counseling

Excerpted from "Pre-Post-Test Counseling," AIDS.gov, October 2010.

General Pre-Test and Post-Test Information

Counseling before and after a human immunodeficiency virus (HIV) test is important because it provides critical information about HIV itself and about the testing process. While counseling services may not be available in all healthcare settings, many testing sites do offer these services. If you would like access to pre-test and post-test counseling, be sure to inquire about the availability of these services at your chosen test site. If they do not have them readily available, the staff may be able to direct you to alternate service providers who do.

Pre-test counseling sessions generally include the following:

- Information about the HIV test—what it tests for, what it might *not* tell you, and how long it will take you to get your results

- Information about how HIV is transmitted and how you can protect yourself from infection

- Information about the confidentiality of your test results

- A clear, easy-to-understand explanation of what your test results mean

Once the results are available, you will usually be given the results in private and in person. Post-test counseling generally includes the following:

- Clear communication about what your test result means.

- HIV prevention counseling, if your results are negative.

- A confirmatory test, called a Western blot test, if your results are positive. The results of that test should be available within two weeks.

If Your HIV Test Is Positive

- Your counselor will discuss what it means to live a healthy life with HIV and how you can keep from infecting others.

- Your counselor will also talk about treatments for HIV and can link you to a physician for immediate care. Getting into treatment quickly is important—it can help you keep your immune system healthy and keep you from progressing to acquired immunodeficiency syndrome (AIDS).

- All HIV-positive test results must be reported to your state health department for data tracking. Many states then report data to the Centers for Disease Control and Prevention (CDC), but no personal information (name, address, etc.) is ever shared when those data are reported.

HIV Pre-Test and Post Test Counseling for Pregnant Women

CDC has outlined these recommendations for HIV counseling and testing of pregnant women:

- All pregnant women should be tested for HIV as early as possible during pregnancy, and HIV screening should be included in the routine panel of prenatal screening tests.

- Patients should be informed that HIV screening is recommended for all pregnant women and that it will be performed unless they decline (opt-out screening).

- If a pregnant woman declines to be tested for HIV, her healthcare providers should explore and address her reasons for declining HIV testing.

- Pregnant women should receive appropriate health education, including information about HIV and its transmission, as a routine part of prenatal care.

- Access to clinical care, prevention counseling, and support services is essential for women with positive HIV test results.

- HIV screening should be repeated in the third trimester of pregnancy for women known to be at high risk for HIV.

- Repeat HIV testing in the third trimester is also recommended for all women in areas with higher rates of HIV or AIDS and for women receiving healthcare in facilities with at least one diagnosed HIV case per thousand pregnant women per year.

Chapter 15

Types of HIV Diagnostic Tests

Chapter Contents

Section 15.1

ELISA/Western Blot Tests

Excerpted from "ELISA/Western Blot Tests for HIV,"
© 2010 A.D.A.M., Inc. Reprinted with permission.

Human immunodeficiency virus (HIV) enzyme-linked immunosorbent assay (ELISA)/Western blot is a set of blood tests used to diagnose chronic infection with HIV.

How the Test Is Performed

Blood is typically drawn from a vein, usually from the inside of the elbow or the back of the hand. The site is cleaned with germ-killing medicine (antiseptic). The healthcare provider wraps an elastic band around the upper arm to apply pressure to the area and make the vein swell with blood.

Next, the healthcare provider gently inserts a needle into the vein. The blood collects into an airtight vial or tube attached to the needle. The elastic band is removed from your arm. Once the blood has been collected, the needle is removed and the puncture site is covered to stop any bleeding.

In infants or young children, a sharp tool called a lancet may be used to puncture the skin and make it bleed. The blood collects into a small glass tube called a pipette, or onto a slide or test strip. A bandage may be placed over the area if there is any bleeding.

How to Prepare for the Test

No preparation is necessary.

How the Test Will Feel

When the needle is inserted to draw blood, some people feel moderate pain, while others feel only a prick or stinging sensation. Afterward, there may be some throbbing.

Why the Test Is Performed

Testing for HIV infection is done for many reasons, including:

- screening people who want to be tested;
- screening people in high-risk groups (men who have sex with men, injection drug users and their sexual partners, and commercial sex workers);
- screening people with certain conditions and infections (such as Kaposi sarcoma, *Pneumocystis* pneumonia);
- screening pregnant women to help prevent them from passing the virus to the baby;
- when a patient has an unusual infection.

Normal Results

A negative test result is normal. However, early HIV infection (termed acute HIV infection or primary HIV infection) often results in a negative test.

What Abnormal Results Mean

A positive result on the ELISA screening test does not necessarily mean that the person has HIV infection. There are certain conditions that may lead to a false positive result, such as Lyme disease, syphilis, and lupus.

A positive ELISA test is always followed by a Western blot test. A positive Western blot confirms an HIV infection. A negative Western blot test means the ELISA test was a false positive test. The Western blot test can also be "indeterminate," in which case additional testing is done to clarify the situation.

Negative tests do not rule out HIV infection. There is a period of time (called the "window period") between HIV infection and the appearance of anti-HIV antibodies that can be measured.

If a person might have acute or primary HIV infection, and is in the "window period," a negative HIV ELISA and Western blot will not rule out HIV infection. More tests for HIV will need to be done.

Risks

Veins and arteries vary in size from one patient to another and from one side of the body to the other. Obtaining a blood sample from some people may be more difficult than from others.

Other risks associated with having blood drawn are slight but may include:

- excessive bleeding;
- fainting or feeling light-headed;
- hematoma (blood accumulating under the skin);
- infection (a slight risk any time the skin is broken).

Considerations

People who are at high risk (men who have sex with men, injection drug users and their sexual partners, commercial sex workers) should be regularly tested for HIV.

If the healthcare provider suspects early (acute or primary) HIV infection, other tests (such as HIV viral load) will be needed to confirm this diagnosis, because the HIV ELISA/Western blot test will often be negative during this window period.

References

Goldman L, Ausiello D, eds. *Cecil Medicine. 23rd ed*. Philadelphia, PA: Saunders Elsevier; 2007: sect XXIV.

Section 15.2

p24 Antigen Tests

"p24 Antigen" © 2010 American Association for Clinical Chemistry. Reprinted with permission. For additional information about clinical lab testing, visit the Lab Tests Online website at www.labtestsonline.org.

Also known as: p24 capsid or core antigen; p24 antigen capture assay

Formal name: p24 antigen

Related tests: HIV antibody; HIV viral load; CD4 and CD8; HIV genotypic resistance testing; HIV phenotypic resistance testing

The Test Sample

What Is Being Tested?

The p24 antigen test detects actual human immunodeficiency virus (HIV) viral protein in blood. The test is generally positive from about one week to three to four weeks after infection with HIV. The p24 protein cannot be detected until about a week after infection with HIV because it generally takes that long for the virus to become established and multiply to sufficient numbers that they can be detected. About two to eight weeks after initial exposure, antibodies are produced in response to HIV infection. Once antibodies are produced, the results of the p24 test will usually be negative although the person may be infected with HIV. The antibodies bind to the p24 protein, causing the p24 antigen to no longer be detected in the blood. At that point, however, the HIV antibody test that is most often used for routine screening will be positive. Later in the course of HIV, p24 protein levels again become detectable if the disease is untreated.

The use of this test has declined somewhat, especially with the increase in use of molecular tests to detect early infections and to screen blood and blood products. However, it is often used in areas where resources are limited and where molecular tests are not as widely available.

Sometimes this test may be combined with a test for HIV antibodies to increase the likelihood of detecting HIV infection in the early stages.

How Is the Sample Collected for Testing?

A blood sample is obtained by inserting a needle into a vein in the arm.

Is Any Test Preparation Needed to Ensure the Quality of the Sample?

No test preparation is needed.

The Test

How Is It Used?

p24 antigen testing may be used to help diagnose early HIV infection. Levels of p24 antigen increase significantly at about one to three weeks after initial infection. It is during this timeframe before HIV antibody is produced when the p24 test is useful in helping to diagnose infection. About two to eight weeks after exposure, antibodies to HIV are produced and remain detectable in response to the infection, making the HIV antibody test the most useful assay to diagnose an infection.

When Is It Ordered?

If the HIV antibody test is negative and you have had a recent exposure to HIV, a p24 test may be ordered to detect the infection. However, this test is not ordered as frequently as it once was since tests that can detect HIV ribonucleic acid (RNA) early in infections (HIV viral load) have become more widely available. Tests for HIV antibody are the most commonly ordered screening test.

What Does the Test Result Mean?

A positive result means that you are infected with HIV.

A negative result may mean that you are not infected with HIV or that the level of p24 is below the detectable limits of the test. If you suspect that you have been exposed or if you are at an increased risk, repeat testing or screening with a different test, such as the HIV antibody test, is recommended.

Is There Anything Else I Should Know?

The p24 test is one of the earlier tests developed to detect HIV infection. Because p24 is only detectable during a short window of time, its utility is limited. However, this test can still be used when other tests are unavailable.

Section 15.3

Rapid Oral HIV Tests

"Rapid Oral HIV Test: Questions and Answers,"
U.S. Department of Veterans Affairs, August 6, 2009.

What Is the Rapid Oral HIV Test?

This test tells if you have human immunodeficiency virus (HIV), the virus that causes acquired immunodeficiency syndrome (AIDS). With the rapid test, results take only twenty minutes.

How Does the Rapid Oral HIV Test Work?

When HIV enters the body, antibodies are produced. The test looks for HIV antibodies in your body.

Who Is at Risk for HIV?

HIV is considered to be a sexually transmitted disease (STD). Anyone who has had sex with someone (vaginal, anal, or oral), male or female, should consider having an HIV test.

Other risk factors include the following:

- Sharing needles or works to inject drugs or vitamins or for tattooing or piercing

- Having sex with an injection drug user

- Having been a sex partner with someone who has HIV

- Being a victim of sexual assault

- Having a sexually transmitted disease (STD)

What Happens When You Agree to Be Tested?

- The test is explained to you by a healthcare provider.
- A healthcare provider will ask you to rub your gums with a special cotton pad.
- Results are ready in twenty minutes.
- You will learn your results and discuss what they mean.
- Your test result will be confidential (results will be discussed only with you).

What Does a Negative Test Result Mean?

This means that HIV antibodies have not been found at this time in your system.

This could mean one of two things:

- You do not have HIV; or
- You have HIV but it can take up to three months for your system to produce enough antibodies to show on a test result. If you have engaged in activities that have put you at risk for HIV infection in the past three months, you should repeat this test in ninety days.

What Does a Positive Test Result Mean?

This means HIV antibodies may be in your system. Positive results must always be confirmed by another test that is sent to the lab.

A confirmed positive test result means the following:

- You have HIV and can give it to other people during vaginal, anal, or oral sex.
- You can give HIV to others if you share needles and works to inject drugs or vitamins or for any other reason.
- A pregnant woman may pass the HIV virus to the fetus in her womb or to the baby during birth or breastfeeding. Medications are available to reduce the risk of transmission.

Why Should You Get Tested?

- Getting diagnosed early can improve your quality of life and improve your treatment options.

- Knowing your HIV status helps you protect yourself and others.

- If you test negative, you may feel less anxious after testing.

- An HIV test is part of routine medical care.

Should You Get an HIV Test?

Deciding whether to get an HIV test may not be easy. Fear and worry are common feelings. Talking with your healthcare provider can help you decide if this test is right for you and how to respond to the results of the test.

HIV health educational material can also explain HIV testing options and answer questions about HIV risk and transmission.

How Are Test Results Delivered?

Your healthcare provider can explain what your test results mean. He or she can give you information about how to protect yourself and others from HIV, no matter what the test results are. If your test result is positive, your healthcare provider can direct you to medical, legal, and emotional support services, as needed.

Section 15.4

HIV Home Test Kits

"Vital Facts About HIV Home Test Kits," U.S. Food and
Drug Administration, January 29, 2008.

Privacy and confidentiality are the main factors that lead people to
choose home testing kits to find out if they are infected with human
immunodeficiency virus (HIV), which causes acquired immunodeficiency syndrome (AIDS).

It is important that consumers know there is only one product currently approved by the U.S. Food and Drug Administration (FDA) and
legally sold in the United States as a "home" testing system for HIV.

This product is a kit marketed as either "The Home Access HIV-1
Test System" or "The Home Access Express HIV-1 Test System." The kit
is a home collection-test system that requires users to collect a blood
specimen and then mail it to a laboratory for professional testing. No
test kits allow consumers to interpret the results at home.

Beware of False Claims

Numerous HIV home test systems that have not been approved by
the FDA are currently being marketed online and in newspapers and
magazines.

Manufacturers of unapproved systems have falsely claimed that
their products can detect antibodies to HIV in blood or saliva samples,
and that they can provide results in the home in fifteen minutes or less.
Some have even claimed that their systems are approved by the FDA
or are manufactured in a facility that is registered with FDA.

The FDA takes appropriate action against people or firms that sell
unapproved and ineffective tests.

About the Approved Product

The FDA-approved Home Access System kits allow people to collect
a blood sample. Using a personal identification number (PIN), they
then mail the sample anonymously to a laboratory for testing. The
PIN can then be used to obtain results.

The kits, manufactured by Illinois-based Home Access Health Corporation, can be purchased at pharmacies, by mail order, or online. They allow testing only for the presence of antibodies of the virus known as HIV-1. They do not provide the ability to test for HIV-2, a less common cause of AIDS.

The Home Access System offers users pre- and post-test, anonymous, and confidential counseling through both printed material and telephone interaction. It also provides the user with an interpretation of the test result.

Checking for Antibodies to HIV

Like most HIV tests, the approved Home Access testing system checks for the presence of antibodies to HIV that are produced once the virus enters the body. The rate at which individuals infected with HIV produce these antibodies differs.

There's a "window period" between the time someone is infected with HIV and the time the body produces enough antibodies to be detected through testing. During this time, an HIV-infected person will still get a negative test result.

According to the FDA's Center for Biologics and Research (CBER), which regulates all HIV tests, detectable antibodies usually develop within two to eight weeks. The average is about twenty-two days.

Still, some people take longer to develop detectable antibodies. Most will develop antibodies within three months following infection. In very rare cases, it can take up to six months to develop detectable antibodies to HIV.

Rapid Tests: A Clinical Option

Consumers do have the option of taking a rapid test, some of which test for both HIV-1 and HIV-2. These tests are run where the sample is collected, and produce results within twenty minutes.

Because HIV testing requires interpretation and confirmation, rapid antibody tests are approved and available only in a professional healthcare setting, such as doctors' offices, clinics, and outreach testing sites.

According to the Centers for Disease Control and Prevention (CDC), there are tests that look for HIV's genetic material directly, but these are not in widespread use. Tests using saliva or urine are also available, although not for "at-home" use.

Chapter 16

Understanding Your Test Results

Chapter Contents

Section 16.1

What Do Your Test Results Mean?

Excerpted from "Post Test Results," AIDS.gov, October 2010.

What Your Test Results Mean: Negative Test Result

Studies have proven that both conventional and rapid human immunodeficiency virus (HIV) tests are highly accurate when they show an HIV-positive result.

But a negative result may not always be accurate. It depends on when you might have been exposed to HIV and when you took the test.

It takes time for seroconversion to occur. This is when your body begins to produce the antibodies an HIV test is looking for—anywhere from two weeks to six months after infection. So if you have an HIV test with a negative result within three months of your last possible exposure to HIV, the Centers for Disease Control and Prevention (CDC) recommend that you be retested three months after that first screening test.

A negative result is accurate only if you have not had any risks for HIV infection in the last six months—and a negative result is good only for past exposure. If you get a negative test result, but continue to engage in high-risk behaviors, you are still at risk for HIV infection.

What Your Test Results Mean: Positive Test Result

If your initial HIV test comes back positive, you will automatically be offered a confirmatory test. If the confirmatory test is also positive, you will be diagnosed as "HIV-positive."

At this point, the person giving you your test results will discuss what having HIV means for you and your health. You will be informed about how the virus can affect you and how to protect others from becoming infected. You will also be informed about resources and treatments available to you. Finally, you will be referred to a medical professional for follow-up treatment.

Next Steps If You Are HIV-Positive

If you are diagnosed with HIV, you should do the following things—even if you don't feel sick:

- Find a doctor or licensed healthcare provider who has experience treating HIV. It is important to maintain a relationship with a healthcare provider you trust. Contact your local health department for a referral if you don't know how to find a provider with HIV experience.

- Get screened for other sexually transmitted diseases (STDs) and for tuberculosis (TB). Undetected co-infections, such as STDs and TB, can cause serious health complications—and having HIV makes you more vulnerable to those complications.

- Maintain a healthy lifestyle. This is crucial for success in treating HIV. Smoking, drinking too much, or taking illegal drugs can weaken your immune system, allowing the virus to replicate and grow.

- Safer sex practices are very important. Condoms are very effective in preventing HIV transmission when used correctly and consistently.

- Tell your partner(s) about your HIV status before you have any type of sexual contact (vaginal, anal, or oral) and don't share needles or syringes.

Section 16.2

Do You Have AIDS?

Excerpted from "Testing HIV Positive—Do I Have AIDS?"
AIDSinfo.gov, December 2009.

I tested HIV-positive. What does this mean? Does it mean I have AIDS?

A positive human immunodeficiency virus (HIV) test result means that you are infected with HIV, the virus that causes acquired immune deficiency syndrome(AIDS). Being infected with HIV does not mean that you have AIDS right now. However, if left untreated, HIV infection damages a person's immune system and can progress to AIDS.

What is AIDS?

AIDS is the most serious stage of HIV infection. It results from the destruction of the infected person's immune system.

Your immune system is your body's defense system. Cells of your immune system fight off infection and other diseases. If your immune system does not work well, you are at risk of serious and life-threatening infections and cancers. HIV attacks and destroys the disease-fighting cells of the immune system, leaving the body with a weakened defense against infections and cancer.

Which disease-fighting cells does HIV attack?

CD4 cells are a type of white blood cell that fights infections. They are also called CD4+ T cells or CD4 T lymphocytes. A CD4 count is the number of CD4 cells in a sample of blood.

When HIV enters a person's CD4 cells, it uses the cells to make copies of itself. This process destroys the CD4 cells, and the CD4 count goes down. As you lose CD4 cells, your immune system becomes weak. A weakened immune system makes it harder for your body to fight infections and cancer.

How will I know if I have AIDS?

AIDS is not a diagnosis you can make yourself; it is diagnosed when the immune system is severely weakened. If you are infected with HIV and your CD4 count drops below 200 cells/mm³, or if you develop an AIDS-defining condition (an illness that is very unusual in someone who is not infected with HIV), you have AIDS.

What are the AIDS-defining conditions?

In December 1992, the Centers for Disease Control and Prevention (CDC) published the most current list of AIDS-defining conditions.[1] The AIDS-defining conditions are as follows:

- Candidiasis
- Cervical cancer (invasive)
- Coccidioidomycosis, cryptococcosis, cryptosporidiosis
- Cytomegalovirus disease
- Encephalopathy (HIV-related)
- Herpes simplex (severe infection)
- Histoplasmosis
- Isosporiasis
- Kaposi sarcoma
- Lymphoma (certain types)
- *Mycobacterium avium* complex
- *Pneumocystis carinii / jiroveci* pneumonia
- Pneumonia (recurrent)
- Progressive multifocal leukoencephalopathy
- Salmonella septicemia (recurrent)
- Toxoplasmosis of the brain
- Tuberculosis
- Wasting syndrome

People who are not infected with HIV may also develop these diseases; this does not mean they have AIDS. To be diagnosed with AIDS, a person must first be infected with HIV.

What is HIV treatment?

HIV treatment is the use of anti-HIV medications to keep an HIV-infected person healthy. Treatment can help people at all stages of HIV disease. Although anti-HIV medications can treat HIV infection, they cannot cure HIV infection. HIV treatment is complicated and must be tailored to you and your needs.

Notes

1. CDC. 1993 Revised classification system for HIV infection and expanded surveillance case definition for AIDS among adolescents and adults. *MMWR* 1992;41(no. RR-17).

Section 16.3

Signs and Symptoms of HIV and AIDS

Excerpted from "Signs and Symptoms," AIDS.gov, October 2010.

HIV-Positive without Symptoms

Many people who are HIV-positive do not have symptoms of HIV infection. Often people begin to feel sick only when they progress toward acquired immunodeficiency syndrome (AIDS). Sometimes people living with HIV go through periods of being sick and then feel fine.

While the virus itself can sometimes cause people to feel sick, most of the severe symptoms and illnesses of HIV disease come from the opportunistic infections that attack a damaged immune system. It is important to remember that some symptoms of HIV infection are similar to symptoms of many other common illnesses, such as the flu, or respiratory or gastrointestinal infections.

Early Stages of HIV: Signs and Symptoms

As early as two to four weeks after exposure to HIV (but up to three months later), people can experience an acute illness, often described as "the worst flu ever." This is called acute retroviral syndrome (ARS), or primary HIV infection, and it's the body's natural response to HIV infection. During primary HIV infection, there are higher levels of virus circulating in the blood, which means that people can more easily transmit the virus to others.

Symptoms can include the following:

- Fever

- Chills

- Rash

- Night sweats

- Muscle aches

- Sore throat

- Fatigue

- Swollen lymph nodes

- Ulcers in the mouth

It is important to remember, however, that not everyone gets ARS when they become infected with HIV.

Chronic Phase or Latency: Signs and Symptoms

After the initial infection and seroconversion, the virus becomes less active in the body, although it is still present. During this period, many people do not have any symptoms of HIV infection. This period is called the "chronic" or "latency" phase. This period can last up to ten years—sometimes longer.

AIDS: Signs and Symptoms

When HIV infection progresses to AIDS, many people begin to suffer from fatigue, diarrhea, nausea, vomiting, fever, chills, night sweats, and even wasting syndrome at late stages. Many of the signs and symptoms of AIDS come from opportunistic infections, which occur in patients with a damaged immune system.

Chapter 17

You and Your HIV/AIDS Healthcare Provider: First Steps

Chapter Contents

Section 17.1

Choosing a Provider

Excerpted from "You and Your Provider," AIDS.gov, October 2010.

Who Provides Human Immunodeficiency Virus (HIV) Care?

Choosing a clinician who will provide your HIV care is a very important step in getting the treatment you need to stay healthy. Providers are medical professionals who work with you to manage your HIV care. Many providers will also manage your primary healthcare needs as well. HIV care providers can include the following:

- Doctors
- Nurse Practitioners
- Nurses
- Physician Assistants

Your primary provider will probably work with a large team of other important healthcare professionals to ensure that you have the best care possible. Other important members of your healthcare team may include the following:

- Social workers
- Psychologists/psychiatrists
- Pharmacists
- Dieticians
- Dentists
- Case managers or other health professionals

Choosing a Provider

Everyone will work together to ensure you have the best plan of care and that all your medical, psychological, and social needs are met.

When choosing and working with a provider, here are some tips to keep in mind:

- It's possible that you will be referred to an HIV specialist by your HIV testing center or your primary healthcare provider. If not, you may want to locate resources in your community that can help you find a HIV service provider. You can always change your provider later if he or she is not a good fit.

- It's important to remember that not all providers are specialists in HIV. It's perfectly fine for you to ask them about their training or experience in treating people living with HIV. A good health-care provider will not be offended or defensive if you ask.

- You are entitled to quality care for your HIV disease. Geography or funding may limit your choices about who your care provider will be, but you have a right to expect treatment from a competent and caring medical professional.

Helping Your Provider Help You

Always be open and honest with your provider about things like the following:

- **Medication:** Have you missed any doses of medication? Have you taken them on time?

- **Side effects:** Are you experiencing any problems with your meds? Have you noticed any changes in your body (e.g., fatigue, weight loss, diarrhea) that might be related to your HIV meds?

- **Sexual activity:** Are you having sexual contact? Are you protecting yourself and your partner(s)?

Be prepared and on time to your provider visits. Bring all the necessary materials (see below) for you and your clinician to review.

If your provider asks you to take other medical tests or gives you a referral to a laboratory or another provider, follow up promptly. These tests and referrals need to be done on time so that you and your healthcare provider have the information and support you both need to manage your care and keep you healthy.

What to Bring to Your Appointment

- A list of any questions you may have about HIV disease, medications, etc. During an appointment, it can be easy to forget questions you meant to ask. Your best bet is to write them down and show them to your provider. Remember: There are no stupid questions!

- If you have gotten information from friends or the internet, it's a good idea to bring this up with your provider too.

- A list of all the medications you are currently taking, including nonprescription ones, like vitamins or other supplements (e.g., omega-3 fish oil), or the medications themselves. It is important for your providers to know this information because interactions between different medications in your body can have serious side effects, or make some of your HIV medications less effective.

- Your most recent lab results, if you have them

Section 17.2

Questions to Ask Your Doctor

Reprinted from "Questions to Ask Your Doctor about Your Diagnosis," "Questions to Ask Your Doctor about HIV Drugs," "Questions to Ask Your Doctor about Combination Therapy," and "Questions to Ask before Joining a Clinical Trial," U.S. Department of Veterans Affairs, December 15, 2009.

Questions to Ask Your Doctor about Your Diagnosis

To help you understand your diagnosis, here is a list of questions to ask your doctor:

- How much experience do you have treating human immunodeficiency virus (HIV) infection and acquired immunodeficiency syndrome (AIDS)?

- What do my lab tests say about the health of my immune system?

- How will you keep track of my immune system's health?

- What can I do to prevent complications, such as opportunistic infections, and stay healthy?

- What are the signs that I might be getting an opportunistic infection or AIDS-related cancer?

- Are there certain daily habits I should change in order to help me stay healthy?

- How much exercise should I aim for?

- How will I know whether I should start taking anti-HIV drugs?

- How can I protect others from getting infected with HIV?

Questions to Ask Your Doctor about HIV Drugs

One of the most important things you can do to make sure you take your medicine correctly is to talk with your doctor about your lifestyle, such as your sleeping and eating schedule. If your doctor prescribes a drug, be sure and ask the following questions (and make sure you understand the answers):

- What dose of the drug should be taken? How many pills does this mean?

- How often should the drug be taken?

- Does it matter if it is taken with food, or on an empty stomach?

- Does the drug have to be kept in a refrigerator?

- What are the side effects of the drug?

- What should be done to deal with the side effects?

- How severe do side effects have to be before a doctor is called?

- Does this medication interact with any other medications I am taking?

During every visit to your doctor, you should talk about whether you are having trouble staying on your treatment plan. Studies show that patients who take their medicine in the right way get the best results: their viral loads stay down, their CD4 counts stay up, and they feel healthier.

Questions to Ask Your Doctor about Combination Therapy

Here are some questions to ask your doctor when discussing taking combination drug therapy:

- How powerful is the combination?
- What are the possible side effects?
- How much is known about the combination?
- How many pills need to be taken, and how often do they need to be taken?
- Will a particular combination interact with other medications?

Questions to Ask before Joining a Clinical Trial

- Why are they doing the study in the first place?
- How long will it last, and where is it taking place?
- What will I have to pay for?
- Will I be able to continue taking the test drug after the trial is over? Who will pay for it?
- Will I have to stop any drugs or other treatments I am now using?

Chapter 18

Navigating the Healthcare System: What You Need to Know

It is important to remember: Human immunodeficiency virus (HIV) treatment is most successful for those people who stay engaged and active in their own care! Here are a few tips and tricks to keep in mind when you are moving through the medical and service system:

- Know your rights!

- As a client of HIV or acquired immunodeficiency syndrome (AIDS) service providers, you are entitled to the same rights as any other patient in the medical system—and those rights include safety, competent medical care, and confidentiality.

- Keep track of all the services you access and be knowledgeable about them.

- If you are living with HIV, you may work with multiple clinicians, including a primary care provider (doctor, nurse, etc.), as well as a case manager, dietician, dentist, social worker, therapist, and other specialist providers.

- In addition to your medical providers, you may benefit from access to food assistance programs, housing or home healthcare programs, or community support groups. It is important to find out what services are available in your local community and, if possible, engage your clinic's staff to help you access these services.

Excerpted from "Navigating the System: What You Need to Know to Work the System," AIDS.gov, October 2010.

- Keep records of your lab tests and other test results and the name of the provider who ordered them for you.

- Keep a written record of your doctor or provider visits, including your questions (and the answers you receive), tests, plan of care, and next appointment.

- Communicate with your providers. Be open and honest. Don't be afraid to ask questions!

- You always know more about your body and the way you are feeling than your provider does—and your provider can do a better job of helping you if you talk about what you are experiencing.

- Ask your care providers for copies of your test and lab results.

- What they don't know *can* hurt you! Be open and honest with them about things that might have an impact on your physical and mental health, including your sex life, changes in your personal life or living situation, your medications (side effects and missed doses), new research you may have done, your frustrations or concerns, etc.

- Let your providers know how they are doing—and be constructive with your criticisms. If you feel your care providers are doing a great job managing your care with you, tell them. Everyone likes to hear positive feedback! And if you are unhappy with your care, try to complain in a constructive way. Give specific examples of things that have made you unhappy with your care—and try to give your provider some positive suggestions on how the two of you can have a more satisfying relationship.

- Ask about clinical trial options!

- Always let your providers know when you are going to miss, reschedule, or be late to an appointment. If you have to cancel an appointment, always reschedule at the time you cancel! This will ensure that you don't forget and that you continue to get the care you need to stay healthy.

- Remember your provider's receptionist probably isn't a clinician, so if you are calling because you need help with a medical issue, the receptionist is unlikely to be able to help you. You will probably need to wait for your provider to call you back. Be sure you leave the information your provider will need to help you—including a detailed description of any symptoms or problems you may be having.

- Be prepared—and on time—for your appointments.

- Keep track of your appointments the same way you keep track of your other events or activities (phone, paper calendar, online calendar, etc.).

- If you are concerned about confidentiality, you could use a code word or activity on your calendar instead. For example, you could enter "late lunch" for your appointments with your doctor or "go to the grocery store" for your meetings with your HIV case manager.

- If possible, arrive a few minutes before your scheduled appointment time. A patient who is even ten minutes late can radically disrupt the schedule of a healthcare provider. Remember—your care providers want to give you all the time they possibly can, and it helps if you are there on time.

- Keep in mind you may have to wait when you arrive at your appointment. Providers don't always have control over what happens in the healthcare environment, and things can change rapidly. There may be someone ahead of you who has an emergency or needs extra attention that day. Be patient—you might be that person sometime!

- Follow up on your labs and get them drawn when your healthcare providers advise you to do so. If they ask you to do a test or a lab before your appointment, try to do so. Providers often ask you do this so they can review your results with you when you come in for your visit.

- Ask for copies of your labs and tests.

- Before you leave, ask when your next appointment will be and get a written reminder from the front desk. This will help you stay on track with your care and protect your health.

- Be prepared for lifelong learning!

- HIV research is constantly evolving and changing. It's important to keep up with new advances in care.

- Learn about your community's resources and become active in your community's HIV services.

- Learn about politics and HIV and how your government (local, state, and federal) responds to HIV issues.

- Read HIV-related publications, including magazines, journals, on-line blogs, and related materials.

Part Four

Treatments and Therapies for HIV/AIDS

Chapter 19

Antiretroviral Treatment

Chapter Contents

Section 19.1

Introduction to HIV and AIDS Treatment

Excerpted from "Introduction to HIV and AIDS Treatment," © 2010
AVERT (www.avert.org). All rights reserved. Reprinted with permission.

What Is HIV Antiretroviral Drug Treatment?

This is the main type of treatment for human immunodeficiency
virus (HIV) or acquired immunodeficiency syndrome (AIDS). It is not
a cure, but it can stop people from becoming ill for many years. The
treatment consists of drugs that have to be taken every day for the
rest of a person's life.

The aim of antiretroviral treatment is to keep the amount of HIV
in the body at a low level. This stops any weakening of the immune
system and allows it to recover from any damage that HIV might have
caused already.

The drugs are often referred to as:

- antiretrovirals;

- anti-HIV or anti-AIDS drugs;

- HIV antiviral drugs;

- ARVs.

What Is Combination Therapy?

Taking two or more antiretroviral drugs at a time is called combination therapy. Taking a combination of three or more anti-HIV
drugs is sometimes referred to as highly active antiretroviral therapy
(HAART).

Why Do People Need to Take More Than One Drug at a Time?

If only one drug was taken, HIV would quickly become resistant to
it and the drug would stop working. Taking two or more antiretrovirals

at the same time vastly reduces the rate at which resistance would develop, making treatment more effective in the long term.

How Many HIV and AIDS Drugs Are There?

There are more than twenty approved antiretroviral drugs but not all are licensed or available in every country. See Table 19.1 for a comprehensive list of antiretroviral drugs approved by the American Food and Drug Administration.

There are five groups of antiretroviral drugs. Each of these groups attacks HIV in a different way.

Table 19.1. The Groups of Antiretroviral Drugs

Antiretroviral drug class	Abbreviations	First approved to treat HIV	How they attack HIV
Nucleoside/Nucleotide Reverse Transcriptase Inhibitors	NRTIs, nucleoside analogues, nukes	1987	NRTIs interfere with the action of an HIV protein called reverse transcriptase, which the virus needs to make new copies of itself.
Non-Nucleoside Reverse Transcriptase Inhibitors	NNRTIs, non-nucleosides, non-nukes	1997	NNRTIs also stop HIV from replicating within cells by inhibiting the reverse transcriptase protein.
Protease Inhibitors	PIs	1995	PIs inhibit protease, which is another protein involved in the HIV replication process.
Fusion or Entry Inhibitors		2003	Fusion or entry inhibitors prevent HIV from binding to or entering human immune cells.
Integrase Inhibitors		2007	Integrase inhibitors interfere with the integrase enzyme, which HIV needs to insert its genetic material into human cells.

NRTIs and NNRTIs are available in most countries. Fusion/entry inhibitors and integrase inhibitors are usually only available in resource-rich countries.

Protease inhibitors are generally less suitable for starting treatment in resource-limited settings due to the cost, number of pills which need to be taken, and the particular side effects caused by protease drugs.

What Does Combination Therapy Usually Consist Of?

The most common drug combination given to those beginning treatment consists of two NRTIs combined with either an NNRTI or a "boosted" protease inhibitor. Ritonavir (in small doses) is most commonly used as the booster; it enhances the effects of other protease inhibitors so they can be given in lower doses. An example of a common antiretroviral combination is the two NRTIs zidovudine and lamivudine, combined with the NNRTI efavirenz.

Some antiretroviral drugs have been combined into one pill, which is known as a "fixed dose combination." This reduces the number of pills to be taken each day.

The choice of drugs to take can depend on a number of factors, including the availability and price of drugs, the number of pills, the side effects of the drugs, the laboratory monitoring requirements, and whether there are co-blister packs or fixed dose combinations available. Most people living with HIV in the developing world still have very limited access to antiretroviral treatment and often only receive treatment for the diseases that occur as a result of a weakened immune system. Such treatment has only short-term benefits because it does not address the underlying immune deficiency itself.

First and Second Line Therapy

At the beginning of treatment, the combination of drugs that a person is given is called first line therapy. If after a while HIV becomes resistant to this combination, or if side effects are particularly bad, then a change to second line therapy is usually recommended.

Second line therapy will ideally include a minimum of three new drugs, with at least one from a new class, in order to increase the likelihood of treatment success.

Section 19.2

Starting Anti-HIV Medications

Excerpted from "Starting Anti-HIV Medications," AIDSinfo.gov,
December 2009.

I am HIV-positive. Do I need to start anti-HIV medications?

Even though you are human immunodeficiency virus (HIV)–
positive, you may not need to start treatment right away. When to
start anti-HIV (also called antiretroviral) medications depends on
the following:

- Your overall health

- How well your immune system is working (CD4 count)

- The amount of virus in your blood (viral load)

You and your doctor will determine the best time to start treatment.

How will I know when to start anti-HIV medications?

It's time to start treatment if any of the following are true:

- You have severe symptoms of HIV infection or are diagnosed
  with acquired immunodeficiency syndrome (AIDS)

- Your CD4 count is below 500 cells/mm^3 (especially below 350
  cells/mm^3)

- You are pregnant

- You have HIV-related kidney disease

- You are being treated for hepatitis B

Some research suggests that it may be helpful to start treatment
early (when CD4 count is above 500 cells/mm^3). You may want to
discuss the risks and benefits of starting treatment early with your
doctor.

If anti-HIV medications can help me stay healthy, why wait to start treatment?

If you and your doctor feel that you are committed to lifelong treatment and prepared to take medications exactly as directed, you may begin treatment at any time. However, if you feel you aren't ready, you may decide to delay treatment. Delaying treatment will give you and your doctor time to work on a plan to handle issues that can affect treatment.

HIV treatment may affect your lifestyle. Some anti-HIV medications must be taken several times a day at specific times. When you start anti-HIV medications you may need to change what and when you eat. You may need to change the time you take other medications.

Taking your medications according to your doctor's directions (treatment adherence) is very important. Skipping doses or not taking anti-HIV medications as prescribed can make it easier for HIV to multiply. Your HIV can become resistant to the anti-HIV medications you take (drug resistance).

What treatment is right for me?

The U.S. Department of Health and Human Services (HHS) provides guidelines on using anti-HIV medications to treat HIV infection. The HHS guidelines recommend starting treatment with a combination (called a regimen) of three anti-HIV medications from at least two different classes. This is called highly active antiretroviral therapy (HAART). The guidelines list recommended HAART regimens. However, the recommended regimens may not be exactly right for everyone. You and your doctor will need to consider your individual needs when choosing a regimen.

Factors to consider in selecting a treatment regimen include the following:

- Your drug resistance testing results
- Results of other laboratory tests
- How many pills you will need to take and how often you will need to take them
- If you will need to take pills with food or on an empty stomach
- How medications in your regimen affect one another
- Other medications you take
- Other diseases or conditions you may have
- If you are pregnant or expect to become pregnant soon

Section 19.3

Recommended HIV Treatment Regimens

Excerpted from "Recommended HIV Treatment Regimens,"
AIDSinfo.gov, December 2009.

When I start treatment, what medications will I take?

Highly active antiretroviral therapy (HAART) is the recommended treatment for human immunodeficiency virus (HIV). HAART means taking a combination (regimen) of three or more anti-HIV (also called antiretroviral) medications from at least two different classes. Anti-HIV medications fall into six classes: non-nucleoside reverse transcriptase inhibitors (NNRTIs), nucleoside reverse transcriptase inhibitors (NRTIs), protease inhibitors (PIs), entry inhibitors, fusion inhibitors, and integrase inhibitors. Each class of medications blocks the virus in a different way. Taking a combination of medications from different classes makes treatment more effective at controlling the virus. It also reduces the risk of drug resistance.

Some of the medications are available as a combination pill of two or more different anti-HIV medications from one or more classes.

Which combination of anti-HIV medications should I take?

For people taking HAART for the first time, the preferred regimens (in alphabetical order) are as follows:

- Atripla® (a combination of three anti-HIV medications in one pill)
- Isentress® + Truvada® (a combination of two anti-HIV medications in one pill)
- Prezista® + Norvir® + Truvada®
- Reyataz® + Norvir® + Truvada®

Women who are planning on becoming pregnant or are in the first trimester of pregnancy should not use Atripla® or Sustiva®. (Sustiva is one of the three drugs in Atripla.) If you are pregnant or expect to become pregnant soon, talk to your doctor about the benefits and risks of taking anti-HIV medications.

A HAART regimen must meet a person's individual needs. There isn't a "best" regimen that works for everyone. If the preferred regimens are not right for you, there are several other treatment regimens. You and your doctor will select a regimen based on your needs.

In general, it's not recommended to include medications from only one class in a regimen. The number of pills you take (and how often you take them) will depend on the HAART regimen you and your doctor choose.

Will I have side effects from the medications I take?

You can have side effects from the medications in your treatment regimen. Possible side effects depend on the anti-HIV medication. People taking the same medications may not have the same side effects.

Most side effects are manageable; however, if side effects become unbearable or life threatening, you may have to change medications. Discuss possible side effects of the medications in your regimen with your doctor or pharmacist.

Side effects that may seem minor, such as fever, nausea, fatigue, or rash, can mean there are serious problems. Always discuss any side effects from your medications with your doctor.

Section 19.4

Deciding Which Drugs to Take

Excerpted from "Treatment," U.S. Department of Veterans Affairs,
December 15, 2009.

Once you and your doctor have decided that you should start taking drugs for human immunodeficiency virus (HIV), your doctor will come up with a personal treatment plan for you. You will find it easier to understand your plan if you learn about the different drugs available and what they do.

What Kinds of Drugs Are Available?

Anti-HIV drugs are also called antiretroviral drugs or antiretrovirals. They work because they attack the HIV virus directly. The drugs cripple the ability of the virus to make copies of itself.

There are several classes of anti-HIV drugs:

- Nucleoside reverse transcriptase inhibitors (NRTIs or "nukes")

- Non-nucleoside reverse transcriptase inhibitors (NNRTIs or "non-nukes")

- Protease inhibitors (PIs)

- Fusion or entry inhibitors

- Chemokine co-receptor antagonists (CCR5)

- Integrase inhibitors

Each group attacks HIV and helps your body fight the infection in its own way. Most of these drugs come as pills, capsules, or coated tablets. Several of these drugs may be combined into one tablet to make it easier to take your medications. These are known as fixed-dose combinations.

The following is a short description of how each group of drugs works and the names of the drugs. A new group of antiretrovirals is on the horizon: integrase inhibitors. Since this group is still in the experimental phase, and not yet widely available, we won't go beyond mentioning it here.

Note: The names of drugs are long and sometimes hard to pronounce. Don't worry! You can always come back and read this again, and you can talk to your doctor about questions you have.

Nucleoside Reverse Transcriptase Inhibitors (NRTIs or Nukes)

The first group of antiretroviral drugs is the nucleoside reverse transcriptase (say "trans-krip-tase") inhibitors (NRTIs).

NRTIs were the first type of drug available to treat HIV. They remain effective, powerful, and important medications for treating HIV when combined with other drugs. They are better known as nucleoside analogues or "nukes."

When the HIV virus enters a healthy cell, it attempts to make copies of itself. It does this by using an enzyme called reverse transcriptase. The NRTIs work because they block that enzyme. Without reverse transcriptase, HIV can't make new virus copies of itself.

The following is a list of the drugs in the NRTI class:

- Emtriva® (emtricitabine)
- Epivir® (3TC, lamivudine)
- Retrovir® (AZT, zidovudine)
- Videx-EC® (ddI, didanosine)
- Viread® (tenofovir)
- Zerit® (d4T, stavudine)
- Ziagen® (abacavir)

Several of the NRTI drugs may be combined into one tablet to make it easier to take your medications. These drugs are known as fixed-dose combinations:

- Combivir® (Retrovir®+ Epivir®)
- Epzicom® (Epivir® + Ziagen®)
- Trizivir® (Retrovir® + Epivir® + Ziagen®)
- Truvada® (Viread® + Emtriva®)

Non-Nucleoside Reverse Transcriptase Inhibitors (NNRTIs or Non-Nukes)

The second type of antiretroviral drugs is the non-nucleoside reverse transcriptase inhibitors (NNRTIs). These drugs are sometimes called non-nucleosides or "non-nukes."

These drugs also prevent HIV from using reverse transcriptase to make copies of itself, but in a different way.

Three NNRTIs are available:

- Rescriptor® (delavirdine)

- Sustiva® (efavirenz)

- Viramune® (nevirapine)

Protease Inhibitors (PIs)

The third group of drugs is the protease (say "pro-tee-ase") inhibitors (PIs).

Once HIV has infected a cell and made copies of itself, it uses an enzyme called protease to process itself correctly so it can be released from the cell to infect other cells. These medicines work by blocking protease.

Nine PIs are available:

- Aptivus® (tipranavir)

- Crixivan® (indinavir)

- Invirase® (saquinavir)

- Kaletra® (lopinavir + ritonavir combined in one tablet)

- Lexiva® (fosamprenavir)

- Norvir® (ritonavir)

- Prezista® (darunavir)

- Reyataz® (atazanavir)

- Viracept® (nelfinavir)

Note: Many PIs are recommended or approved for use only with low-dose Norvir, which "boosts" their effect.

Fusion or Entry Inhibitors

The fourth group of antiretrovirals is called fusion or entry inhibitors.

These medicines work by stopping the HIV virus from getting into your body's healthy cells in the first place.

Only one fusion inhibitor is available at present, and it needs to be injected:

- Fuzeon® (enfuvirtide, T-20)

Chemokine Co-receptor Antagonists (CCR5)

To infect a cell, HIV must bind to two types of molecules on the cell's surface.

One of these is called a chemokine co-receptor. Drugs known as chemokine co-receptor antagonists block the virus from binding to the molecules:

* Selzentry™ (maraviroc)

Which Drugs Should You Take?

Now that you have learned a little about the types of drugs that are available and how they work, you may be wondering how your healthcare provider will know which medicines you should take.

Anti-HIV drugs are used in combination with one another in order to get the best results. The goal is to get the viral load as low as possible for as long as possible.

Anti-HIV medicines do different things to the virus—they attack it in different ways—so using the different drugs in combination works better than using just one by itself.

Except in very special circumstances, anti-HIV drugs should never be used one or two at a time. Using only one or two drugs at a time can fail to control the viral load and let the virus adapt (or become resistant) to the drug. Once the virus adapts to a drug, the drug won't work as well against the virus, and maybe it won't work at all.

Experts haven't come up with one combination of HIV medications that works best for everyone. Each combination has its pluses and minuses.

When drugs are used together, it is called combination therapy (or HAART, highly active antiretroviral therapy).

Combination Therapy

So, how will your doctor know which combination to choose? You and your doctor can consider the options, keeping certain things in mind, such as possible side effects, the number of pills you'll need to take, and how the drugs interact with each other.

Chapter 20

HIV/AIDS Treatment Adherence

What Is Treatment Adherence?

What Is Adherence?

Adherence refers to how closely you follow a prescribed treatment regimen. It includes your willingness to start treatment and your ability to take medications exactly as directed.

Is Adherence Important for Human Immunodeficiency Virus (HIV) Treatment?

Yes! Adherence is a major issue in HIV treatment for two reasons:

- Adherence affects how well anti-HIV medications decrease your viral load. When you skip a medication dose, even just once, the virus has the opportunity to reproduce more rapidly. Keeping HIV replication at a minimum is essential for preventing acquired immunodeficiency syndrome (AIDS)–related conditions and death.

- Adherence to HIV treatment helps prevent drug resistance. When you skip doses, you may develop strains of HIV that are resistant to the medications you are taking and even to medications you have not yet taken. This may leave you with fewer treatment options should you need to change treatment

Excerpted from "What Is Treatment Adherence?" and "Adhering to My HIV Treatment Regimen," AIDSinfo.gov, December 2009.

regimens in the future. Because drug resistant strains can be transmitted to others, engaging in risky behavior can have especially serious consequences.

Although there are many different anti-HIV medications and treatment regimens, studies show that your first regimen has the best chance for long-term success. Taking your anti-HIV medications correctly (adherence) increases your odds of success.

Why Is Adherence Difficult for Many People with HIV?

HIV treatment regimens can be complicated; most regimens involve taking multiple pills each day. Some anti-HIV medications must be taken on an empty stomach, while others must be taken with meals or before or after doses of other medications. This can be difficult for many people, especially for those who are sick or are experiencing HIV symptoms or negative side effects caused by their medications.

Other factors that can make it difficult to adhere to an HIV treatment regimen include the following:

- Experiencing unpleasant side effects to your medications (such as nausea)
- Sleeping through doses
- Traveling away from home
- Being too busy
- Feeling sick or depressed
- Forgetting to take medications

What Can I Do to Adhere to My Treatment Regimen?

There are many things you can do to better adhere to your treatment regimen.

One of the most important things you can do when starting a treatment regimen is to talk with your doctor about your lifestyle. He or she will then be able to prescribe a regimen that works best for you. Topics you should address with your doctor include the following:

- Your work, sleep, eating, and travel schedules
- Possible side effects of medications
- Other medications you are taking and their possible interaction with anti-HIV medications

- Your level of commitment to following an HIV treatment regimen

- Not being able to afford the medications

Many people adhere well to their treatment early on but find adherence becomes more difficult over time. Talk with your doctor about adherence during every visit. Your commitment to a treatment plan is critical; studies show that patients who take their medications correctly achieve the best results.

Adhering to My HIV Treatment Regimen

What Should I Do Before I Begin Treatment?

Before you begin an HIV treatment regimen, there are several steps you can take to help you with adherence:

- Talk with your doctor about your treatment regimen.

- Get a written copy of your treatment plan that lists each medication; when and how much to take; and if it must be taken with food, on an empty stomach, or before or after doses of other medications.

- Understand how important adherence is.

- Be honest about personal issues that may affect your adherence. Adherence may be harder for people dealing with substance abuse or alcoholism, unstable housing, mental illness, or other life challenges.

- Consider a "dry run." Practice your treatment regimen using vitamins, jellybeans, or mints. This will help you determine ahead of time which doses might be difficult to take correctly.

- Develop a plan that works for you.

Many people find it helpful to identify the activities they normally do at the times they will be taking their medication. People who arrange their medication schedule around their daily routines adhere to their treatment plans better than those who do not.

How Can I Maintain Adherence After I Start Treatment?

- Take your medication at the same time each day.

- Put a week's worth of medication in a pillbox at the beginning of each week.

- Use timers, alarm clocks, or pagers to remind you when to take your medication.

- Keep your medication in the place where you will take it. You may want to keep backup supplies of your medication at your workplace or in your briefcase or purse.

- Keep a medication diary. Write the names of your medications in your daily planner, then check off each dose as you take it.

- Plan ahead for weekends, holidays, and changes in routine.

- Develop a support network of family members, friends, or co-workers who can remind you to take your medication. Some people also find it helpful to join a support group for people living with HIV infection.

- Monitor your medication supply. Contact your doctor or clinic if your supply will not last until your next visit.

What Should I Do If I Have Problems Adhering to My Treatment Regimen?

It is important that you tell your doctor right away about any problems you are having with your treatment plan. If you are experiencing unpleasant side effects, your dose may need to be adjusted or you may need a change in your regimen. Missed doses may be a sign that your treatment plan is too complicated or unrealistic for you to follow. Talk with your doctor about other treatment options. Your doctor needs to stay informed to help you get the most out of your treatment regimen and to provide workable treatment options.

Chapter 21

HIV/AIDS Treatment Interruptions

The reasons why someone may want to take a break from therapy can vary from treatment fatigue to struggling with adherence issues to avoiding side effects. Various structured treatment interruptions (STIs) have been studied since the late 1990s with mixed results. Taken as a whole, STI research suggests that their risks greatly outweigh their possible benefits.

A General Caution on STIs

Taking an STI involves going off human immunodeficiency virus (HIV) therapy for a period of time in a strategic way. This is usually paired with more frequent lab tests and health check-ups. Taking an STI is considered experimental since no conclusive data can recommend it as standard care.

Should you wish to try an STI, you should only do so with the full support of your doctor(s) who are experienced with them. Most STIs are generally unsafe and some may only be safe for certain people.

Someone who takes an STI may face the typical symptoms seen in acute infection. These can occur within the first few weeks after starting one. Symptoms are flu-like and can include fever, muscle aches, swollen lymph nodes, and rash.

"Structured Treatment Interruptions," © 2010 Project Inform. Reprinted with permission. For more information, contact the National HIV/AIDS Treatment Hotline, 1-800-822-7422, or visit www.projectinform.org.

It's important to check CD4 counts and HIV levels before and after the STI as well as resume HIV therapy and prevent opportunistic infections (OIs) as needed.

The Most Notable Research to Date

The Salmeterol Multicenter Asthma Research Trial (SMART) study compared two strategies in nearly six thousand people worldwide: continued treatment vs. regularly interrupted treatment as guided by CD4 counts. The researchers expected that by keeping people off their meds for periods of time, there would be lower rates of certain conditions like heart disease.

The opposite was true. SMART was stopped early when its data showed that people who interrupted treatment had higher rates of illness and death. Some believe these results are so bad that STIs have been proven to be risky and should be avoided in most cases. Others feel that SMART raises some concerns, but studying other STIs should still continue.

SMART isn't the only study to highlight the dangers of STIs. Others—like PART, DART (Development of Anti-Retroviral Therapy in Africa), and TRIVICAN—have shown similar results. However, one Swiss study found that STIs may be safe for people who started HIV therapy at higher CD4 counts.

Using an STI to Reinvigorate the Immune Response

HIV disease progression may be due in part to the loss of a potent type of immune cell, called a CTL, or HIV-specific cytotoxic lymphocyte. These cells seek out and destroy HIV-infected cells. Some findings indicate that some people who stay well for many years without HIV therapy maintain their CTLs, while those who progress more rapidly do not.

Research was designed to study how STIs could preserve, restore, or enhance the body's natural immune responses in both early and established HIV infections. These included giving treatment within the first few weeks or months after acute HIV infection followed by an STI as well as STIs taken with therapeutic vaccines.

By starting and stopping therapy at regular intervals, it was hoped that with each STI the immune system would become more able to control HIV on its own. However, the results were the opposite of what was expected. Those who had started therapy just before or after acute infection had fairly weak responses with CTLs. They were boosted somewhat during the STI but then surprisingly they decreased back to lower levels after restarting therapy. Similar results were found in several other studies in people with long-term infection.

Other studies combined STIs with immune therapies or therapeutic vaccines. The hope here was that these therapies, when used with an STI, would provide the needed "lift" to bring on a stronger immune response. Again, the results were not promising. Therefore, people who hope to "boost" their immune systems should not look to STIs as an answer.

Using an STI to Help People with Treatment Fatigue

Treatment fatigue is when a person is "tired" of taking HIV medicines due to physical or emotional tiredness. For those who wish to take an STI for this reason, the data are somewhat conflicting. Several factors can help predict when a person may have a poorer outcome:

- Low CD4 count before first starting therapy (below 200)
- High HIV level before first starting therapy (above 55,000)
- Poor control of virus while on therapy or other signs of drug resistance
- History of opportunistic infections

Several studies used CD4 counts and HIV levels as a guide for when to restart therapy after one STI. Nearly all were done in people who had reached undetectable HIV levels in their last twelve months or beyond and CD4 counts above 350 in their last six months.

In most studies, at least one in three of the people could stay off therapy for at least one year. However, the average time off therapy for the others ranged from eight to twelve weeks. Some were able to control their HIV levels during the first STI; others needed two or three of them. It should be noted that people on STIs had large drops in their CD4 counts (on average by half). These decreases could be dangerous when CD4s drop below 200, especially without preventive medicine for OIs.

Also, most studies were unable to measure meaningful improvements in cholesterol and triglycerides in people on STIs. Dropout rates also tended to be higher among those on STIs. This indicates that STIs may actually be harder to manage than taking pills every day.

For people who wish to take an STI due to treatment fatigue, certain guidelines can be followed. Careful monitoring by your doctor is critical during this time. People should check to see if their insurance will cover the additional lab tests.

Testing your HIV level and CD4 count should be done before the STI and three months after, if not sooner. You and your doctor should decide beforehand what factors would lead you to resume therapy, at least using the federal guidelines as a guide. Also, resistance tests should be done when HIV levels are at their highest.

If your CD4 count was ever below 200, or you ever had an OI, it's risky to take an STI to deal with treatment fatigue. People taking an STI usually see their CD4 counts fall fairly quickly to pre-treatment levels.

Some data show it may be safe for people who started therapy early in their infection to go off treatment safely. Swiss researchers looked at people who began taking HIV drugs when their CD4 counts were over 500. They had the option to stop or continue their HIV treatment. The researchers found no evidence of harm in those on STIs.

However, other research suggests the opposite. An analysis from SMART found that people who restarted their meds when the study was stopped continued to have higher rates of heart, liver, and kidney problems compared to those on continuous treatment.

Using an STI Before Starting Third Line Therapy

When a person tries to create a new regimen which may contain drugs that had failed before, the regimen is often referred to as third line or salvage or even rescue therapy. Some studies looked at using STIs before starting third line therapy hopefully to improve these drugs' suppression of HIV.

The reason for this is that when a person goes off therapy to which HIV has become resistant, the new virus will revert to what is called wild-type. This is the strain that reproduces most easily and responds to HIV therapy. Therefore, a drug that had stopped working before could sometimes regain some of its potency.

A Barcelona study found that a three-month STI before starting third line therapy did not provide any advantage. However, the French giga-HAART study, using a shorter STI, showed that people taking an STI had larger reductions in HIV than those without an STI.

San Francisco researchers conducted a similar study using a four-month STI before starting salvage therapy to others who started their regimens immediately. In contrast to the French study, these results showed no benefits in viral response. In fact, people on the STI were more likely to develop an OI or die.

Using an STI to Reduce the Costs and Side Effects of Therapy

Another form of STI studied was one designed mainly to cut the time a person spent on treatment. This was the basis for SMART, and several other studies. As mentioned, SMART found higher rates of heart and other problems as well as poorer quality of life for people on STIs. Another study, where volunteers went off and on therapy every fourteen days, resulted in some of them developing drug-resistant virus and losing control of their HIV levels.

Another small study, this time with cycles of seven days off and on therapy, resulted in fewer side effects and better quality of life for people on STIs. Their HIV levels were also well controlled. However, a similar study in Thailand conflicted with these results, so it's impossible to state for certain whether STIs of this type work.

A Final Word on STIs

It's fair to say that the trend in research has been solidly against STIs for some time now. While it may be safe for people who began therapy with high CD4 counts, for most people the research suggest the risks of STIs probably outweigh their benefits.

Some have called for an outright halt to all STI research. Project Inform does not share this belief. The burdens of lifelong treatment are significant, as is the challenge of adherence. If safer ways of managing STIs can be developed, then they should be studied. We should remain hopeful and examine every piece of new information as the possible thread that will lead us one day to a cure.

Chapter 22

Monitoring HIV/AIDS Treatment Success

Chapter Contents

Section 22.1

Viral Load Test

Excerpted from "Viral Load," AIDS.gov, October 2010.

What Is "Viral Load"?

When healthcare providers discuss your "viral load," they are talking about the level of human immunodeficiency virus (HIV) in your blood. Knowing your viral load helps your provider to monitor your HIV disease, decide when to start treatment, and determine whether or not your HIV medications are working once you begin taking them.

There is usually a relationship between your viral load and the number of CD4 cells you have. Typically, if your viral load is high, your CD4 count will be low—making you more vulnerable to opportunistic infections. The antiretroviral medications you may take for your HIV disease work to keep HIV from reproducing in your body. This lowers your viral load and protects your immune system.

"Normal" Viral Load

There really is no such thing as a "normal" viral load. People who aren't infected with HIV have no viral load at all, so there's no "normal" range for reference, as there is with many other lab tests (including CD4 counts).

Viral load testing looks for the number of virus particles in a milliliter of your blood. These particles are called "copies."

The goal of HIV treatment is to help move your viral load down to undetectable levels. In general, your viral load will be declared "undetectable" if it is under 40 to 75 copies in a sample of your blood (the exact number depends on the lab performing the test).

Changes in Viral Load

Your viral load changes over time. Typically, after you are first infected with HIV, your viral load will be extremely high—sometimes numbering in the millions in one blood sample. But your immune system responds and eventually brings your viral load back to a set point.

In general, your viral load continues to remain at low levels early in the course of your HIV disease, once the initial infection period has passed. It does begin to increase over time, however—eventually destroying more and more CD4 cells, until your CD4 count begins to show major damage to your immune system. At this point, treatment becomes necessary.

Viral Load Testing—When and How Often?

Your HIV healthcare provider will probably order a viral load test at your first visit after you are diagnosed, in order to establish a baseline level. After that, you will probably have a viral load test every three to six months, before you begin a new HIV medication, and two to eight weeks after starting or changing therapies.

The trend of your viral load (whether it's rising or falling) over time is what's really important—not an individual test result.

Viral Load and Beginning HIV Treatment

For most healthcare providers, your CD4 count will be the major factor in deciding whether to recommend that you begin treatment for your HIV disease. Federal HIV treatment guidelines recommend that you begin treatment when your CD4 count falls below 350 cells/mm³.

But because of the strong association between increased viral load and increased destruction of CD4 cells, some providers may decide to start treatment based on your viral load alone.

Viral Load and Transmission of HIV

Studies have found that having a low viral load greatly decreases the risk that you will pass HIV to someone else through sexual contact.

But having a low viral load does not guarantee that you won't transmit HIV to someone else. Even when the viral load in your blood is undetectable, HIV can still exist in semen, vaginal and rectal fluids, breast milk, and other parts of your body.

You should continue to take steps to prevent HIV transmission, even when your viral load is undetectable. You can protect your partner(s) by using condoms consistently and correctly for all sexual contact.

Section 22.2

CD4 Test

Excerpted from "CD4 Count," AIDS.gov, October 2010.

What Is a CD4 Cell or T-Cell?

CD4 cells or T-cells are the "generals" of the human immune system. These are the cells that send signals to activate your body's immune response when they detect "intruders," like viruses or bacteria.

Because of the important role these cells play in how your body fights off infections, it's important to keep their numbers up in the normal ranges. This helps to prevent human immunodeficiency virus (HIV)–related complications and opportunistic infections.

The Name Game

You may have noticed that your healthcare providers often use the terms "T-cell" and "CD4 cell" interchangeably. When talking in terms of HIV, these two names mean the same thing. They both refer to the same type of cell. While there are many different types of T-cells, these particular cells have a specific receptor site on their surface called the CD4 receptor site. HIV uses this particular receptor to latch on to the T-cell, making it a prime target for infection.

It's All About the Numbers!

Ok, it's not all about the numbers—but your CD4 count is one of the most important things to consider when you and your healthcare provider are deciding the best way—and time—to treat your HIV disease.

A normal CD4 count can range from 500 cells/mm³ to 1,000 cells/mm³. So if your CD4 count is within that range, the Centers for Disease Control and Prevention (CDC) do not generally recommend that you start treatment for your HIV disease, unless there are other concerns (pregnancy, young age, constitutional symptoms, acute retroviral syndrome, etc.).

The guidelines from the U.S. Department of Health and Human Services suggest starting treatment when your CD4 count falls to 350 cells/mm^3 or below. This is because opportunistic infections typically begin to affect people whose CD4 counts are below that level. (This is why a CD4 count is often used to determine the stages of HIV disease.)

Recent research has indicated that it may be easier to maintain higher CD4 counts if you start HIV treatment before your CD4 counts drop below 350 cells/mm^3. You should discuss when to begin treatment with your healthcare provider and choose the approach that is best for you.

The Basics

- A normal CD4 count ranges from 500 to 1,000 cells/mm^3.

- When your CD4 count is 350 cells/mm^3 or less, it's time to consider treatment.

- A CD4 count of fewer than 200 cells/mm^3 is one of the qualifications for a diagnosis of acquired immunodeficiency syndrome (AIDS).

- Your CD4 count can vary from day to day. It can also vary depending on the time of day your blood is drawn and on whether you have other infections or illnesses, like the flu or sexually transmitted diseases (STDs).

- Typically, your healthcare provider will check your CD4 counts every three to six months.

Section 22.3

Drug Resistance Test

Excerpted from "Resistance Test,"
AIDS.gov, October 2010.

What Is "Resistance?"

"Resistance" occurs when the medicines you may be taking for your human immunodeficiency virus (HIV) disease can't stop the virus from making more copies of itself—a process known as replication.

What Causes Resistance?

Resistance is caused by the way HIV makes new copies of itself.

If you aren't being treated for your HIV disease, it can make billions of new virus particles every day.

But that replication process isn't perfect. HIV multiplies so quickly that it makes a lot of genetic mistakes in the new copies. If these imperfect copies of the virus are able to go on to create copies of themselves, they are known as mutations.

Mutations are good for viruses—but they can be bad news for people living with HIV. That's because HIV medications may not work on mutations. We say that HIV is "drug-resistant" when it can multiply quickly in your body, even though you are taking medications to stop that from happening.

Preventing Resistance

The best way to prevent resistance is to keep HIV from replicating. If it isn't reproducing, the virus can't mutate and make new strains of HIV that are drug-resistant.

That's what antiretroviral drugs do—they keep HIV from reproducing. And that's why it's important to take all your HIV medications on time and consistently. When you do that, your medications can do a better job of keeping the virus under control and keep it from mutating into strains that won't respond to treatment.

Testing Positive and Resistant

Drug-resistant HIV can be passed from one person to another. That's one reason why it's important to have drug resistance testing soon after you test positive for HIV—you need to know as soon as possible if your particular strain of HIV is drug-resistant, so that you and your providers can make the best choices for your care.

Testing for Resistance

There are two types of resistance tests: a genotypic assay and a phenotypic assay. These are scientific terms that describe the way each test measures resistance.

Genotypic assays look directly at the genetic material of the HIV in your blood and give you information about the HIV drugs your virus is resistant to. Genotypic assays are the most common and widely used resistance tests. They usually take about one to two weeks to come back from the lab. They are less expensive than phenotypic assays.

Phenotypic assays actually measure how well the virus responds to medications in a controlled environment, such as a laboratory. It typically takes two to three weeks to get your results. It is easier for care providers to interpret those results. Phenotypic assays are used if you have multiple HIV mutations and/or multiple forms of treatment have not worked for you.

Chapter 23

HIV/AIDS Treatment Side Effects

Chapter Contents

Section 23.1

Common
Side Effects

Excerpted from "Side Effects Guide," U.S.
Department of Veterans Affairs, December 15, 2009.

Overview

Almost all medicines have side effects, including medicines for human immunodeficiency virus (HIV). Always let your doctor know if your side effects are severe, especially if you are finding it difficult to stay on your treatment plan.

The following is information on some common side effects and tips on how to deal with them.

Anemia

Anemia means you have a low red blood cell count. The red blood cells take oxygen to different parts of the body, and when your body is short of oxygen, you feel tired.

Many people with HIV have anemia at some point. HIV can cause it; so can some of the anti-HIV drugs.

To see if you have anemia (a symptom of anemia is feeling tired, fatigued, or short of breath), your healthcare provider can do a simple blood test. If you are anemic, food or other medicines can help.

Quick Tips: Anemia

If you find out you have anemia, your doctor will prescribe a treatment according to the cause of the anemia. Some of these treatments include the following:

- Changing medications

- Taking iron, folate, or vitamin B_{12}

- Changing your diet

Diarrhea

Diarrhea is common in people with HIV, and it can be caused by some anti-HIV medicines. Diarrhea can range from being a small hassle to being a serious medical problem. Talk to your healthcare provider if diarrhea goes on for a long time, if it is bloody, if it is accompanied by fever, or if it worries you.

Quick Tips: Diarrhea

What to try:

- Try the BRATT diet (bananas, rice, applesauce, tea, and toast).

- Eat foods high in soluble fiber. This kind of fiber can slow the diarrhea by soaking up liquid. Soluble fiber is found in oatmeal, grits, and soft bread (but not in whole grain).

- Try psyllium husk fiber bars (another source of soluble fiber). You can find these at health food stores.

- Ask your doctor about taking calcium pills.

- Drink plenty of clear liquids.

Dry Mouth

Certain HIV medicines can cause dry mouth, making it difficult to chew, swallow, and talk.

Treating dry mouth can be simple—start by drinking plenty of liquids during or between meals. If your dry mouth is severe or doesn't go away, talk to your doctor about prescribing a treatment for you.

Quick Tips: Dry Mouth

- Rinse your mouth throughout the day with warm, salted water.

- Carry sugarless candies, lozenges, or crushed ice with you to cool the mouth and give it moisture.

- Try slippery elm or licorice tea (available in health food stores). They can moisten the mouth, and they taste great!

- Ask your doctor about mouth rinse and other products to treat your dry mouth.

Fatigue

Many people feel tired, especially when they are stressed or their lives are busier than usual. Symptoms of being tired can include: having a hard time getting out of bed, walking up stairs, or even concentrating on something for very long.

If the tiredness (or fatigue) doesn't go away, even after you have given your body and mind time to rest, this tiredness can become a problem. It can get worse if you don't deal with it.

Quick Tips: Fatigue

- Get plenty of rest.

- Go to sleep and wake up at the same time every day. Changing your sleeping habits too much can actually make you feel tired.

- Try to get some exercise.

- Keep prepackaged or easy-to-make food in the kitchen for times when you're too tired to cook.

- Follow a healthy, balanced diet. Your healthcare provider may be able to help you create a meal plan.

- Talk to your doctor about the possibility that you have anemia. Anemia means that you have a low red blood cell count, and it can make you feel tired.

Hair Loss

Many people lose their hair as they get older, or when they are going through a very stressful time in their lives.

You can also lose your hair from taking certain medications, including those used to treat HIV.

Quick Tips: Hair Loss

- To stop any more hair loss, stay away from doing such things as dyeing, perming, and straightening your hair.

- If losing your hair is very upsetting for you and causing anxiety, you may want to talk to you doctor about whether you can try something like Rogaine®, which is a medicine that helps your hair to regrow.

- Since stress can make hair loss worse, try to reduce stress and anxiety in your life.

Headaches

The most common cause of headaches is tension or stress, something we all have from time to time. Medications, including anti-HIV drugs, can cause them, too.

Headaches usually can be taken care of with drugs you can buy without a prescription, such as aspirin. You can also help to prevent future headaches by reducing stress.

Quick Tips: Headaches

For on-the-spot headache relief, try some of these suggestions:

- Lie down and rest in a quiet, dark room.
- Take a hot, relaxing bath.
- Give yourself a "scalp massage"—massage the base of your skull with your thumbs and massage both temples gently.
- Check with your doctor about taking an over-the-counter pain reliever, such as aspirin.

To prevent headaches from happening again, try the following:

- Avoid things that can cause headaches, like chocolate, red wine, onions, hard cheese, and caffeine.
- Reduce your stress level.

Nausea and Vomiting

Certain medications used to treat HIV can cause nausea. They make you feel sick to your stomach and want to throw up. This usually goes away a few weeks after starting a new medication.

Call your doctor if you vomit repeatedly throughout the day, or if nausea or vomiting keeps you from taking your medication.

Quick Tips: Nausea and Vomiting

What to try:

- Eat smaller meals and snack more often.
- The BRATT Diet (bananas, rice, applesauce, tea, and toast) helps with nausea and diarrhea.
- Leave dry crackers by your bed. Before getting out of bed in the morning, eat a few and stay in bed for a few minutes. This can help reduce nausea.

- Try some herbal tea—such as peppermint or ginger tea.

- Sip cold, carbonated drinks such as ginger ale or Sprite.

- Open your windows when cooking so the smell of food won't be too strong.

- Talk with your healthcare provider about whether you should take medicine for your nausea.

- If you do vomit, be sure to "refuel" your body with fluids such as broth, carbonated beverages, juice, or popsicles.

Pain and Nerve Problems

HIV itself and some medications for HIV can cause damage to your nerves. This condition is called peripheral neuropathy. When these nerves are damaged, your feet, toes, and hands can feel like they're burning or stinging. It can also make them numb or stiff.

You should talk to your doctor if you have pain like this.

Quick Tips: Pain and Nerve Problems

- Massaging your feet can make the pain go away for a while.

- Soak your feet in ice water to help with the pain.

- Wear loose-fitting shoes and slippers.

- When you're in bed, don't cover your feet with blankets or sheets. The bedding can press down on your feet and toes and make the pain worse.

- Ask your doctor about taking an over-the-counter pain reliever to reduce the pain and swelling.

Rash

Some medications can cause skin problems, such as rashes. Most rashes come and go, but sometimes they signal that you are having a bad reaction to the medication.

It's important that you check your skin for changes, especially after you start a new medication. Be sure to report any changes to your healthcare provider.

Quick Tips: Rash

- Avoid extremely hot showers or baths. Water that is too hot can irritate the skin.

- Avoid being in the sun. Sun exposure can make your rash worse.

- Keep medications such as Benadryl® on hand in case you develop a rash. Ask your doctor for suggestions.

- Try using unscented, non-soapy cleansers for the bath or shower.

- A rash that blisters, or involves your mouth, the palms of your hands, or the soles of your feet, or one that is accompanied by shortness of breath, can be dangerous: contact your doctor right away.

Weight Loss

Weight loss goes along with some of these other side effects. It can happen because of vomiting, nausea, fatigue, and other reasons.

Talk with your healthcare provider if you're losing weight without trying, meaning that you're not on a reducing diet.

Quick Tips: Weight Loss

- Be sure to keep track of your weight, by stepping on scales and writing down how much you weigh. Tell your doctor if there are any changes.

- Create your own high-protein drink by blending together yogurt, fruit (for sweetness), and powdered milk, whey protein, or soy protein.

- Between meals, try store-bought nutritional beverages or bars (such as Carnation Instant Breakfast®, Benefit®, Ensure®, Scandishake®, Boost High Protein®, NuBasics®). Look for ones that are high in proteins, not sugars or fats.

- Spread peanut butter on toast, crackers, fruit, or vegetables.

- Add cottage cheese to fruit and tomatoes.

- Add canned tuna to casseroles and salads.

- Add shredded cheese to sauces, soups, omelets, baked potatoes, and steamed vegetables.

- Eat yogurt on your cereal or fruit.

- Eat hard-boiled (hard-cooked) eggs. Use them in egg salad sandwiches or slice and dice them for tossed salads.

- Add diced or chopped meats to soups, salads, and sauces.

- Add dried milk powder, whey protein, soy protein, or egg white powder to foods (for example, scrambled eggs, casseroles, and milkshakes).

Section 23.2

Hepatotoxicity and Lactic Acidosis

"Risk to Your Liver (Hepatotoxicity)," from AIDSmeds.com.
Reprinted with permission. Copyright © 2010 CDM Publishing, L.L.C.

Introduction

The liver is one of the largest and most important organs in the human body. It is located behind the lower right section of your ribs and carries out numerous functions that your body requires to remain healthy. These are just a few of the liver's many functions:

- Storing important nutrients from the food that you eat.

- Building necessary chemicals that your body needs to stay healthy.

- Breaking down harmful substances, like alcohol and other toxic chemicals.

- Removing waste products from your blood.

For human immunodeficiency virus (HIV)–positive people, the liver is of major importance, as it is responsible for making new proteins needed by the immune system, helps the body to resist infection, and processes many of the drugs used to treat HIV and acquired immunodeficiency syndrome (AIDS)–related infections. Unfortunately, these same medications can also damage the liver, which can prevent the liver from performing all of its necessary tasks and can eventually cause damage to the liver.

"Hepatotoxicity" is the official term for liver damage caused by medications and other chemicals. This section has been prepared to help readers better understand hepatotoxicity, including the ways in which medications can cause liver damage, the factors that can increase the risk of hepatotoxicity, and some of the ways in which you can monitor and protect the health of your liver. If you have questions or concerns about hepatotoxicity, particularly as it relates to the antiretroviral (ARV) drugs you are taking, do not be afraid to discuss them with your doctor.

How Do ARV Drugs Cause It?

Even though HIV drugs are intended to do your health good, the liver recognizes these medications as toxic compounds. After all, they are not naturally produced by the body and do contain some chemicals that could potentially cause damage to your body. Working with the kidneys and other organs, the liver processes these drugs to render them safer. In the process, the liver can become "overworked," which can lead to liver damage.

There are actually two ways that HIV meds can lead to liver damage.

Direct Damage to Liver Cells

Liver cells, called hepatocytes, play a vital role in the functioning of the liver. If these cells begin working too hard to remove chemicals from the blood, or if they are harmed by other infections (e.g., hepatitis C virus), abnormal chemical reactions can occur that can damage these cells. There are actually three ways in which this can happen:

- **Taking a very high dose of a drug:** If you were to swallow a high dose of an ARV drug or another medication (i.e., taking many pills when you are supposed to take one or two), this can cause immediate and sometimes severe damage to liver cells. Almost any drug, if an overdose is taken, can cause this type of liver damage.

- **Taking standard doses of medication for a long period of time:** If you take medications on a regular basis for a long period of time, there is also a risk of damage to these liver cells. This usually occurs after several months or years of taking certain medications. Protease inhibitors have the ability to cause damage to liver cells if they are used for long periods of time.

- **An allergic reaction:** When we hear the term "allergic reaction," we often think of itchy skin or runny eyes. However, allergic reactions can also take place in the liver. If you are allergic to a particular drug, your immune system can cause your liver to become inflamed as a result of interactions between key liver proteins and the drug. If the drug is not stopped, the inflammation can worsen and can cause serious damage to the liver. Two HIV drugs known to cause such allergic reactions (sometimes referred to as "hypersensitivity") in HIV-positive people are Ziagen® (abacavir) and Viramune® (nevirapine). Allergic reactions such as these usually occur within a few weeks or months after the drug is started and either may or may not be accompanied by other allergy-related symptoms (e.g., fever or a rash).

- **Non-allergic liver damage:** Some drugs can cause liver damage without an allergic reaction or use at high doses. Two particular HIV drugs that can cause serious liver damage, though in relatively small numbers of people, are Aptivus® (tipranavir) and Prezista® (darunavir). People with hepatitis B virus (HBV) or hepatitis C virus (HCV).

Lactic Acidosis

Nucleoside reverse transcriptase inhibitors (NRTIs) are not processed by the liver; they are removed from the bloodstream and from the body by the kidneys. Thus, many experts once speculated that these drugs would not likely cause damage to the liver. But we now know that these drugs can damage "cellular mitochondria," the "powerhouses" inside cells that convert nutrients into energy. This can cause levels of lactate, a cellular waste product, to become elevated. If these levels become too high, a condition called lactic acidosis can occur, which can result in liver problems, including a buildup of fat in and around the liver and liver inflammation.

How Do I Find Out If My ARV Drugs Are Causing Liver Damage?

The best indicator of hepatotoxicity is an increase in certain liver enzymes that circulate in the bloodstream. The most important enzymes are AST (aspartate aminotransferase), ALT (alanine aminotransferase), alkaline phosphatase, and bilirubin. These four enzymes are normally checked as a part of a "chem screen," a panel of tests that your doctor probably orders every time you have blood drawn to check your CD4 cells and viral load.

If you or your doctor has any reason to suspect that a drug you are taking has been causing liver injury, then a blood test should be performed. It is always best to detect hepatotoxicity in its early stages so that steps can be taken to prevent it from getting worse and to allow the liver to heal.

Most of the time, hepatotoxicity takes several months or years to develop and usually begins with mild increases in either AST or ALT that progresses to more serious increases. Generally speaking, if your AST or ALT levels are elevated but are no higher than five times the normal range (e.g., AST above 43 IU/L but below 215 IU/L or ALT above 60 IU/L but below 300 IU/L), you have mild to moderate hepatotoxicity. If your AST is higher than 215 IU/L or your ALT is above 300 IU/L, you have severe hepatotoxicity, which can lean to permanent liver damage and serious problems.

Fortunately, as stated above, the vast majority of doctors order chem screens on a regular basis (every three to six months) and are usually able to catch mild to moderate hepatotoxicity (which is often reversible) before it progresses to severe hepatotoxicity. However, some drugs, such as Ziagen® (abacavir) and Viramune® (nevirapine), can result in an allergic reaction in the liver that can cause liver enzymes to increase sharply soon after the medication is started. In turn, it is very important that your doctor check your liver enzymes every two weeks for the first three months if you begin taking either of these medications.

Increased liver enzymes can rarely be felt. In other words, you may not have any physical symptoms, even if your liver enzymes are elevated. Thus, it is very important that you and your doctor monitor your liver enzymes on a regular basis using blood tests. However, symptoms can occur in people with severe hepatotoxicity and these symptoms are very similar to those associated with viral hepatitis (e.g., hepatitis B or hepatitis C). Symptoms of hepatitis include:

- anorexia (loss of appetite);
- malaise (feeling unwell);
- nausea;
- vomiting;
- light-colored stools;
- unusual tiredness/weakness;
- stomach or abdominal pain;
- jaundice (yellowing of the skin or whites of the eyes);
- loss of taste for cigarettes.

If you are experiencing any of these symptoms, it is very important that you speak with your doctor or another healthcare provider.

Does Hepatotoxicity Occur in Everyone Taking ARV Drugs?

No, it does not. There have been a number of studies looking at the percentage of patients who develop hepatotoxicity, according to the different ARV medications they are taking. One particular study, conducted by researchers at the National Institutes of Health, looked at rates of hepatotoxicity among 10,611 HIV-positive people participating in twenty-one government-funded clinical trials conducted between 1991 and 2000. Overall, 6.2 percent of the clinical trial participants experienced severe hepatotoxicity. Among the participants who took a non-nucleoside reverse transcriptase inhibitor (either Viramune®, Sustiva®, or Rescriptor®) in combination with two nucleoside analogues, severe hepatotoxicity occurred in 8.2 percent. Among the participants who took a protease inhibitor in combination with two nucleoside analogues, severe hepatotoxicity occurred in 5 percent.

Unfortunately, clinical trials do not always reflect what is going to happen in the real world. Many clinical trials only follow participants for a year—and we know that HIV-positive people will need to take these medications for many years, which can increase the risk of hepatotoxicity. What's more, most clinical trials enroll patients who don't have other conditions that can further increase the risk of hepatotoxicity. For example, it is believed that women and people over the age of fifty are at a higher risk of developing hepatotoxicity. Obesity and heavy alcohol use can also increase the chances of hepatotoxicity occurring. There is also a very real concern that HIV-positive people who are co-infected with hepatitis B or hepatitis C are more likely to experience hepatotoxicity than those who are only infected with HIV.

I Have HIV and Hepatitis C. Can I Use ARV Medications?

Yes. If you have chronic hepatitis C or hepatitis B—two viral infections that can cause the liver to become inflamed and damaged—you can take HIV medications. However, it is important to understand that there may be a higher risk of liver damage occurring if you have either of these infections and are taking ARV medications.

While there have been a number of studies looking at rates of hepatotoxicity among people co-infected with both HIV and hepatitis C or hepatitis B who are taking HIV drugs, the results often conflict with one another. For example, one study conducted by the San Francisco Community Health Network demonstrated that Viramune® (nevirapine) was the only anti-HIV medication to significantly increase the risk of hepatotoxicity in people co-infected with HIV and either hepatitis C or hepatitis B. But there have also been study results suggesting that Viramune is no more or less likely to cause hepatotoxicity in co-infected patients than other anti-HIV medications, although it's still important to watch out for liver enzyme increases during the first three months of Viramune treatment.

As for the protease inhibitors, there have been a few studies demonstrating that Norvir® (ritonavir) is the most likely to cause hepatotoxicity in HIV-positive people co-infected with hepatitis C or hepatitis B. However, Norvir is rarely used at the approved dose (600 mg twice a day)—much lower doses of Norvir are usually used (100 or 200 mg twice a day), as it is now most frequently prescribed to boost other protease inhibitor levels in the bloodstream. This, in turn, likely decreases the risk of hepatotoxicity in people who are only infected with HIV or co-infected with HIV and either hepatitis C or hepatitis B. Extra caution is also suggested when people with HBV or HCV use either Aptivus® or Prezista®, especially if they have even moderate liver damage already.

If one thing is clear, it is that people who are co-infected with HIV and either hepatitis C or hepatitis B should work closely with their doctors to come up with safe and effective treatment plans. For example, many experts now believe that, if you have HIV and hepatitis C, you should consider starting hepatitis C treatment while your CD4 cell counts are high, before treatment is needed for HIV. Successfully treating or controlling HCV is, perhaps, the best way to reduce the risk of hepatotoxicity once ARV medications are started.

It is also important to monitor your liver carefully while taking ARV medications. You'll want to find out the levels of your liver enzymes before you begin taking anti-HIV medications. Even if they are higher than normal because of either hepatitis C or hepatitis B, you can then monitor your levels closely while on treatment.

Are There Ways to Reverse or Prevent Hepatotoxicity?

If you have been told that your ARV medications are causing liver toxicity, you and your doctor will likely want to figure out which drug—or which combination of drugs—are causing your liver enzymes to increase. Working together, you and your doctor can then determine if it's necessary to stop the offending drug(s), with a possible switch to new medications that are less likely to cause liver toxicity.

Fortunately, taking proper care of your liver is not limited to avoiding or switching certain HIV medications. The next few parts of this section review some of the most important things that you can do to protect your liver while you are taking anti-HIV medications.

What's the Deal with Alcohol?

There's no shortage of information concluding that heavy alcohol use —generally defined as more than five drinks a day—can cause liver damage. It's also known that heavy alcohol use can worsen liver disease in people with hepatitis C and hepatitis B. Although it's still not known if light or moderate drinking—no more than one to two drinks a day—is harmful to the liver, especially in people taking medications on a regular basis. Most physicians, however, recommend that people with more severe liver damage avoid alcohol. If you drink alcohol, it is very important that you discuss this with your doctor. It's also important to note that the American Liver Association recommends no more than one drink a day. Some medications, such as Flagyl® (used to treat some parasitic infections), should not be combined with alcohol, and most experts advise staying away from alcohol completely if you have hepatitis.

What about My Diet?

Yes, absolutely. The liver is not only responsible for processing medications—it must also process and detoxify the liquids and foods we drink and eat on a daily basis. In fact, between 85 and 90 percent of the blood that leaves the stomach and intestines contains nutrients from the liquids and foods we consume for further processing by the liver. As a result, a well-balanced diet is a terrific way to help take some of the stress off the liver and to help it remain healthy. Here are some tips to consider:

- Eat plentiful amounts of fruits and vegetables, especially dark green leafy vegetables and orange- and red-colored fruits and vegetables.

- Cut down on fats that may put a lot of stress on the liver, such as dairy products, processed vegetable oils (hydrogenated fats), deep-fried foods, foods that are not fresh and contain rancid fats, preserved meats, and fatty meats.

- Concentrate on eating "good fats," which contain essential fatty acids. These are found in cold pressed vegetable and seed oils, avocados, fish, flaxseed, raw nuts and seeds (must be fresh), and legumes. Not only are good fats believed to be easier for the liver to process, they can help build healthy cell membranes around the liver cells.

- Do your best to avoid artificial chemicals and toxins such as insecticides, pesticides, artificial sweeteners (especially aspartame), and preservatives. You should also be careful regarding the coffee you drink. Many nutritionists recommend no more than two cups a day and should be brewed from ground natural coffee, not instant coffee powders. A recent study, however, suggested that moderate coffee intake actually had positive effects on the liver.

- Consume a diverse range of proteins from grains, raw nuts, seeds, legumes, eggs, seafood, and if desired, free range chicken and lean fresh red meats. If you are a vegetarian, you may want to consider supplements such as vitamin B_{12}, taurine, and carnitine to avoid poor metabolism and fatigue.

- Drink large amounts of fluids, especially water. Drinking at least eight glasses of water a day is a must, especially if you're taking ARV medications.

- Be wary of raw fish (sushi) or shellfish. Sushi can harbor bacteria that may harm the liver and shellfish can contain the hepatitis A virus, which can cause serious liver problems in people who have not received the hepatitis A vaccine. Also take care to avoid wild mushrooms. Many types of wild mushrooms contain toxins that can cause serious damage to the liver.

- Be cautious of iron. Iron, a mineral found in meat and fortified cereals, can be toxic to the liver, especially in people who have hepatotoxicity or infections that can cause hepatitis. Foods and cooking equipment—such as iron skillets—high in iron should be used sparingly.

There are a number of vitamins and minerals that have been shown to be healthful to the liver and many nutrition experts recommend that people at risk for liver toxicity seek out these foods at the grocery market. These include:

- **Vitamin K:** Green leafy vegetables and alfalfa sprouts are a great source of this vitamin.

- **Arginine:** The liver can sometimes have a difficult time processing protein. This can cause ammonia levels to increase in the bloodstream. Arginine, which is found in beans, peas, lentils, and seeds, can help detoxify ammonia.

- **Antioxidants:** Antioxidants work by neutralizing highly reactive, destructive compounds called free radicals, which are produced in abundance by highly active organs (such as the liver, especially when it is processing drugs on a daily basis). Foods high in antioxidants include vegetables and fruits like carrots, celery, beets, dandelion, apples, pears, and citrus. Selenium, a powerful antioxidant, can be found in brazil nuts, brewers yeast, kelp, brown rice, liver, molasses, seafood, wheat germ, whole grains, garlic, and onions.

- **Methionine:** A detoxifying agent found in beans, peas, lentils, eggs, fish, garlic, onions, seeds, and meat.

What about Nutritional Supplements and Herbs?

Some complementary and alternative therapies (CAMS) have been suggested to help prevent or control liver damage. The complementary therapy that has been researched and used most frequently in liver disease is milk thistle (*Sylibum marianum*), but studies have yet to determine conclusively that it can prevent, halt, or reverse liver damage in people with hepatitis. The National Center for Complementary and Alternative Medicine (NCCAM) at the National Institutes of Health (NIH) concludes that there is not sufficient evidence to recommend milk thistle for hepatitis C or other causes of liver damage. The HCV Advocate, an nonprofit organization for people living with HCV, recommends that milk thistle is probably safe and that no one should be discouraged from using it, provided that they inform their provider that they are taking it, that they are aware of any possible drug interactions, and that they do not use it as a substitute for hepatitis C treatment.

N-acetyl-cysteine (NAC), is another CAM that is often used to treat liver toxicity from overdoses of acetaminophen (Tylenol®). There are not, however, conclusive studies of NAC in treating other types of liver damage.

It is important to remember that simply because these complementary therapies can be purchased without a prescription, this does not mean that they are always safe to take. Some complementary therapies have their own side effects. Also, consumer protection groups who have done spot checks of various herbs and supplements have frequently found that herbs and supplements have either much less or much more of the active ingredients than stated on the bottles. Be sure to check with your healthcare provider before starting any complementary therapy.

Some herbs that have been associated with liver damage, and that the HCV Advocate recommends avoiding, include: Blue-green algae, borage (*Borago officinalis*), Bupleurum, chaparral (*Larrea tridentata*), comfrey (*Symphytum officinale* and *S. uplandicum*), Dong Quai (*Angelica polymorpha*), germander (*Teucrium chamaedrys*), Jin Bu Huan (*Lycopodium serratum*), kava, mistletoe (*Phoradendron leucarpum* and *Viscum album*), pennyroyal (*Mentha pulegium*), sassafras (*Sassafras albidum*), shark cartilage, skullcap (*Scutellaria lateriflora*), and valerian. This list does not include every herb with known or suspected liver toxicities.

Section 23.3

Hyperglycemia

"Diabetes," © 2010 The Well Project (www.thewellproject.org).
Reprinted with permission.

What Is Diabetes?

Diabetes and pre-diabetes are serious conditions in which people have high levels of glucose in their blood. Almost twenty-four million Americans have diabetes and at least fifty-seven million have pre-diabetes.

Glucose is a type of sugar. It is used as fuel by the body. When you eat, your body converts the food into glucose. The glucose then goes into your bloodstream and is carried throughout the body to provide energy to all of your cells. In order for glucose to get into your cells, you need insulin. Insulin is a hormone made by the pancreas.

If your body has a problem making or using insulin, glucose can't get into your cells. As a result, glucose stays in the blood and the cells do not get enough. A diagnosis of pre-diabetes or diabetes is made when glucose stays at higher than normal levels (also called hyperglycemia).

There are several types of diabetes.

Type 1 Diabetes

- The pancreas no longer makes any insulin.

- You must take insulin every day to survive.

- Usually begins in childhood or adolescence.

Type 2 Diabetes

- Your pancreas makes some insulin (but usually not enough), and the body doesn't respond to the insulin normally.

- Some people with type 2 diabetes are able to control it with diet and exercise, many others need diabetes medication, and some need insulin.

- Most common form of diabetes, usually occurring after age forty-five.

Gestational Diabetes

- Occurs in some women during pregnancy

Pre-Diabetes

- Blood glucose levels are higher than normal but not high enough for a diagnosis of diabetes.

- Having pre-diabetes puts you at increased risk for developing type 2 diabetes.

- Type 2 diabetes can often be prevented or delayed by making changes to your diet and increasing exercise.

Symptoms of Diabetes

Symptoms of diabetes include:

- extreme thirst;
- need to urinate frequently;
- unexplained weight loss;
- hunger;
- blurry vision;
- irritability;
- tingling or numbness in the hands or feet;
- difficulty healing;
- extreme fatigue.

Symptoms typically occur when glucose levels have gotten very high. If you are diagnosed while diabetes is in its early stages, you may not have any symptoms.

Glucose Tests

Since there are not always obvious symptoms of diabetes, it's important to have regular lab tests to check if your glucose levels are high. The most common glucose tests are:

- **Fasting glucose test:** Measures the glucose in a blood sample taken when you have not had anything to eat or drink (except water) for at least eight hours.

- **Random glucose test:** Measures the glucose in a blood sample taken when you have been eating on your usual schedule.

- **Glucose tolerance test:** You take a fasting glucose test and are then given a drink with a measured amount of glucose in it. Several more glucose measurements are taken at specific time intervals after you have had the drink.

To find out if you have diabetes or pre-diabetes, it is generally recommended that you have a fasting glucose test. A glucose tolerance test may be ordered to help diagnose diabetes and as a follow-up to a high fasting glucose level.

A diagnosis of diabetes can be made based on any of the following test results, confirmed by retesting on a different day:

- A fasting blood glucose level of 126 milligrams per deciliter (mg/dL) or higher

- A random blood glucose level of 200 mg/dL or higher, along with symptoms of diabetes

- A glucose tolerance test level of 200 mg/dL or higher

In January of 2010, the American Diabetes Association recommended another test called A1C as an additional way to diagnose diabetes and pre-diabetes. The A1C test is already used to monitor blood glucose levels. One advantage of this test is that it doesn't require fasting.

Who Is at Risk for Diabetes?

Anyone can get diabetes. However, certain factors may increase your risk, such as:

331

- taking protease inhibitors (PIs);
- being over forty;
- being overweight or obese;
- a family history of the disease;
- a poor diet;
- not exercising regularly;
- a lot of fat around the belly;
- hepatitis C or liver damage;
- high cholesterol;
- high blood pressure.

What Problems Can Diabetes Cause?

Diabetes can lead to serious illness and even death. Adults with diabetes are at high risk for heart disease. In fact, at least 65 percent of people with diabetes die from heart disease or stroke.

Some of the other possible complications of diabetes are:

- blindness;
- kidney failure;
- blood vessel disease that requires an amputation;
- nerve damage (neuropathy).

How Are Diabetes and Pre-Diabetes Treated?

Although diabetes can be a very serious disease, it can be treated. It is important to manage diabetes by checking glucose and keeping it under control. Many people control their glucose levels by keeping their weight down, changing their diet, and increasing exercise.

A healthy diet for people with diabetes involves reducing sugar and starchy foods (carbohydrates), such as bread, potatoes, rice, and corn. See a registered dietitian to help you plan your meals. Many acquired immunodeficiency syndrome (AIDS) service organizations have registered dietitians on staff who will see you free of charge.

Sometimes, despite diet and exercise, glucose can't be controlled without the help of medications and/or insulin. There are a number of medications available that lower blood glucose levels. Because the medications act in different ways, they may be used together.

Some of the diabetes medications may interact with human immunodeficiency virus (HIV) drugs. To reduce the chance of drug interactions, make sure your healthcare provider is aware of all the medications you take.

Pre-Diabetes

People with pre-diabetes are likely to develop type 2 diabetes within ten years, unless they take action. The good news is that if you have pre-diabetes, you can do a lot to prevent or delay diabetes.

Studies have shown that people can lower their risk of developing diabetes by losing weight through diet and increased physical activity. One study found that diet and exercise leading to 5 to 7 percent weight loss (about ten to fourteen pounds in a person who weighs two hundred pounds) lowered the rate of type 2 diabetes by nearly 60 percent. Study participants lost weight by cutting fat and calories in their diet and by exercising (mostly walking) at least thirty minutes a day, five days a week.

HIV and Diabetes

High glucose levels can be a side effect of HIV drugs. Specifically, the protease inhibitors (PIs) can make it difficult for insulin to get glucose into the cells. This is called insulin resistance. It can lead to pre-diabetes and diabetes.

Some studies show that HIV-positive women on PIs are three times more likely to develop diabetes than HIV-positive women on non-PI drug combinations or HIV-negative women. In fact, up to 6 percent of all people on PIs have diabetes.

If you need to take PIs for your HIV treatment, be aware of this possible side effect. Get monitored at regular medical checkups for glucose. If you have high glucose levels, your healthcare provider may recommend that you change your HIV drugs. Some studies have shown that switching to a combination that does not include a PI can help bring these levels under control. Switching is not an option for everyone and you should speak to your healthcare provider before stopping any HIV drugs.

Many women, whether or not they are HIV-positive, develop gestational diabetes during pregnancy. This is of particular concern to HIV-positive women who must take PIs to prevent transmitting HIV to their unborn babies. Women who take PIs during pregnancy should have their glucose levels monitored very closely.

Some HIV-positive people experience lipodystrophy. Lipodystrophy includes a number of health problems including high glucose levels as well as unwanted changes in body fat and increases in fat (cholesterol and triglyceride) levels in the blood. These conditions have been linked with diabetes, heart disease, and strokes.

Taking Care of Yourself

Since HIV-positive people may already have a number of risk factors for diabetes, as well as heart disease and stroke, it is important to be aware of all of these conditions.

Have regular medical checkups and lab work that includes a glucose test. As well as checking and, if necessary, managing glucose levels, monitor other factors that can contribute to the risk of heart disease and strokes. These include high blood pressure and cholesterol and triglyceride levels.

If you have high blood pressure, make sure it is treated. A healthy diet and exercise can help with high cholesterol and triglyceride levels as well as high glucose. Finally, giving up smoking is one of the best things you can do for your heart and your health.

HIV-positive people with diabetes can work with their healthcare providers to achieve good diabetes control as well as management of HIV and other health concerns. Keeping diabetes under control (or decreasing your risk of getting diabetes) involves lifestyle changes. While this is difficult, it will give you the best chance of good overall health.

Section 23.4

Hyperlipidemia

Excerpted from "Hyperlipidemia," Aidsinfo.gov, October 2005.
Reviewed by David A. Cooke, M.D., FACP, November 2010.

What is hyperlipidemia?

Hyperlipidemia is an increase in the amount of fat (such as cholesterol and triglycerides) in the blood. These increases can lead to heart disease and pancreatitis.

Which anti-HIV (human immunodeficiency virus) medications can cause hyperlipidemia?

Some protease inhibitors (PIs) can raise blood lipid (fat) levels. Some PIs, such as Norvir®, are more likely to cause hyperlipidemia than other PIs. Sustiva® is a non–protease inhibitor drug that can also raise blood lipid levels.

Other factors can increase your risk of developing hyperlipidemia. Risks you can control include your alcohol intake, physical activity, and diet. Other risks include hypothyroidism, diabetes, and genetic factors. Oral contraceptives (birth control pills) can also increase triglycerides and total cholesterol.

What are the symptoms of hyperlipidemia?

Hyperlipidemia has no symptoms. The only way your doctor can diagnosis it is through laboratory tests. Your doctor should order a lipid profile when you start anti- HIV medication. Once your baseline lipid levels are determined, your doctor should monitor your levels every three to four months, or at least once a year.

What can I do if I have hyperlipidemia?

There are several things you can do to control your cholesterol and triglyceride levels. You can switch to a low-fat diet and control your weight. Your doctor may refer you to a dietician for help with your diet. Regular aerobic exercise has been shown to lower cholesterol. Quitting smoking and avoiding or limiting alcohol can also lower your cholesterol. Keeping your blood pressure under control is critical; you may need to take medication to lower your blood pressure.

What medications are used to treat hyperlipidemia?

You and your doctor may decide that you should take a cholesterol-lowering medication. This might be a medication from the statin group. Examples of statins are Lipitor® (atorvastatin) and Pravachol® (pravastatin). If statins are not effective, another medication from a group called fibrates might be added. Lopid® (gemfibrozil) and TriCor® (fenofibrate) are drugs from the fibrate group. All of these medications can cause serious side effects and should be taken only as directed by your doctor.

Will I need to change my HIV treatment regimen?

If your hyperlipidemia is severe or you do not respond to other treatments, you and your doctor may decide to change your anti-HIV medications. One option may be to replace your PI(s) with an anti-HIV medication from a different class; this might mean changing your entire regimen.

Section 23.5

Lipodystrophy

"Lipodystrophy," by Jean Kressy, MS, RN, with Christine
Wanke, MD, and Jül Gerrior, RD. © 2009 Tufts University School
of Medicine. Reprinted with permission.

What is lipodystrophy?

Lipodystrophy, also called fat redistribution syndrome, is a condition that often occurs in human immunodeficiency virus (HIV)–positive people and is characterized by changes in body shape and metabolism. Body shape changes may include the accumulation and/or loss of fat, which can affect appearance. Metabolic changes may include increased resistance to insulin and abnormally high levels of blood cholesterol and triglycerides. These do not all necessarily occur together; each may occur separately or in any combination.

What causes lipodystrophy?

Health experts are not sure why HIV-positive people develop lipodystrophy, but they think it may be related to antiretroviral medications they take to control their disease. In addition to medications, factors including a person's age, gender, weight, genetic predisposition, length of time he or she has been HIV-positive, and severity of the disease may be linked to the development of lipodystrophy.

What body shape changes can occur with lipodystrophy?

Fat accumulation. The most visible signs of lipodystrophy and the ones that people may notice first are deposits of fat at various sites on their bodies. The two places where fat generally accumulates are the back of the neck (called "buffalo hump") and around the abdomen (truncal obesity). Increased breast size, especially in women, may also occur. However, the changes in fat distribution are not necessarily the same in everyone.

Fat loss. Loss of body fat, called lipoatrophy, is another characteristic of lipodystrophy that affects appearance. The most common places where people lose fat are in their cheeks, making their faces look thinner, and in their buttocks, arms, and legs. When fat loss occurs in the arms and legs, veins may be more visible.

The loss of body fat that occurs with lipodystrophy is not the same as the weight loss that happens with wasting. People with wasting lose weight as well as muscle and fat. In lipodystrophy, there are alterations in body fat but not necessarily a change in weight. Some people with lipodystrophy experience both fat accumulation and fat loss. In some instances, body shape changes may affect a person's ability to perform daily activities, such as exercising, sleeping, and even breathing.

What metabolic changes can occur with lipodystrophy?

Insulin resistance. Insulin, a hormone produced by the pancreas, is responsible for transporting sugar (also called glucose) from the blood into the cells, where it is used for energy. Normally after eating, the amount of glucose in the blood increases; this signals the pancreas to secrete insulin, which in turn prompts the cell to absorb the glucose. In short, insulin is the substance that allows cells to absorb glucose from the blood. Once it enters the cells, glucose is used by the cells as fuel. In insulin resistance, either insulin is not doing its job or the cells are unable to absorb glucose. The result is that glucose may continue to rise in the blood, and if not treated, can lead to diabetes. Insulin resistance may be related to some of the antiretroviral medications used to treat HIV, and/or to a genetic predisposition in the individual.

Dyslipidemia. Dyslipidemia, or higher than normal amounts of lipids (cholesterol and/or triglycerides) in the blood, is another metabolic change which often occurs in HIV-positive people with lipodystrophy. It also may be related to some of the antiretroviral medications used to treat the disease, and/or to genetic predisposition.

In general, anyone with dyslipidemia may be more likely to develop cardiovascular disease. However, studies show that unless HIV-infected people with high blood lipids have other risks that increase heart disease, such as smoking, obesity, or high blood pressure, their chances of heart attack are no greater than HIV-negative people.

How is lipodystrophy treated?

Although lipodystrophy includes a variety of body shape and metabolic changes, a single intervention can often control more than one symptom. For example, small research studies have shown that when people with lipodystrophy eat more fiber, they may lose some abdominal fat and may become less resistant to insulin. Exercise also provides more than one benefit; in addition to losing fat, people who exercise may have lower triglycerides and may be less insulin resistant.

Diet. Instead of focusing on specific foods, some physicians advise people with lipodystrophy to follow an eating plan based on the Mediterranean diet. The diet, also recommended to healthy people and those at risk for heart disease, is low in fat, especially saturated fat, and refined sugars (such as candy, soft drinks, cakes, cookies, ice cream) and alcohol, and high in fiber-rich whole grains, fruits, and vegetables. Fat, especially saturated fat, increases blood cholesterol and refined sugars, and alcohol increase triglycerides. Fiber, on the other hand, may control insulin resistance and may help decrease abdominal fat.

Nutrition experts say that the kind of fat eaten is as important as the amount. Omega-3 fatty acids, for instance, are recommended, but saturated fats (fatty meat, poultry with skin, butter, whole-milk dairy foods, and coconut and palm oils) should be limited. In addition to saturated fats, trans fats, found in some stick margarines and Crisco®, which are solid at room temperature, should be avoided. Many packaged foods, especially baked goods, contain trans fats to prolong their shelf lives. Read labels; if one of the ingredients has the word "hydrogenated," it means it contains trans fats. When choosing fats, look for tub or soft margarines, which do not contain trans fats, and unsaturated oils like canola, corn, and olive. Because fish is an excellent source of heart-healthy omega-3 fatty acids, nutrition experts recommend eating fish regularly. Although all seafood contains omega-3 fatty acids, the best sources are fatty fish like salmon, albacore tuna, and mackerel.

Fiber and nutrient-packed whole grains, legumes, and fruits and vegetables, the cornerstones of Mediterranean eating, should play leading roles in a healthful diet. If you're not used to eating fruits and vegetables, the recommended five servings of fruits and/or vegetables a day may seem overwhelming—but once you get into the habit, it's very achievable. In addition to snacking on fruits and eating vegetables and salads with meals, fruits and vegetables are easy to add to everyday foods. For example, slice a banana on breakfast toast or cereal, stir berries into a cup of yogurt, layer sandwiches with tomato or roasted pepper, stir a can of beans into a pot of vegetable soup or store-bought spaghetti sauce, tweak the proportion of meat and vegetables in a stew in favor of the vegetables, or make yourself a fruit smoothie. When shopping for whole grains, read labels and look for the words, "bran" or "whole-grain" or "whole-wheat" on the label.

Exercise. Progressive resistance exercises (weight training), which are recommended to build muscles in HIV-positive people with wasting, may reduce triglycerides, decrease insulin resistance, and decrease abdominal fat in people with lipodystrophy. Regular weightlifting and push-up routines, either in a gym or at home, are excellent, but if this is not possible, incorporate activities like walking, gardening, or housecleaning into your day. Any activity that gets you up and moving counts.

Aerobic exercises, which raise pulse rate and increase blood flow to muscles, including the heart, are also recommended for people with lipodystrophy. Moderate to vigorous aerobic exercise, such as fast walking, running, or using a treadmill, combined with resistance exercises, have increased strength and fitness, improved blood cholesterol and insulin resistance, and reduced fat in HIV-positive people without negatively affecting their viral loads or CD4 counts.

For people who are not used to exercising, experts suggest they start slowly and gradually increase the amount of the time they exercise. For some people a regular routine works best; others like to incorporate exercise into their daily schedules or to combine it with a regular workout. The bottom line is to exercise in any way that works for you. Anyone with concerns about cardiovascular disease or over the age of forty-five should consult with their physician before beginning an exercise program.

Medications. Although antiretroviral medications may be linked to the development of lipodystrophy, there are no data that suggest that stopping the medications improves body shape changes. Instead physicians may recommend diet, exercise, and medicines targeted to the body shape and metabolic changes associated with lipodystrophy.

Growth hormone. Growth hormone, used to treat HIV-positive people with wasting, may also be given to people with lipodystrophy, although it is not currently approved for this use. In research studies, growth hormone has successfully lowered blood triglycerides and reduced abdominal fat and fat behind the neck. However, once growth hormone is stopped, the abnormalities return. Furthermore, because growth hormone may worsen insulin resistance, it's not for everyone with lipodystrophy. Investigators need to learn more about its safety over a long time, and like all drugs, growth hormone has multiple side effects.

Testosterone. Because testosterone replacement has been used to reduce fat in HIV-negative men, researchers are studying its potential for treating lipodystrophy. However, at the moment it is not being used to reverse the fat accumulation that occurs in lipodystrophy.

Metformin. Metformin, which is used to treat diabetes, is also being prescribed for people with lipodystrophy. In individuals with abnormal glucose tolerance, metformin may improve insulin resistance, and may result in weight loss, including abdominal fat loss. Other benefits may include a drop in blood pressure and a decrease in blood triglycerides. Patients taking metformin are monitored by their physicians for side effects; there is particular concern about liver toxicity.

Anyone who is concerned that he or she may have changes associated with lipodystrophy should discuss this with their healthcare provider. It may be possible for them to refer you to an appropriate research study or to a specialist who has an interest in the management of the syndrome, if they do not have particular expertise in this area.

Section 23.6

Mitochondrial Toxicity

"Mitochondrial Toxicity," Fact Sheet #556. © 2010 AIDS InfoNet. Reprinted with permission. InfoNet fact sheets are updated frequently. Please visit the website at http://www.aidsinfonet.org for the newest version.

What are mitochondria?

Mitochondria (my-toe-con´-dree-a) are small "organs" in our cells. They are the cell's power plant. They use oxygen, fat, and sugar to produce adenosine triphosphate (ATP). This process is called "cellular respiration." When the cell needs energy, it breaks down molecules of ATP to release the stored energy.

The more energy the cell needs, the more mitochondria it contains. One cell can have anywhere from a few mitochondria up to thousands. The highest numbers are found in nerve, muscle, and liver cells.

Some scientists believe that mitochondria are the key to aging. As we grow older, our mitochondria collect more and more mutations. Our cells have a way to check for mistakes (mutations) when they multiply, but mitochondria don't.

What is mitochondrial toxicity?

Mitochondrial toxicity (MT) is damage that decreases the number of mitochondria. If there are too few mitochondria in a cell, it might stop working properly. It's not clear how much loss of mitochondria can occur before there is loss of cell function.

What are the signs of MT?

One of the most common signs of MT is muscle weakness (myopathy). If muscle cells can't get enough energy through cellular respiration, they have to get energy without oxygen. This "anaerobic" energy production creates lactic acid as a waste product.

Lactic acid can cause sore muscles. For example, the soreness people feel after running a marathon is caused by a buildup of lactic acid.

Some people with MT have very high levels of lactic acid in their blood. This rare condition is called lactic acidosis. There is a blood test for lactic acid levels, but experts disagree on how to interpret the results. Physical exertion before the blood test—including climbing stairs or walking quickly—can increase lactic acid levels and throw off the test results.

It's difficult to know if you have MT. However, you can look for the following signs of lactic acidosis:

- Nausea
- Vomiting
- Severe fatigue
- Recent weight loss
- Rapid, deep breathing
- Cramps, muscle aches, and numbness or tingling
- Muscle weakness that rapidly gets worse

Lactic acidosis can be fatal. See your healthcare provider immediately if you have these symptoms.

MT may also cause nerve damage. It has been linked to kidney damage and hearing loss. Some researchers believe it might also contribute to fat redistribution in people taking antiretroviral medications (ARVs).

How do ARVs cause?

Mitochondria have an enzyme that helps them multiply. This enzyme is called polymerase gamma, or "pol gamma." It is very similar to human immunodeficiency virus's (HIV's) reverse transcriptase enzyme. Unfortunately, this means that the drugs we use to inhibit reverse transcriptase can also inhibit pol gamma. When this happens, fewer new mitochondria are produced.

The nucleoside analog reverse transcriptase inhibitors (AZT, 3TC, ddI, d4T, and abacavir) all inhibit pol gamma to some degree. MT is more likely to occur the longer you take these drugs.

Different medications build up in different parts of the body. This could explain how MT caused by different drugs can lead to side effects in different parts of the body.

We know that MT can cause muscle weakness in people taking AZT. It is probably the cause of "fatty liver" (hepatic steatosis) and high levels of lactic acid that can be caused by all of the nukes. Unfortunately, there is very little research on how much mitochondrial damage each ARV causes to different parts of the body. We also don't know which combinations of drugs cause the most MT.

Researchers know how to measure the number of mitochondria in different cells, compared to normal. However, they don't know how many mitochondria a cell can lose before there are problems.

What's next?

Unfortunately, there is very little research on MT caused by nukes. Laboratory and animal studies show that MT can cause nerve damage. But there are no human studies.

Over the next few years, researchers will study MT. They will work on tests to identify it. They will also study the link between MT and various side effects. Some researchers believe that certain vitamins and minerals can help mitochondria overcome the effects of ARVs.

In the meantime, people with HIV need to know the symptoms of lactic acidosis, a rare side effect that can be fatal.

Section 23.7

Osteonecrosis, Osteoporosis, and Osteopenia

"Bone Disease," © 2010 The Well Project (www.thewellproject.org).
Reprinted with permission.

The Importance of Healthy Bones

Bones play many important roles in your body. They support you and help you to move. They protect your brain, heart, and other organs from injury. Bones also store minerals such as calcium and phosphorous.

Bones are living tissue and change during your life. Every day, your body removes old bone and adds new bone in its place. In young people, more bone is added than removed. After age thirty, more bone is removed than added. This makes the bones lighter and more fragile, putting them at greater risk for injury.

Many people have weak bones and don't know it. That is because bone loss often happens over a long period of time and doesn't hurt. For many people, a broken bone is the first sign that they have a bone disorder.

Bone Disease and Human Immunodeficiency Virus (HIV)

Being HIV-positive puts you at higher risk for bone disease. Experts don't know why this happens. It could be due to HIV itself, HIV drugs, or HIV-positive people getting older. HIV-positive people have unusually high rates of three kinds of bone diseases.

Osteoporosis

Osteoporosis happens when too much bone gets broken down and not enough put back. This causes lower bone density, also called bone mineral density (BMD), which means there are lower-than-normal levels of minerals in the bones. Bones become weak and are more likely to break. People with osteoporosis most often break bones in the wrist, spine, and hip.

Osteopenia

Like osteoporosis, osteopenia is caused by a loss of bone minerals that leads to lower-than-normal bone density. It is a less serious condition; however, people with osteopenia are at higher risk of developing osteoporosis over a five- to ten-year period.

Osteonecrosis (avascular necrosis)

Osteonecrosis means bone death. It is caused by a loss of blood supply to the bone. It usually affects the head of the femur, the part of the thighbone that connects it to the hip.

Risk Factors

In addition to HIV and HIV drugs, there are other things can put you at risk for bone disease.

Risk Factors You Can Control

- **Diet:** Getting too little calcium and vitamin D
- **Exercise:** Not exercising and not being active
- **Low body weight:** Being too thin
- **Tobacco use:** Smoking cigarettes
- **Alcohol and coffee intake:** Drinking a lot of alcohol and/or caffeine
- **Testosterone levels:** Low testosterone levels in men
- **Use of certain medicines:** Long-term use of medicines including glucocorticosteroids (drugs such as prednisone and cortisone), thyroid hormones, anticonvulsants (anti-seizure medications), heparin, pentamidine, and ketoconazole

Risk Factors You Cannot Control

- **Age:** Your chances of getting osteoporosis increase as you get older.
- **Gender:** Women have a greater chance of getting osteoporosis because they have smaller bones.
- **Menopause:** Women lose bone due to hormone changes that happen after menopause.

- **Ethnicity:** White and Asian women are at higher risk; Hispanic and African-American women are also at risk, but less so.

How to Know if you have Bone Problems

Osteoporosis and Osteopenia

Bone mineral density (BMD) tests are the only way to find out if you have osteoporosis or osteopenia. The most widely used BMD test is a dual energy x-ray absorptiometry (DEXA) scan. A DEXA scan is an easy and painless test.

Osteonecrosis

Osteonecrosis causes pain in the joints, usually in the hip area. At first the pain might only occur when you put weight on the joint. In more severe cases the pain could be constant. A magnetic resonance imaging (MRI) scan can spot early stages. X-rays and other scans can detect advanced osteonecrosis.

Diet and Healthy Bones

Even though you cannot control some of the things that lead to bone disease, you can control your diet. The mineral calcium makes up a large part of your bones. This means that if you do not get enough calcium in your diet, your bones may get weaker.

Calcium is found naturally in some foods, and it is added to others. Some foods that contain calcium are:

- milk;
- yogurt;
- cheese;
- calcium-fortified orange juice;
- tofu;
- salmon with the bones.

Most HIV-positive people still need to take calcium pills every day even if they eat dairy products like milk, cheese, and yogurt. A registered dietitian or other trained healthcare provider can help you decide if you should take calcium supplements. If so, it may be a good idea to take calcium pills with vitamin D in them, since your body cannot use calcium without vitamin D. According to the National Osteoporosis Foundation (NOF):

- Adults under age fifty need 1,000 mg of calcium and 400–800 IU of vitamin D daily.

- Adults fifty and over need 1,200 mg of calcium and 800–1,000 IU of vitamin D daily.

Talk to your healthcare provider before taking any supplements and do not take more than these amounts unless your healthcare provider tells you to.

Exercise and Healthy Bones

If you don't have joint pain, it is also important to exercise on a regular basis. When you exercise your muscles pull against your bones, which helps keep them healthy and strong. The best kind of exercise to keep your bones strong is exercise that uses weight, such as:

- walking (you can use ankle weights);
- working out with weights or weight machines;
- stair climbing;
- hiking;
- aerobics;
- jogging.

If you can't do high-impact weight-bearing activities, try lower-impact ones. For example, try walking or stair climbing instead of jogging. If you haven't exercised regularly for a while, check with your healthcare provider before beginning a new exercise program.

Once you have your healthcare provider's approval, start your exercise routine slowly. Every two weeks make your routine five minutes longer. In the end, you should be working out three to seven times a week, about twenty to sixty minutes each time.

Drugs to Treat Osteoporosis

Diet and exercise are best at keeping bone disease from occurring. They can also be helpful if you already have osteopenia or osteoporosis, but in some cases, your healthcare provider may also recommend treatment with medication.

347

Make sure to ask your healthcare provider about how to take the medication, possible side effects, and whether there are any interactions with HIV drugs you take. Some of the osteoporosis medications that are commonly used include the following.

Bisphosphonates

Drugs like Fosamax® (alendronate), Boniva® (ibandronate), and Actonel® (risedronate) are widely used to treat and prevent osteoporosis. It is important to get enough calcium and vitamin D when you are taking a bisphosphonate.

Hormones

- **Estrogen:** In women, replacing the hormone estrogen has shown to significantly decrease the number of fractures. Sometimes estrogen is combined with another hormone called progesterone. However, there is an increased risk of developing other diseases including certain cancers. Because of this, the US Food and Drug Administration (FDA) recommends using other osteoporosis medications and, if estrogen/progesterone are used, the lowest possible doses should be considered.

- **Testosterone:** Testosterone therapy may be useful to slow or reverse decreased bone density and strength in men.

- **Miacalcin® (calcitonin):** This naturally occurring hormone slows bone loss and increases bone density in the spine.

- **Forteo® (teriparatide):** Forteo is a parathyroid hormone that has been shown to rebuild bone and increase bone mineral density, especially in the spine.

Selective Estrogen Receptor Modulators (SERMs)

Evista® (raloxifene) is in a class of osteoporosis drugs called SERMs. Evista was developed to work like estrogen therapy, but with fewer side effects.

Protect Your Bones

HIV-positive women, especially those who have gone through menopause, need to be particularly careful about bone health. Speak to your healthcare provider and follow these steps to help protect your bones:

- Ask your healthcare provider if you need a DEXA scan.

- Follow a diet with plenty of calcium and vitamin D.

- Seek the advice of a registered dietitian if you need help choosing the right foods.

- Take calcium supplements, if needed (talk to your healthcare provider first).

- Ask your healthcare provider what exercises are safe for you, and start doing them.

- Stop smoking and reduce your intake of caffeine and alcohol.

- Tell your healthcare provider if you are experiencing joint pain, especially in the hip area.

Section 23.8

Peripheral Neuropathy

"Peripheral Neuropathy," Fact Sheet # 555. © 2009 AIDS InfoNet. Reprinted with permission. InfoNet fact sheets are updated frequently. Please visit the website at http://www.aidsinfonet.org for the newest version.

What Is Peripheral Neuropathy?

Peripheral neuropathy (PN) is a disease of the peripheral nerves. These are all the nerves except for those in the brain and spinal cord.

About 30 percent of people with human immunodeficiency virus (HIV) develop PN. Some PN is a breakdown of the nerve endings (axons) that send sensations to the brain. Sometimes, PN is damage to the coating of nerve fibers (myelin). This affects the transmission of pain signals to the brain.

PN can be a minor nuisance or a disabling weakness. It is usually a feeling of pins and needles, burning, stiffness, or numbness in the feet and toes. It can also be tickling sensations, unexplained pain, or sensations that seem more intense than normal. PN symptoms can come and go. Serious PN can cause difficulty walking or standing.

What Causes PN?

PN can be caused by HIV infection of nerve cells, by drugs used to treat HIV or other health problems, or other factors. Risk factors for PN include higher HIV viral load, diabetes, age greater than fifty, and heavy alcohol use. Other risk factors are the use of cocaine or amphetamines, cancer treatments, thyroid disease, or deficiency of vitamin B_{12} or vitamin E. A study in 2009 found that Hispanics may have a higher rate of PN. The researchers suggest follow-up studies.

Several HIV drugs can cause PN. The most important are the "d" drugs; ddI (didanosine, Videx®) and d4T (stavudine, Zerit®). Hydroxyurea, which is sometimes combined with antiretroviral drugs, increases the risk of PN.

Zidovudine (Retrovir®), abacavir, non-nucleoside reverse transcriptase inhibitors (NNRTIs), and protease inhibitors do not appear to cause PN.

How Is PN Diagnosed?

No laboratory testing is needed to diagnose PN. The signs and symptoms are enough. Special tests may be needed to find the cause of PN. These tests measure tiny electrical currents in nerves and muscles. The amount or speed of these electric signals drops with different types of PN. However, many patients with PN are not diagnosed correctly.

How Is It Treated?

Talk to your healthcare provider about discontinuing any drugs that might be causing PN. Drug-induced PN normally goes away totally if the drugs are stopped when PN first appears. However, this can take as long as eight weeks. If you continue to take the drugs, the nerve damage might become permanent.

Non-Drug Treatments

Some simple things can reduce the pain of PN:

- Wear looser shoes.
- Don't walk too far.
- Don't stand for too long a time.
- Soak your feet in ice water.

A recent study showed the benefit of smoking marijuana to relieve PN pain.

Drug Treatments

No drug has been approved to repair nerve damage. Some health-care providers use drugs developed to treat seizures, such as gabapentin (Neurontin®) or phenytoin (Dilantin®). Antidepressants such as amitriptyline may also help.

L-acetyl-carnitine (also called acetyl-l-carnitine or acetyl carnitine) has shown initial good results.

Treatment depends on how serious the symptoms of PN are:

- **Mild symptoms:** Ibuprofen can be used.

- **Moderate symptoms:** Amitriptyline or nortriptyline can be used. These anti-depressants increase the brain's transmission of nerve signals. Other treatments include Neurontin®, an anticonvulsant drug; and a gel containing the anesthetic lidocaine.

- **Severe symptoms:** Narcotic pain relievers such as codeine or methadone can be used. The anti-seizure medication pregabalin (Lyrica®) is also used to reduce PN pain.

Other drugs being used for PN include patches or creams for local treatment. These contain the anesthetic lidocaine, or capsaicin, the chemical that gives hot chili peppers their heat.

Nutrient Therapies

Nutrient therapies have been studied for PN caused by diabetes:

- **B vitamins:** Several B vitamins are useful in treating diabetic neuropathy. These include biotin, choline, inositol, and thiamine. They appear to improve nerve function.

- **Alpha-lipoic acid:** This may help protect nerves from inflammation.

- **Gamma linolenic acid:** Found in evening primrose oil, this has reversed nerve damage in some diabetics.

- **Magnets:** A recent study found that socks containing magnets relieved diabetic neuropathy in most cases. However, they were less effective for foot pain due to other causes.

The Bottom Line

Peripheral neuropathy is a disease of the nervous system. It causes strange sensations, especially in the feet, legs, and fingers, and can cause pain. The pain might be mild, or so severe that it prevents someone from walking.

Tell your healthcare provider immediately if you have any signs of PN. You will probably stop taking any drugs that can cause PN. If that doesn't take care of the problem, you may be tested to see what's causing the PN. There are different treatments for different causes of PN.

Drugs can be used to control the pain of PN, and several nutrient therapies might help repair nerve damage.

Section 23.9

Skin Rash

Excerpted from "Skin Rash," Aidsinfo.gov, October 2005.
Updated by David A. Cooke, MD, FACP, November 2010.

What kinds of skin rash can anti-HIV medications cause?

Anti-HIV (human immunodeficiency virus) medications can cause mild skin rashes as well as serious, even life-threatening rashes. The vast majority of skin rashes are mild to moderate. They usually appear within a few weeks of starting a new medication, and often go away with continued use of the medication. However, because some rashes can be serious, you should contact your doctor if you notice a skin rash. He or she will advise you about how best to manage the rash.

Which anti-HIV medications cause skin rash?

Skin rash may occur with medications from any of the three main HIV drug classes: non-nucleoside reverse transcriptase inhibitors (NNRTIs), nucleoside reverse transcriptase inhibitors (NRTIs), and protease inhibitors (PIs).

NNRTIs cause the majority of skin rashes, with Viramune® (nevirapine) causing the most severe rashes. If you and your doctor decide to use Viramune in your HIV treatment regimen, you will likely be instructed to take only one pill a day for the first fourteen days, then to increase to two pills a day. This dosing schedule may decrease your risk of developing a severe skin rash. Women appear to be at higher risk for developing Viramune- associated skin rashes than men.

NRTIs may also cause skin rashes. Ziagen® (abacavir) may cause a rash that is a symptom of a severe drug hypersensitivity (allergic) reaction. If you develop a rash while taking Ziagen, notify your doctor right away. If you and your doctor decide that you need to stop taking the drug, you should never again take Ziagen; any exposure to the drug could result in an even more severe hypersensitivity reaction.

Agenerase® (amprenavir) and Aptivus® (tipranavir) are the PIs most likely to cause skin rash. Lexiva® (fosamprenavir) is converted into Agenerase® (amprenavir) in the body, and can probably cause the same issues. Women taking birth control pills that contain estrogen may be more likely to develop a rash when taking Aptivus. If you are allergic to sulfa drugs, your doctor should monitor you carefully if you start taking Agenerase or Aptivus as part of your HIV treatment regimen. Another PI, Prezista® (darunavir), is also known to cause life-threatening rashes in some cases.

Selzentry® (maraviroc) is a medication from the CCR5 antagonist class used in specialized situations. This may cause a rash, which usually occurs in the setting of serious liver toxicity.

What characterizes a severe skin rash?

Severe skin rashes cause significant damage to the skin and can result in serious complications, even death. The severe skin rashes that may occur with the use of anti- HIV medications are Stevens-Johnson syndrome (SJS) and toxic epidermal necrolysis (TEN), which are two different forms of the same kind of skin rash. TEN differs from SJS in the extent of skin damage—TEN involves at least 30 percent of the total body skin area. Both SJS and TEN are severe conditions that must be treated by a doctor.

What are the symptoms of SJS and TEN?

The symptoms of SJS and TEN include the following:

- Flat or raised red spots on the skin that develop blisters in the center

- Blisters in the mouth, eyes, genitals, or other moist areas of the body

- Peeling skin that results in painful sores

- Fever

- Headache

- General ill feeling

Are there any other drug-associated skin rashes I should know about?

Another rare but life-threatening rash occurs as part of the DRESS syndrome (drug rash with eosinophilia and systemic symptoms). DRESS is characterized by a drug-related rash with eosinophilia and whole-body symptoms, such as fever, blood abnormalities, and organ inflammation.

How are skin rashes treated?

If you have a mild or moderate skin rash, you and your doctor may decide to change the medications in your HIV treatment regimen. Alternatively, your doctor may treat you with an antihistamine drug while you continue on the same HIV treatment regimen. Be sure to talk with your doctor before stopping or making any changes to your medications.

In cases of severe rash (SJS, TEN, or DRESS), your doctor will stop your anti-HIV medication and may admit you to the hospital. While in the hospital, you may be treated with intravenous (IV) fluids and medications such as anti-inflammatories and antibiotics. Patients with TEN and significant skin loss may need to be in a hospital's burn unit for specialized care.

If you have a severe rash while taking anti-HIV medications, you and your doctor must identify which medication caused the rash, and you should never take that medication again, even as part of a future HIV treatment regimen. Exposure to the problem medication could result in an even more severe, and perhaps fatal, drug reaction. Be aware that if you experienced a reaction to a drug in a particular class (for example, an NNRTI), you may be at risk of a serious reaction to another drug in that class. This is referred to as cross-hypersensitivity.

Chapter 24

Other HIV/AIDS Treatment Complications

Chapter Contents

Section 24.1

Drug Interactions

"What's in Your Medicine Cabinet?" © 2005 Center for AIDS
(www.centerforaids.org). Reprinted with permission. Revised by
David A. Cooke, MD, FACP, November 2010.

What are drug interactions?

Human immunodeficiency virus (HIV) treatment usually involves three or more medications taken in combination.

HIV-positive people may also take additional meds to treat opportunistic infections (OIs) and other conditions associated with HIV/AIDS (acquired immunodeficiency syndrome), or to manage drug side effects. As a result, drug interactions are possible between the HIV meds and these other kinds of meds. A drug interaction occurs when one med affects how the body processes or reacts to another med. This is true even for meds sold over-the counter (OTC) without a doctor's prescription. Also, street drugs, methadone, alternative and complementary ("natural") therapies, and even certain foods may cause drug interactions with HIV meds. Some of these interactions have little effect, while others can lead to severe toxicities, loss of HIV suppression, or the emergence of drug-resistant virus.

What causes drug interactions?

Drug interactions fall into two broad categories: pharmacodynamic and pharmacokinetic. Pharmacodynamic interactions are those related to the combined activity of two or more drugs when used together. For example, sometimes the effects are additive or "synergistic," while other times the two drugs may be negative or "antagonistic." This can make either or both drugs more or less effective. Pharmacokinetic interactions occur when one agent changes the blood concentration of another:

- **Pharmacodynamics:** What a drug does to the body

- **Pharmacokinetics:** What the body does to a drug

Drug interactions are not the same in all people. Several factors can influence pharmacokinetics, including sex, age, race/ethnicity, pregnancy, hormone levels, body size, alcohol use, and coexisting conditions such as liver or kidney problems. For instance, individuals may possess genetic differences that affect expression of specific liver proteins (or "enzymes") used to process medications. One example of this includes the CYP450 enzymes in the liver.

The impact of liver disease is of special concern because a substantial proportion of HIV-positive people have chronic hepatitis B or C co-infection, which can lead to liver damage including fibrosis and cirrhosis (scarring). When the liver is damaged—as a result of viral hepatitis, heavy alcohol use, drug toxicity, or some other cause—its ability to process drugs may be impaired, potentially leading to higher than normal drug levels in the blood. The vast majority of drug interactions involving HIV meds are pharmacokinetic and the result of a change in the absorption, distribution, metabolism, or elimination of either the HIV medication itself or the concurrently administered medication.

How does this involve HIV meds?

Most of the HIV meds currently taken belong to one of the following families: nucleoside reverse transcriptase inhibitors (NRTIs or "nukes"), non-nucleoside reverse transcriptase (NNRTIs or "non-nukes"), and protease inhibitors (PIs). The cytochrome P450 (CYP450) enzyme system is responsible for turning drugs from active to inactive metabolites that are excreted by the body. Both PIs and NNRTIs can affect the CYP450 system. Therefore, metabolic drug interactions are most common and problematic when prescribing combinations that include these kinds of HIV meds. Numerous isoenzymes in the CYP450 family have been identified, and those responsible for the elimination of the majority of HIV meds are CYP3A4, CYP1A2, and CYP2D6:

- **NRTIs :** NRTIs are prone to pharmacodynamic interactions such as additive and synergistic toxicities, but because they are primarily eliminated by the kidneys, not the liver, they have little impact on the CYP450 system. As such, NRTIs have few known pharmacokinetic interactions with NNRTIs or PIs. AZT (zidovudine, Retrovir®) is processed by glucuronyl transferases in the liver, and agents that affect levels of these enzymes can raise or lower AZT blood levels. In the NRTI class of meds, only abacavir (Ziagen®) is broken down by the same enzyme that metabolizes alcohol; so taking alcohol may raise abacavir levels.

Tenofovir (Viread®) can have high failure rates if it is combined with didanosine and lamivudine, so this particular combination should be avoided.

- **NNRTIs:** All four approved NNRTIs affect the CYP450 system: nevirapine (Viramune®) is a CYP3A4 inducer (making it process drugs more quickly), delavirdine (Rescriptor®) is a CYP3A4 inhibitor (making it process drugs more slowly), and efavirenz (Sustiva®) combines both effects. Etravirine (Intelence®) is an inducer of CYP3A4, and an inhibitor of CYP2C9 and CYP2C19. The NNRTIs also induce and/or inhibit other isoenzymes that play less important roles in drug interactions.

- **PIs:** As a class, the PIs raise the most concern related to drug interactions. All approved PIs are metabolized by the CYP3A4 isoenzyme and are CYP3A4 inhibitors, but some are stronger inhibitors than others and have additional side effects. In fact, ritonavir (Norvir®) is known for its difficult side effects, but because it is a potent inhibitor of CYP450, it has since been used in low doses to achieve better levels of other PIs. This is the idea behind "boosted" PIs—now commonly done when people take PIs as part of their HIV combination therapy. Certain protease inhibitors such as darunavir (Prezista®) and tipranavir (Aptivus®) are approved for use only in combination with ritonavir, and lopinavir is only available as a lopinavir-ritonavir combination tablet (Kaletra®).

While most HIV therapy consists of drugs from the above three classes, there are a few other types of antivirals used in selected patients. These drugs are invariably given in combination with other drugs, and can also have some significant interactions:

- **Fusion Inhibitors**: At present, there is only one fusion inhibitor available, enfuvirtide (Fuzeon®). It is not metabolized by the CYP450 system, so it has few drug interactions. However, it is known to increase levels of tipranavir/ritonavir (Aptivus®), which may increase the risk of side effects from the PIs.

- **Integrase Strand Transfer Inhibitors**: There is only one drug of this class currently available, raltegravir (Isentress®). It does not appear to alter the metabolism of other medications. However, its effect is reduced by etravirine (®) and rifampin, and increased by omeprazole (Prilosec®). Dose adjustments must be made if it is combined with these medications.

- **CCR5 Antagonists:** The sole drug of this class, maraviroc (Selzentry®), is metabolized by CYP3A4, and significant dosing adjustments need to be made if it is prescribed with other drugs that induce CYP3A4.

What about drugs used to treat OIs?

Several different kinds of meds may be used to treat OIs. The azoles, macrolides, and rifamycins can interact not only with HIV meds, but also with each other. Because of this complexity, the care of HIV-positive people who require treatment for multiple OIs should be managed by experienced physicians.

How do acid-lowering drugs interact?

Medications that neutralize stomach acid can interfere with the absorption of drugs like atazanavir (Reyataz®) and tipranavir (Aptivus®) that require an acid environment. Such medications are often taken to relieve acid reflux, or "heartburn." Over-the-counter antacids (such as TUMS® or Maalox®) and buffered medications work for only a short time, making it possible to use them one to two hours after taking acid-dependent drugs. Other types of acid lowering agents are much longer-acting. Proton pump inhibitors, which block the production of stomach acid, can alter gastric pH for twenty-four hours or longer. These include omeprazole (Prilosec®, Zegerid®), esomeprazole (Nexium®), lansoprazole (Prevacid®), pantoprazole (Protonix®), rabeprazole (AcipHex®), and dexlansoprazole (Kapidex®, Dexilant®).

What if you are taking cholesterol-lowering medications?

One class of commonly used cholesterol-lowering agents, the "statins," are metabolized by the CYP450 system and their concentrations can be increased by PIs (particularly ritonavir). But not all statins are equal. In its 2000 and 2003 reports, the Cardiovascular Disease Focus Group of the Adult AIDS Clinical Trials Group recommended that people on combination HIV therapy should start with low doses of pravastatin (Pravachol®), atorvastatin (Lipitor®), or fluvastatin (Lescol®), which appear to interact least with HIV meds. While the above guidelines do not address them, rosuvastatin (Crestor®) and pitavastatin (Livalo®) also have fewer interactions with most HIV medications.

The panel advised against use of lovastatin (Mevacor®) or simvastatin (Zocor®), which can reach dangerously high levels when used with PIs. Such high levels of statins might cause severe side effects including rhabdomyolysis (muscle damage) and kidney failure.

What about other meds?

PIs can increase blood levels of meds used to treat migraine headaches (ergot alkaloid derivatives such as Cafergot® and Migranal®), so co-administration of these drugs should be avoided. Levels of calcium-channel blockers (for example, diltiazem and verapamil) may also increase in the presence of CYP3A4 inhibitors (like PIs). These drugs are used to treat conditions such as angina (chest pain), high blood pressure, and cardiac arrhythmias.

PIs can also interact dangerously with immunosuppressive drugs such as tacrolimus (Prograf®), which are used to prevent organ rejection after a transplant. Levels of the erectile dysfunction drugs sildenafil (Viagra®), vardenafil (Levitra®), and tadalafil (Cialis®) may be increased when used with PIs, so a dose reduction of these drugs is recommended. In women using oral contraceptives containing ethynyl estradiol or other forms of estrogen, concurrent use of efavirenz, nevirapine, nelfinavir (Viracept®), ritonavir, or lopinavir/ritonavir (Kaletra®) may decrease hormone levels—enough to cause unintentional pregnancies.

Recreational and street drugs. Evidence suggests that ritonavir can increase blood concentrations of ecstasy (methylenedioxymethamphetamine [MDMA], "X"), which is metabolized by the CYP2D6 isoenzyme. Elevated ecstasy levels may cause heightened agitation, seizures, increased heart rate, and/or cardiac arrest. Other forms of amphetamine, including crystal meth ("speed," "crank," "Tina"), share the same processing pathway and may have similar interactions. However, cocaine, also a stimulant, has not been reported to interact with HIV meds. Ritonavir, other PIs, efavirenz, and nevirapine appear to reduce plasma concentrations of opiates (for example, heroin and numerous prescription pain-relievers), which may lead to withdrawal symptoms or inadequate pain relief.

Herbal remedies. Herbal remedies and nutritional supplements are not closely regulated like medications, and it is not always easy to determine the exact ingredients or amounts of various substances in these products. To reduce the risk of interactions, people with HIV should inform their healthcare providers about any alternative or complementary therapies they are using or considering. A clear example of why this is important is the herbal remedy St. John's wort, which is used to relieve depression. Studies have shown that St. John's wort induces both CYP3A4 and P-glycoproteins (which help clear drugs out of cells in the body). This was associated with significantly decreased indinavir (Crixivan®) concentrations in one study. Low levels of HIV meds can lead to the development of viral resistance to those meds. Garlic inhibits CYP3A4 activity, and a study showed that high-dose garlic supplements reduced saquinavir (Invirase®) levels. Another herbal remedy that could interact pharmacokinetically with HIV med is milk thistle (and its derivative, silymarin). Also, while grapefruit juice does affect CYP3A4 activity in the intestines, it does not appear to cause major interactions with PIs or NNRTIs.

How can drug interactions be prevented?

People with HIV should inform their healthcare team (general practitioners, specialist physicians, nurses, and alternative/complementary therapy providers) about all the medicinal products they are using: prescription drugs, OTC meds, recreational or street drugs, and alternative or complementary therapies including herbs and nutritional supplements. When considering a regimen change, do some research and ask about potential interactions. Discuss potential interactions with your healthcare provider. Pharmacists, who specialize in drugs and their pharmacokinetics, can be also an excellent resource.

Section 24.2

Immune Reconstitution Inflammatory Syndrome

It's a mouthful of a phrase, but immune reconstitution inflammatory syndrome (IRIS) is a serious condition that can be challenging to diagnose and treat. The main concern with IRIS is the inflammation that it causes. Though research is beginning to sort out the condition, it is still not well understood or predicted.

It's not clear who will more likely experience IRIS, though it most often occurs shortly after the start of human immunodeficiency virus (HIV) therapy in people with more damaged immune systems. More study needs to tease out its risk factors and to find screening tools to help predict and manage the condition.

What Is Inflammation?

Inflammation means to "put on fire," and it's a complex response that results when your body attacks germs or repairs damaged tissue. A simple example of it is the redness, swelling, and soreness that emerges around a cut as it heals. For your immune system to repair the damage and clear any infection that's present, cells and fluids are recruited to the site of the damage. This shows up as swelling, redness, and pain.

Inflammation can appear nearly anywhere in your body—in the liver, in lymph nodes, in nerve fibers, and even in areas outside organs like your immune system. Inflammation can be acute or chronic.

Acute inflammation lasts a short amount . . . a normal process that promotes healing. By contrast, chronic inflammation persists over time. Here, cells and tissues are healed and destroyed at the same time. It's thought to be unhealthy and possibly linked to serious diseases like heart disease and Alzheimer disease.

What Is IRIS?

IRIS can occur shortly after a person starts HIV therapy for the first time. It can also occur in people who restart their meds after a time being off them. IRIS happens when your immune system recovers too quickly. It can start to "overwork" and respond to other infections that may or may not have been diagnosed before starting therapy, even ones that may have been under control.

This results in inflammation throughout the body, sometimes flaring up as severe disease. IRIS is a paradoxical situation because, as your immune system does its job, the inflammation that occurs actually makes your symptoms worse. For some, these symptoms can be life threatening. Though most cases of IRIS resolve after a few weeks, the symptoms may be mistaken by you or your doctor as HIV disease progression or another condition.

Most people who start their first regimens do not develop IRIS. And of those who do, many cases resolve on their own. However, it's wise to report these symptoms to your health provider as soon as possible.

When IRIS does occur, it happens more often in people with tuberculosis (TB) and other mycobacterial infections, accounting for about two in five of the total IRIS cases. Some chronic conditions, particularly autoimmune disorders like rheumatoid arthritis, lupus, or Grave disease, may become aggravated by IRIS.

List of Known Infections That Contribute to IRIS

- CMV, or cytomegalovirus
- Cryptococcal meningitis, or cryptococcosis
- Eosinophilic folliculitis
- Hepatitis B and C
- Herpes, or HSV
- Herpes zoster, or shingles (VZV)
- Human papillomavirus, or HPV
- Kaposi sarcoma, or HHV8
- MAC, or *Mycobacterium avium* complex
- PCP, or *Pneumocystis jiroveci* pneumonia
- PML, or progressive multifocal leukoencephalopathy
- TB, or *Mycobacterium* tuberculosis

Who Is at Risk?

In general, people with poorer immune systems before starting HIV therapy are most at risk for IRIS. You and your doctor should be aware that IRIS is possible after starting therapy; especially if you know that another infection was or is present and even under control. Possible risk factors are listed below. The more of these risks you have, the more likely that IRIS can result:

- CD4s below 100 before starting HIV therapy.

- Starting HIV therapy for the first time, or restarting therapy after a time off meds.

- Large drops in HIV levels (2.5 logs or more) due to therapy (IRIS has been seen in people with drops of 1.0 log).

- Diagnosis of another infection before starting therapy. The closer that is to starting therapy, the higher the risk.

- Starting on protease inhibitors boosted with Norvir® (some evidence).

How Is It Diagnosed?

A differential diagnosis is normally used to identify IRIS. This is when the diagnosis is narrowed down from a list of possibilities until one emerges as the best. This diagnosis will consider the failed treatment of the current infection, a possible new infection or malignancy, and drug side effects (especially with hepatitis).

IRIS tends to occur when there's a large drop in HIV levels (viral loads). An example of this would be going from 100,000 copies of HIV down to about 500 in just a few weeks, which shows a strong response to therapy but an increased risk for IRIS. So closely checking HIV levels is an important way to help diagnose possible IRIS.

Other tests can also assist the diagnosis, such as white blood count and C-reactive protein, which show inflammation. The higher the levels, the more likely major inflammation is taking place.

What Are the Symptoms?

Symptoms of IRIS can vary and can be dangerous. They usually appear within two to six weeks of starting HIV therapy. For some, the symptoms may improve and resolve on their own. For others, they may persist or get worse and become life threatening. In any of these cases, these symptoms should be told to your health provider.

Common symptoms include fever, swollen lymph nodes, skin lesions and rashes, changes in breathing, pneumonia, hepatitis, abscesses, and eye inflammation. Although less common, some people can experience short-term mental changes, like memory problems. Though IRIS can react to a specific infection like TB, IRIS symptoms may not appear like the symptoms originally did for the TB, or other infections.

IRIS symptoms are mostly different than and should not be confused with the possible side effects from starting HIV drugs, like fever or skin rash. If drug side effects do occur, they usually appear soon after starting your meds. Within a few weeks your body usually readjusts to them and they go away. However, drug side effects may overlap IRIS symptoms, which makes it challenging to diagnose IRIS.

How Do You Treat IRIS?

No standard of care is currently in place for treating IRIS, so the best way to treat it is unknown at this time. However, it's important to address the condition as soon as symptoms appear. Treatment options are based mostly on case reports and other anecdotal data.

Treating IRIS usually starts by treating the active infection, like TB or herpes. HIV therapy is usually continued as well, unless IRIS becomes life threatening. The goal here is to stop the mounting inflammation. You may be prescribed nonsteroidal anti-inflammatory drugs (NSAIDs) and/or corticosteroids.

Starting HIV therapy while an active infection persists is a controversial issue, and it may be dangerous. However, there are not a lot of data to help guide this type of decision. In fact, several studies show that the closer another infection is diagnosed before starting HIV therapy, the more likely IRIS will occur.

Therefore, deciding to start therapy can be especially troubling for you and your doctor if the infection becomes severe or if your immune system doesn't respond. Still, if the immune system is stable and other health markers suggest treating the actual infection, holding off on starting HIV therapy may be the best option until the active infection has been resolved.

Special Concerns for People Living with HIV

Before starting HIV therapy, especially if you have a severely damaged immune system (low CD4 count and high HIV level), it may be wise to aggressively diagnose any possible infections. Some may appear as though they're well under control, such as TB disease. Some may have resolved many months or even years ago.

However, other infections may have occurred without you noticing their symptoms, like herpes or HPV. This is called a subclinical infection. Talking to your doctor, doing a thorough medical history, and checking a full range of blood tests can go a long way in diagnosing other possible infections.

What Can Help to Ask about at a Doctor's Visit?

- Am I at risk for IRIS? How many risk factors do I have?

- What types of symptoms should I be aware of? What should I do if I have them?

- How do I tell the difference between IRIS symptoms and side effects from the HIV drugs?

- Can starting HIV therapy make my herpes (or other infection) worse? How do we manage that?

What Does Recent Research Show?

Asthma medicine

A type of immune chemical, called a leukotriene, causes different types of inflammation. Drugs that reduce these levels in the body, called leukotriene inhibitors, are commonly used to treat asthma. Since it's thought that leukotriene inhibitors affect other inflammation in the body, they may be useful for treating IRIS.

Encouraging results have been reported by doctors in London who used a common asthma medicine, Singulair® (montelukast), to treat IRIS in a fifty-nine-year-old man. After five months off therapy, he restarted with a protease inhibitor boosted with Norvir®. IRIS appeared a few weeks later as a skin rash, and prednisone was used. His health improved somewhat but the rash returned along with a fever and rapid heartbeat. Singulair was prescribed and within five days his symptoms had settled.

Although this case does not prove that this therapy would work for everyone, it may open up new research into using these drugs to treat IRIS. If this turns out to be true, then already approved drugs may be easily adapted to treat the condition.

Gene Markers

Finding ways to diagnose earlier who will develop IRIS will allow for better strategies for its prevention and treatment. One study at the

Conference on Retroviruses and Opportunistic Infections (CROI) 2008 reported results of twenty-eight people with and thirty-eight without recent cryptococcal meningitis who started HIV therapy. Researchers looked at eighty-five genes that were related to inflammation. Results showed that using certain gene markers may help predict IRIS before it becomes a problem, but more study is needed.

Immune Markers in TB Disease

One study at CROI 2008 reported disappointing results of finding immune markers that would adequately predict IRIS in TB disease. A Thai study showed that IL-12 and serum IL-2, among other markers, did not show differences between those who did and did not develop IRIS. However, a second study reported that they're looking at other markers, such as regulatory and effector T cells, monocytes, and macrophages.

Chapter 25

HIV/AIDS Treatment Failure

Chapter Contents

Section 25.1

What Is Treatment Failure?

Excerpted from "HIV Treatment Failure," AIDSinfo.gov,
December 2009.

What is treatment failure?

Treatment failure happens when the anti-HIV (human immunodeficiency virus) medications you take can't control your infection. There are three types of treatment failure: virologic failure, immunologic failure, and clinical progression.

Virologic failure happens when anti-HIV medications can't reduce the amount of virus in the blood. (While taking medications, viral load doesn't drop or it repeatedly rises again after having dropped.)

Immunologic failure happens when the immune system doesn't respond to anti-HIV medications. (While taking medications, CD4 count doesn't rise or it drops.)

Clinical progression happens when a person has symptoms of HIV disease despite taking anti-HIV medications.

The three types of treatment failure may happen alone or together. In general, virologic failure happens first, followed by immunologic failure, and then clinical progression. They may happen months to years apart.

What are risk factors for treatment failure?

Factors that can increase the risk of treatment failure include the following:

- Previous treatment failure

- Drug resistance

- Poor treatment adherence

- Anti-HIV medications poorly absorbed by the body

- Other illnesses or conditions

- Poor health before starting treatment

- Side effects of medications or interactions with other medications
- substance abuse leading to poor treatment adherence

What happens if my treatment fails?

Your doctor will do many things to understand why your treatment failed. He or she will evaluate your treatment history, medication side effects, and your physical condition. Tell your doctor if you often forget to take your medications or if you have problems taking them as directed. Not taking medications as prescribed is one of the main reasons for treatment failure.

You and your doctor may decide to choose a new treatment regimen to better control your infection. Drug resistance testing will help you and your doctor select a new regimen.

What is drug resistance testing?

Drug resistance testing shows if your HIV is resistant to any anti-HIV medications. Resistance testing is done in a laboratory using a sample of your blood. The results of drug resistance testing provide information about which anti-HIV medications will be most effective.

Your doctor will help you find ways to adhere to your new regimen. Taking your medications as prescribed will reduce the chance of treatment failure on your new regimen. Tell your doctor if you can't tolerate your medications because of side effects or if you can't take them according to directions. Don't stop taking your medications or skip pills on your own. Talk to your doctor. He or she can help you find the best regimen and the best ways to take your medications as prescribed.

Section 25.2

Changing Your HIV Treatment Regimen

Excerpted from "Changing My HIV Treatment Regimen,"
AIDSinfo.gov, December 2009.

How will my doctor and I know what medications to use next?

Before changing your treatment regimen, your doctor will try to find out why your current regimen is not working. Your doctor will evaluate your adherence to the regimen, the regimen's tolerability, and drug interactions. Whether you and your doctor decide to change your regimen and what new medications you will take will depend on why your current regimen is failing.

What is adherence?

Adherence refers to how closely you follow (adhere to) your treatment regimen. If your regimen is failing because you cannot adhere to it, you and your doctor should discuss why you are having difficulty taking your medication and what you can do to improve your adherence. Your doctor may change your regimen to reduce the number of pills you take or how often you take them.

What is tolerability?

Tolerability refers to how many and what types of negative side effects you experience while taking your medications. If the side effects are severe, you may need to change your regimen. Your doctor will ask you what side effects you have and how long you have had them. You and your doctor will decide whether to treat the side effects or to change your anti- HIV (human immunodeficiency virus) medications.

What are drug interactions?

Anti-HIV medications may interact with other medications you are taking. This may reduce the effectiveness of the medications or increase the risk of negative side effects. You and your doctor should review all of your medications, including over-the-counter medications and herbal remedies. You should also review whether your medications should be taken with food or on an empty stomach.

When should I consider changing regimens?

If your regimen is failing and you and your doctor have ruled out adherence, tolerability, and drug interactions, you should consider changing your regimen. Before changing anti-HIV medications, talk with your doctor about the following things:

- Anti-HIV medications you have taken before

- The strength of the new medications your doctor recommends

- Possible side effects of the new medications

- How well you will be able to adhere to the new regimen

- The number of anti-HIV medications that you have not yet used

Your doctor will confirm that your regimen is failing with at least two viral load tests and three CD4 counts. You should also be tested for drug resistance while you are taking the failing regimen.

In general, your new treatment regimen should include three or more medications. You and your doctor will choose the medications based on your medication history, results of resistance testing, and side effects you have experienced. If you have already taken many of the U.S. Food and Drug Association (FDA)–approved anti-HIV medications, your doctor may recommend a new medication currently under investigation. You may be eligible to participate in a clinical trial using these medications or new treatment strategies. For more information about participating in a clinical trial, ask your doctor.

Section 25.3

Salvage Therapy

"Salvage Therapy," Fact Sheet #408. © 2009 AIDS InfoNet. Reprinted
with permission. InfoNet fact sheets are updated frequently. Please visit
the website at http://www.aidsinfonet.org for the newest version.

What Is Salvage Therapy?

Antiretroviral therapy (ART) sometimes needs to be changed. This
usually happens when the viral load increases instead of staying very
low. This treatment failure almost always means that human immunodeficiency virus (HIV) has developed resistance to the antiretroviral
drugs (ARVs) someone is taking. Then HIV can multiply even when
someone is taking ART. Treatment failure is also often caused by skipping doses (poor adherence).

Before the use of triple combinations of antiretroviral drugs (ARVs)
many healthcare providers changed ART at the first sign of an increase
in viral load. Patients were given just one new ARV at a time. This
approach is called "sequential monotherapy" or "virtual monotherapy."
The goal was just to keep the patient alive for a few more months.

We now know that this is not the best way to control viral load. If
the virus is only exposed to one new drug, it's much easier for the virus
to develop resistance.

As a patient's virus accumulates more and more resistance mutations, it becomes harder to choose ARVs that can control it. When there
are no good treatment options, ART for these patients is referred to
as "salvage therapy." The number of people with HIV in the United
States who need salvage therapy is unknown, but is estimated to be
between twenty thousand and forty thousand.

How Can You Avoid Salvage Therapy?

The best way to avoid salvage therapy is to make each regimen of
ART last as long as you can. Be sure to miss as few doses as possible.
Learn about the pattern of resistance of your virus. Ask your health-
care provider about any changes in your ART.

If possible, you should always have two or more "active drugs" in your ART regimen. An active drug is one that is expected to work against HIV based on the mutations in your virus. Your healthcare provider will need to review the results of a resistance test. This can be a genotypic test or a phenotypic test.

Remember, the best way to get into trouble is to just add one new drug at a time to failing ART. That will set you up for resistance to the new drug in a very short time.

When Does Someone Need Salvage Therapy?

Once HIV has acquired several resistance mutations, the chances of serious HIV disease are higher. This is especially true for patients with low CD4 counts. You may need to make immediate changes if:

- you are losing weight;
- your CD4 count is dropping;
- you have serious side effects;
- you have increasing symptoms.

However, if your health and CD4 count are stable, you can go onto a "holding regimen" while you wait for new drugs to be developed. Do not stop taking medications to prevent opportunistic infections (OIs). The drugs you need to take to prevent OIs are based on your CD4 count.

What Is a "Holding Regimen"?

If you don't have at least two active ARVs to use, you need to pre-serve your CD4 count and keep your viral load as low as possible. You also want to preserve your treatment options. This normally means stopping any ARVs that are only partly effective so that your virus doesn't develop more resistance to them. This would make them totally ineffective. However, stopping all ARVs can be harmful.

On the other hand, stopping non-nucleoside reverse transcriptase inhibitors (NNRTIs; delavirdine, nevirapine, or efavirenz) does not lead to increases in viral load or drops in CD4 cells. There's no benefit to keeping an NNRTI in a holding regimen. It appears that stopping protease inhibitors is less risky than stopping nukes (reverse transcriptase inhibitors.)

It can be scary to wait until you have two active ARVs available. The alternative is to "use up" a new ARV and lose its benefits quickly due to viral resistance.

Getting Access to New Drugs

You may not have to wait until new drugs are approved before you can use them. You may have access to a clinical trial of a drug in development. Some ARVs become available through an expanded access program long before they are approved. Currently the NNRTI etravirine (TMC125) and the integrase inhibitor raltegravir (Isentress®) are available in expanded access. Sometimes these programs continue after approval for patients with special needs.

Remember that you want to be able to combine a new drug with at least one other active drug. You should review clinical trials carefully with your healthcare provider to make sure you're not exposed to sequential monotherapy. This is most likely if you get assigned to a "placebo" arm and don't receive the new drug being studied.

The best option is being able to use a drug in a new class. Your virus will almost certainly not have any resistance mutations to a fusion or attachment inhibitor, or an integrase inhibitor. Right now, you might have access to T-20 (Fuzeon®, enfuvirtide) which is a fusion inhibitor. There are also clinical trials of attachment inhibitors and integrase inhibitors and other ARVs.

The Bottom Line

There are more options today for people with advanced HIV disease than at any time in the past. Treatment can have excellent results, even for people whose virus is resistant to most existing ARVs. An experienced healthcare provider is very important in helping you decide when to change treatment and when to wait.

Chapter 26

Alternative and Complementary Therapies for HIV/AIDS

Alternative and complementary medicine is quite popular among people living with human immunodeficiency virus (HIV). For example, around one-half of HIV-positive Americans report recent use.[1] Many HIV-positive people say they feel better after using alternative and complementary medicine, and it is likely that some of these treatments are indeed beneficial, although unproven according to conventional Western medicine.

What Are Alternative and Complementary Medicines?

Alternative and complementary medicine is the name generally given to those medical and healthcare systems, practices, and products that are not presently considered to be part of conventional Western medicine. Well-known examples include herbal and other nutritional supplements, acupuncture, aromatherapy and homeopathy.

Alternative medicine is used in place of conventional medicine.

Complementary medicine is used together with conventional medicine.

The more ancient forms of complementary and alternative medicine are also known as traditional medicine.

What Are These Therapies Used For?

In relation to HIV, alternative therapies are most commonly used in areas where it is difficult to access Western medicine. In the absence of antiretroviral treatment, people seek other ways to delay the onset of AIDS, or to treat opportunistic infections. In sub-Saharan Africa, for example, traditional healers outnumber medically qualified doctors eighty-to-one.[2] Traditional healers also usually provide immediate treatment, whereas clinics may have lengthy waiting lists and tests for eligibility.

Most people living with HIV in developed countries have ready access to antiretroviral therapy and conventional treatments for opportunistic infections. Because these treatments are so effective, there is less demand for alternative HIV medicine, except perhaps for addressing relatively minor infections, or when antiretroviral treatment cannot any longer be taken, for example because of drug resistance. Many instead look to complementary medicine as a way to prevent or relieve acquired immunodeficiency syndrome (AIDS) treatment side effects, some of which are not easily treatable with conventional medicine. There is also demand for complementary therapies that might boost immunity, relieve stress, or improve general health and wellbeing.

The people who distrust and avoid Western medicine for HIV include not only individuals, but also some governments. For example, senior politicians in South Africa have promoted unproven therapies while at times disparaging antiretroviral drugs. In Gambia, the president himself has treated patients with an herbal mixture he claims is an AIDS cure.

Do Alternative and Complementary Therapies for HIV and AIDS Work?

Western medicine embraces all approaches shown to be safe and effective in rigorous scientific trials. By definition, complementary and alternative medicine consists of therapies that are unproven, at least by the standards of Western medicine. Given the many therapies in existence, there can be little doubt that some of them do what they are supposed to. Many others are likely to be ineffective or can even be harmful. In the absence of good scientific trials, it is impossible to be certain which is which.

Still it can be argued that, from a scientific point of view, some things are more likely to work than others. Acupuncture, for example, appears to alter brain activity,[3] and there is quite good evidence that it can help relieve postoperative nausea.[4,5] Herbal medicines, too, are scientifically plausible: some 25 percent of modern drugs were derived from plants first used traditionally.[6] Scientists have already identified one plant extract that acts like an antiretroviral drug;[7] it is entirely possible that there are others.

At the other end of the scale are therapies that seem to defy the known laws of science. The most notorious of these is homeopathy, which few scientists see as credible and the World Health Organization recommends should not be used to treat HIV.[8] Homeopathic remedies are so diluted that none of the active ingredient remains.

Yet even if a medicine has no specific effects on an illness, this doesn't necessarily mean it is worse than nothing. It is widely accepted that patients' beliefs about a treatment, and the quality of the doctor-patient relationship, can influence health outcomes. This is what is known as the placebo effect. For example, one trial[9] divided irritable bowel syndrome sufferers into three groups: the first received no treatment, the second underwent sham acupuncture (placebo), and the third got fake acupuncture plus a forty-five-minute consultation with a friendly doctor. The proportions of patients reporting moderate or substantial improvement were 3 percent (no treatment), 20 percent (placebo only), and 37 percent (placebo plus interaction). This effect may well account for some of the reported benefits of alternative and complementary medicine, as suggested in an editorial that accompanied the study: "Is it possible that the alternative medical community has tended historically to understand something important about the experience of illness and the ritual of doctor-patient interactions that the rest of medicine might do well to hear? . . . The meanings and expectations created by the interactions of doctors and patients matter physically, not just subjectively."[10]

Even if it fails to ease symptoms, the treatment experience may have nonspecific effects such as boosting self-confidence and relieving anxiety. Group therapies—such as yoga—are particularly good for meeting new people, who may be able to share knowledge of other treatment options.

Why Is There Such a Lack of Evidence?

Supporters of complementary and alternative medicine propose a number of reasons why their therapies have not been subjected to thorough testing. For one thing, major medical trials are highly expensive; if there is no prospect of a patent then there is less of an incentive to invest in research. Reliable, ethical trials also require a considerable amount of expertise. Many scientists with the necessary skills are reluctant to investigate therapies they think are implausible.

Yet it is misleading to suggest that no research takes place. The U.S. government has an agency (National Center for Complementary and Alternative Medicine [NCCAM]) dedicated to complementary and alternative medicine, and in 2008 allocated nearly $300 million to this field (around 1 percent of all federal funding for medical research). Potential HIV therapies investigated in government-sponsored trials include acupuncture, yoga, Reiki, and distant healing.[11]

Although practitioners of complementary and alternative medicine generally voice support for scientific research, they are often unwilling to accept negative findings. In 2005, medical journal *The Lancet* published the most thorough review of homeopathy trials ever conducted.[12] Having analyzed more than one hundred trials related to a wide range of illnesses, the authors concluded, "there was no convincing evidence that homeopathy was superior to placebo."

Homeopaths united in objecting to the methodology of both the trials and the review.[13] Some even suggested that placebo-controlled randomized trials (regarded as the gold standard of medical science) were inappropriate for testing their system of healing.[14]

Potential for Harm

Some forms of complementary and alternative medicine can cause harmful side effects. Words like "natural" and "traditional" are certainly no guarantee of safety.

Herbal or nutritional therapies (notably St. John's wort) may also interact with other medications, making them less effective or worsening their side effects.

In general, herbal remedies and dietary supplements are not covered by the strict regulations that govern pharmaceutical drugs. Quality is inconsistent even among popular commercial formulations; tests have shown that the concentrations of active ingredients can vary greatly from the amounts listed on the packaging.[15]

The standard of complementary and alternative practitioners is similarly uneven. Although some countries regulate certain types of practitioners (such as osteopaths in the United States and United Kingdom), many people practice without any formal qualifications.

Even if a therapy carries little risk of direct physical harm, it may still turn out to be a waste of time and money. Relying on alternative medicine instead of scientifically proven treatment can have very serious consequences. Once HIV has severely weakened the immune system, antiretroviral drugs are less likely to be lifesaving.

Advice for Those Seeking Complementary Medicine

HIV-positive people have a long history of taking control of their own healthcare decision-making. Those interested in complementary medicine can take steps to maximize their chances of success.

The Canadian AIDS Treatment Information Exchange (CATIE) suggests ten questions for assessing a new therapy:[16]

- What am I hoping to get out of this therapy?

- Do other HIV-positive people use it?

- Am I able to talk to any of these other people about their experiences?

- Is there any research or additional information about this therapy?

- What are the side effects, if any?

- What sort of commitment do I have to make to use this treatment?

- Where can I get this treatment, and will it be regularly available?

- How much of this treatment is too much and what are the early signs of taking too much?

- Does this treatment interact with anything else I'm taking?

- How much does it cost?

Careful research is needed to answer these questions. Good sources of information include reference books on complementary medicine (available in many libraries), medical journals (which can be searched using the PubMed website), and the publications of reputable health organizations. Many AIDS organizations and other bodies, including NCCAM, will answer inquiries over the phone or online.

As already discussed, all forms of complementary medicine are unproven; each individual must make their own assessment of likely risks and benefits based on the available data. The most reliable evidence comes from large human trials—preferably randomized trials in which the treatment is compared to a placebo. Personal testimonies and laboratory findings should be given less weight, especially if they appear only in promotional material. Anyone who makes sensational claims (such as being able to cure many unrelated diseases with a single therapy), or who attacks conventional treatment, is probably a quack and best avoided.

If you have done your research and wish to try a complementary therapy, the next step is to talk to your personal doctor or HIV specialist. This is important because there may be a risk of interactions with other medications.

Some medical doctors have received training in complementary medicine. If your doctor lacks such expertise then it may be sensible to also find a complementary practitioner, ideally one with experience in treating people with HIV. Help finding a practitioner may be obtained from your doctor, an AIDS service organization, or a professional body such as the Institute for Complementary Medicine in the United Kingdom, or the American Holistic Medical Association in the United States. There are many practitioners available; it is worth taking the time to find one you trust and feel comfortable with. Look for experience, qualifications, and references you can verify.

When purchasing an herbal medicine or nutritional supplement, try to choose a reputable seller and manufacturer. Large, long-established companies are generally the most trustworthy because they have more to lose from selling poor-quality goods. If possible, look for a company that submits its products for independent quality testing.

Having started a new treatment, it is a good idea to keep a diary of your symptoms. This will help you assess whether the therapy is having the desired outcome, or whether it may be causing unwanted side effects.

List of Common Complementary and Alternative Therapies

Complementary and alternative therapies can be divided into five main categories. The list below contains a few of the most popular examples.

Whole Medical Systems

- Naturopathic medicine (mostly practiced in the West; includes diet modification, herbal medicine, acupuncture, and massage)

- Traditional Chinese medicine (includes herbal medicine, acupuncture, and massage)

- Ayurveda (ancient Indian healing system; includes diet modification, herbal medicine, cleansing therapies, massage, meditation, and yoga)

- Homeopathy (most commonly prescribes extremely diluted solutions of natural substances)

Mind-Body Medicine

- Relaxation techniques, meditation, and visualization
- Spirituality and prayer
- Yoga (may incorporate spirituality, meditation, and body postures)
- Tai Chi (a Chinese martial art incorporating meditation and breathing exercises)
- Qigong (includes meditation, body postures, and breathing exercises)
- Aromatherapy (uses remedies derived from plants that are inhaled, applied to the skin, or used internally)

Biologically Based Practices

- Vitamins and minerals
- Herbal remedies
- Animal-derived extracts
- Prebiotics and probiotics (aim to encourage the growth of beneficial microbes)

Manipulative and Body-Based Practices

- Massage
- Chiropractic (invented in America; manipulates the spine)
- Osteopathy (invented in America; manipulates the spine, joints, and muscles; American osteopathic physicians are also trained in conventional medicine)
- Shiatsu (traditional form of Japanese massage therapy)
- Reflexology (invented in America; applies pressure to the feet, hands, or ears)
- Rolfing (named after American Ida Pauline Rolf; manipulates soft tissue)

Energy Medicine

- Acupuncture (involves inserting fine needles into the body)
- Reiki (practitioners claim to channel healing energy through their palms)

- Therapeutic touch and distant healing (practitioners claim to manipulate energy "biofields" with their hands)

- Bioelectromagnetic-based therapies (involve unconventional use of sound, light, magnetism, and other forms of electromagnetic radiation)

African Traditional Healers and HIV

Sub-Saharan Africa is the region worst affected by AIDS; it is also a region in which most people turn first to traditional healers when they fall ill. There is potential for traditional healers to play an important role in responding to the epidemic.

Although few have been scientifically tested, there can be little doubt that some of the remedies given by traditional healers are effective in treating HIV-related opportunistic infections and drug side effects. However, in common with all forms of medicine, these therapies may also do harm through side effects, drug interactions, or delaying use of conventional treatment. In addition, the reuse of implements for rituals such as scarification, tattooing, and circumcision can transmit infections, including HIV. Some African healers blame illness on witchcraft, which can lead to ostracism of those accused.

Collaboration between traditional healers and Western doctors has the potential to improve safety, for example by encouraging better hygiene. Training can also assist traditional healers in identifying illnesses beyond their capacity to treat, hastening referral to a clinic when necessary. In South Africa, the Traditional Health Practitioners Act includes a council to oversee and provide training to traditional health practitioners to protect the interests of the patient. As yet, the act has not been fully enforced; there have been calls to implement the act alongside a robust system of scientific testing of "remedies."[17]

Traditional healers are respected within their communities, and know how to convey health information in a culturally appropriate manner. They are ideally placed to teach HIV prevention, distribute condoms, conduct counseling, encourage HIV testing, and set up support groups for affected people.

Yet although traditional healers are generally eager to learn from other health workers, experience has shown it is not easy to establish successful collaboration.[18] Traditional theories of disease causation are very different to those of Western science. Traditional healers— suppressed during the colonial era, and often demonized in the media—are understandably suspicious of authority. Many are reluctant to reveal details of their remedies for fear that their ideas will be stolen. Likewise, conventional doctors are inclined to be prejudiced against treatments that lack scientific foundation. These are not the only difficulties: "How can healers give their clients a diagnosis of AIDS when it means possibly losing their business? How can a traditional healer—the traditional advocate of a clan's fertility—counsel an HIV-positive woman who wants to have a child? And how can a traditional healer turn away a sick patient who has become dependent on his or her care and support?"[19]

It may take months or even years to establish mutual trust, confidence, and respect. Success depends on being sensitive to the local context, and cooperation must be on equal terms, regardless of level of education. Rather than trying to change traditional belief systems, research has shown it is better to stress what is common to both forms of medicine, and to establish a common language.[20]

The best way to maximize the reach of training is to first identify and train a group of the most influential and respected healers, who can each then train many others. This method, however, requires ongoing support if it is to be sustainable.[21]

Despite the challenges, a number of organizations—such as THETA in Uganda and Tanga AIDS Working Group (TAWG) in Tanzania—have demonstrated the benefits of collaborating with traditional healers in HIV prevention and care.[22] Much could be gained from replicating these programs more widely.

References

1. Hsiao A.F. et al (1 June 2003) "Complementary and alternative medicine use and substitution for conventional therapy by HIV-infected patients," *JAIDS* 33(2).

2. Mills E. et al (17 June 2006) "The challenges of involving traditional healers in HIV/AIDS care" *Int J STD & AIDS* 17(6).

3. Lewith G.T. et al (September 2005) "Investigating acupuncture using brain imaging techniques: the current state of play" *Evidence-based complementary and alternative medicine* 2(3).

4. Lee A and Done M. L. (2004) "Stimulation of the wrist acupuncture point P6 for preventing postoperative nausea and vomiting."

5. Lee A et al (September 2006) "Publication bias affected the estimate of postoperative nausea in an acupoint stimulation systematic review" *Journal of Clinical Epidemiology* 59(9),

6. World Health Organisation (May 2003) "Fact Sheet No. 134: Traditional Medicine."

7. Eiznhamer D.A. et al (November–December 2002) "Safety and pharmacokinetic profile of multiple escalating doses of (+)-calanolide A, a naturally occurring nonnucleoside reverse transcriptase inhibitor, in healthy HIV-negative volunteers" *HIV Clinical Trials*.

8. Mashta, O. (2009, 24th August), "WHO warns against using homeopathy to treat serious diseases" *British Medical Journal* 339(b3447).

9. Kaptchuk T. J. et al (3 May 2008) "Components of placebo effect: randomised controlled trial in patients with irritable bowel syndrome" *BMJ* 336(7651).

10. Spiegel D. and Harrington A. (3 May 2008) "What is the placebo worth?" *BMJ* 336(7651).

11. NCCAM: All Clinical Trials.

12. Shang A. et al (27 August 2005) "Are the clinical effects of homoeopathy placebo effects? Comparative study of placebo-controlled trials of homoeopathy and allopathy." *Lancet* 366(9487).

13. The Society of Homeopaths press release (19 September 2005) "Universal Condemnation for *The Lancet*'s Stance on Homeopathy."

14. Chatfield K. and Relton C. (September 2005) "Are the clinical effects of homeopathy placebo effects?—A full critique of the article by Shang et al."

15. Harkey M. R. et al (June 2001) "Variability in commercial ginseng products: an analysis of 25 preparations" *American Journal of Clinical Nutrition* 73(6).

16. CATIE (2004) "A Practical Guide to Complementary Therapies for People Living With HIV."

17. TAC (Dec 2009) "Equal Treatment Magazine."

18. Kayombo E. J. et al (26 January 2007) "Experience of initiating collaboration of traditional healers in managing HIV and AIDS in Tanzania" *Journal of ethnobiology and ethnomedicine* 3:6.

19. UNAIDS (2000) "Collaboration with traditional healers in HIV/AIDS prevention and care in sub-Saharan Africa—A Literature Review."

20. UNAIDS (2006) "Collaborating with Traditional Healers for HIV Prevention and Care in sub-Saharan Africa: suggestions for Programme Managers and Field Workers."

21. Mills E. et al (June 2006) "The challenges of involving traditional healers in HIV/AIDS care" *Int J STD & AIDS* 17(6).

22. UNAIDS (2000) "Collaboration with traditional healers in HIV/AIDS prevention and care in sub-Saharan Africa—A Literature Review."

Chapter 27

Medical Marijuana for HIV/AIDS

How is medical marijuana used by people with human immunodeficiency virus (HIV) and acquired immunodeficiency syndrome (AIDS)?

Medical marijuana is commonly used to relieve nausea, vomiting, and appetite loss sometimes caused by HIV infection or by medications used to treat HIV. Research has consistently found that these side effects are the leading reason patients interrupt or discontinue antiretroviral therapy (ART).

Has medical marijuana been studied in HIV/AIDS patients?

Yes. Although foot-dragging by federal authorities delayed needed research for years, two clinical trials have been completed and more are underway. Other information is available from observational studies. Results thus far have been consistently positive. A landmark study conducted at San Francisco General Hospital looked at the safety of medical marijuana use by patients on stable ART regimens and showed no adverse effects on viral load, CD4, or CD8 count, while the patients using marijuana gained more weight than those receiving a placebo.[1] An observational study published in January 2005 found that patients experiencing ART-related nausea adhered to their drug regimens more consistently if they used marijuana.[2] A study published in the journal *Neurology* in February 2007 reported that smoked marijuana "effectively relieved chronic pain from HIV-associated sensory neuropathy," with few side effects.[3]

I've heard that marijuana may be harmful to the immune system. Is it a danger to people with HIV/AIDS?

Such claims are based on test tube studies, often using enormous doses, rather than on studies of actual patients. In the San Francisco General Hospital study described above, patients using medical marijuana not only showed no signs of immunological damage, they actually gained more CD4 and CD8 cells than those receiving a placebo.

What do leading HIV/AIDS experts say about medical marijuana?

Leading HIV/AIDS organizations overwhelmingly believe seriously ill patients should be allowed to use medical marijuana without fear of arrest. The American Academy of HIV Medicine has stated, "When appropriately prescribed and monitored, marijuana/cannabis can provide immeasurable benefits for the health and well-being of our patients."[4] Other supportive organizations include AIDS Action, Gay Men's Health Crisis, National Association of People With AIDS, AIDS Project Los Angeles, AIDS Foundation of Chicago, Test Positive, Aware Network, AIDS Project Rhode Island, the New York State AIDS Advisory Council, Project Inform, San Francisco AIDS Foundation, and many others.

Do other medical and public health experts agree?

Yes. In a 1999 report commissioned by the White House, the National Academy of Sciences' Institute of Medicine wrote, "Nausea, appetite loss, pain, and anxiety are all afflictions of wasting and all can be mitigated by marijuana."[5] The American Public Health Association, American Nurses Association, and the state medical societies of New York, California, and Rhode Island are just a few of many medical organizations supporting legal access to medical marijuana. Prominent individuals supporting medical marijuana access include former U.S.

Surgeon General Dr. Joycelyn Elders, San Francisco Director of Health Dr. Mitch Katz, and Dr. Kenneth Mayer, director of Brown University's AIDS program.

What is the legal status of medical marijuana?

Twelve states—Alaska, California, Colorado, Hawaii, Maine, Montana, Nevada, New Mexico, Oregon, Vermont, Washington, and Rhode Island—permit medical use of marijuana if certain legal requirements are followed. Unfortunately, federal law still classifies marijuana as having no medical use and as being too dangerous to use even under medical supervision—the same category as phencyclidine (PCP) and heroin. This is unscientific and harmful to people with HIV/AIDS and other serious illnesses.

Notes

1. Abrams, D. et al, "Short-Term Effects of Cannabinoids in Patients with HIV-1 Infection," *Annals of Internal Medicine*, Aug. 19, 2003.

2. deJong, B.C. et al, "Marijuana Use and Its Association with Adherence to Antiretroviral Therapy Among HIV-Infected Persons with Moderate to Severe Nausea," *Journal of Acquired Immune Deficiency Syndromes*, January 1, 2005.

3. American Academy of HIV Medicine, letter to New York Assemblyman Richard Gottfried, Nov. 11, 2003.

4. Abrams D.I. et al, "Cannabis in painful HIV-associated sensory neuropathy," *Neurology*, February 13, 2007.

5. Joy, J., Watson, S. and Benson, J., "Marijuana and Medicine: Assessing the Science Base," National Academy Press, 1999.

Chapter 28

HIV/AIDS Treatments in Development

Chapter Contents

Section 28.1

Acne Drug Prevents HIV Breakout

© 2010 Johns Hopkins Medicine Office of Corporate Communications.
Reprinted with permission.

Johns Hopkins scientists have found that a safe and inexpensive antibiotic in use since the 1970s for treating acne effectively targets infected immune cells in which human immunodeficiency virus (HIV), the virus that causes acquired immunodeficiency syndrome (AIDS), lies dormant and prevents them from reactivating and replicating.

The drug, minocycline, likely will improve on the current treatment regimens of HIV-infected patients if used in combination with a standard drug cocktail known as HAART (highly active antiretroviral therapy), according to research published now online and appearing in print April 15, 2010, in the *Journal of Infectious Diseases*. "The powerful advantage to using minocycline is that the virus appears less able to develop drug resistance because minocycline targets cellular pathways not viral proteins," says Janice Clements, Ph.D., Mary Wallace Stanton Professor of Faculty Affairs, vice dean for faculty, and professor of molecular and comparative pathobiology at the Johns Hopkins University School of Medicine.

"The big challenge clinicians deal with now in this country when treating HIV patients is keeping the virus locked in a dormant state," Clements adds. "While HAART is really effective in keeping down active replication, minocycline is another arm of defense against the virus."

Unlike the drugs used in HAART, which target the virus, minocycline homes in on, and adjusts T cells, major immune system agents and targets of HIV infection. According to Clements, minocycline reduces the ability of T cells to activate and proliferate, both steps crucial to HIV production and progression toward full-blown AIDS.

If taken daily for life, HAART usually can protect people from becoming ill, but it's not a cure. The HIV virus is kept at a low level but isn't ever entirely purged; it stays quietly hidden in some immune cells. If a person stops HAART or misses a dose, the virus can reactivate out of those immune cells and begin to spread.

The idea for using minocycline as an adjunct to HAART resulted when the Hopkins team learned of research by others on rheumatoid arthritis patients showing the anti-inflammatory effects of minocycline on T cells. The Hopkins group connected the dots between that study with previous research of their own showing that minocycline treatment had multiple beneficial effects in monkeys infected with simian immunodeficiency virus (SIV), the primate version of HIV. In monkeys treated with minocycline, the virus load in the cerebrospinal fluid, the viral ribonucleic acid (RNA) in the brain, and the severity of central nervous system disease were significantly decreased. The drug was also shown to affect T cell activation and proliferation.

"Since minocycline reduced T cell activation, you might think it would have impaired the immune systems in the macaques, which are very similar to humans, but we didn't see any deleterious effect," says Gregory Szeto, a graduate student in the Department of Cellular and Molecular Medicine working in the Retrovirus Laboratory at Hopkins.

"This drug strikes a good balance and is ideal for HIV because it targets very specific aspects of immune activation."

The success with the animal model prompted the team to study in test tubes whether minocycline treatment affected latency in human T cells infected with HIV. Using cells from HIV-infected humans on HAART, the team isolated the "resting" immune cells and treated half of them with minocycline. Then they counted how many virus particles were reactivated, finding completely undetectable levels in the treated cells versus detectable levels in the untreated cells.

"Minocycline reduces the capability of the virus to emerge from resting infected T cells," Szeto explains. "It prevents the virus from escaping in the one in a million cells in which it lays dormant in a person on HAART, and since it prevents virus activation it should maintain the level of viral latency or even lower it. That's the goal: Sustaining a latent non-infectious state."

The team used molecular markers to discover that minocycline very selectively interrupts certain specific signaling pathways critical for T cell activation. However, the antibiotic doesn't completely obliterate T cells or diminish their ability to respond to other infections or diseases, which is crucial for individuals with HIV.

"HIV requires T cell activation for efficient replication and reactivation of latent virus," Clements says, "so our new understanding about minocyline's effects on a T cell could help us to find even more drugs that target its signaling pathways."

The research was supported by grants from the National Institutes of Health. Authors of the paper, in addition to Clements and Szeto, are Angela K. Brice, Sheila A. Barber, and Robert F. Siliciano, all of Johns Hopkins. Also, Hung-Chih Yang of National Taiwan University Hospital.

Section 28.2

Gene Therapy Shows Promise against HIV

A new study is among the first to hint that gene therapy could become a weapon against the virus that causes acquired immunodeficiency syndrome (AIDS).

However, any treatment remains far from being ready for use by patients, and would likely be expensive, experts said.

Still, the research is "a step in the direction of using gene therapy" to treat human immunodeficiency virus (HIV) patients, said Dr. Pablo Tebas, co-author of a new study and associate professor of medicine at the University of Pennsylvania.

Existing AIDS drugs allow many patients to live fairly normal lives despite being infected with HIV. But they can cause a variety of side effects, and some patients become immune to them over time.

"The next big challenge is going to be: Can you cure the infection or control it to a level that allows patients to not take these expensive and complex medications that can be toxic?" Tebas said.

One possible solution is to help the body fight off HIV without the use of drugs. That's where gene therapy comes in, Tebas said. "Can you make the patient resistant so they can control HIV on their own?"

In the new study, the Pennsylvania team tested a gene therapy approach in which scientists first remove immune cells from patients, tinker with their genes, and then put them back into the bodies of the patients.

Eight HIV-infected people took part in the study. After the genetically modified cells were placed back into the patients, "we stopped HIV treatment and tried to see what happened," Tebas said.

The findings were reported in February 2010 at the Conference on Retroviruses and Opportunistic Infections in San Francisco.

The levels of HIV fell below the expected levels in seven of the eight patients, the team found. Signs of the virus disappeared altogether in one patient, although that happens sometimes—it's not an indication that the disease is cured—and the researchers aren't sure why it happened in this case.

"We need to understand why it happened and see if we can reproduce that in the general population," Tebas said.

It's still early in the development of the treatment: the current research is in phase 2 of the customary three phases of research that new medical treatments go through.

If gene therapy does become a treatment for HIV patients, it may be best for those who aren't doing well on existing antiretroviral drugs, said John Rossi, chairman of the molecular and cellular biology department at the Beckman Research Institute of City of Hope Medical Center near Los Angeles.

"There are thousands of people who are completely resistant to all the drugs that are out there, and this is one more option they could have," Rossi said.

But the cost of the treatment would probably be high, he added, perhaps reaching around $20,000. And it's not clear how long the treatment would last, he said, since the immune cells aren't permanent.

Section 28.3

Immune Therapies

"Immune Therapies in Development," Fact Sheet #480. © 2009 AIDS InfoNet. Reprinted with permission. InfoNet fact sheets are updated frequently. Please visit the website at http://www.aidsinfonet.org for the newest version.

Immune Stimulators

We can think of most antiviral drugs as "offense," attacking the virus to slow down its multiplication. Another approach to treating human immunodeficiency virus (HIV) infection is "defense," strengthening the immune response of people who are infected. This section describes new immune stimulators being developed.

Cytokines

Some of these treatments use the body's own chemical messengers (cytokines) to increase the immune system's response to HIV. Different cytokines carry different messages to cells of the immune system. Some cytokines tell a cell to start multiplying; others can tell a cell to self-destruct.

Interferon exists in the body in several forms. Hemispherx Biopharma is testing Ampligen®, a form of interferon, in Phase II and Phase III trials. It is supposed to activate some of the cell's own defenses against viruses.

The best-known cytokine is interleukin-2 (IL-2, aldesleukin, Proleukin®) by Novartis. It is currently in Phase III trials. Bayer Corporation is studying Bay 50-4798, a modified recombinant form of IL-2, in Phase II trials.

Interleukin-7 is being developed by Cytheris Corporation as a general immune system booster. CYT107 is in Phase I/II trials and showed positive interim results. It increased both CD4 and CD8 cell counts. It is given in three weekly injections.

Multikine® by Cel-Sci Corporation, is a mixture of several different cytokines. It is in Phase I human trials.

Tumor necrosis factor alpha (TNF-a) is an immune system protein that is over-produced in immune disorders. Advanced Biotherapy is studying a TNF-a blocker in a Phase I trial.

Vaccine-Like Treatment

Another approach to stimulating the immune system is similar to vaccination, except that it is used in people who are already infected with HIV. HRG214 by Virionyx is a genetically engineered group of antibodies to HIV. It is called a "passive immuno-therapeutic pharmaceutical." HRG214 is in Phase I/II trials.

A recent study of ALVAC vaccine plus Remune® found a delay in viral load rebound when treatment was interrupted.

A recent study showed that a combination of vaccines against HIV and interleukin-2 (IL-2) increased immune responses to HIV and allowed some people to stop antiviral therapy for up to a year.

AGS-004 by Argos takes a sample of a patient's virus and extracts ribonucleic acid (RNA). The RNA is loaded into dendritic cells that are administered to the patient, stimulating an immune response to the virus. It is in Phase 2a trials. DermaVir® is applied as a skin patch. It is in Phase I/II trials. Another new therapeutic vaccine is VIR201. It is in Phase I/IIa trials.

Other Immune Modulators

- AVR118 by Advanced Viral Research showed good results against AIDS wasting and anorexia in a Phase I/II study.

- Cytolin® by Cytodyn is designed to improve the immune system's ability to fight HIV. It is given as an intravenous infusion Cytolin is in Phase II trials.

- HspE7 by StressGen Biotechnologies is being tested in Phase II and Phase III trials for tumors related to human papillomavirus (HPV).

- Immunitin® (HE2000) by Hollis-Eden Pharmaceuticals is a new drug that works on an infected person's immune system. It is designed to strengthen the "humoral" immune response which is responsible for producing antibodies. HE2000 is being tested in Phase II trials.

- IR103 is a combination of Remune® by the Immune Response Corporation, which stimulates an immune response to HIV, and Amplivax® by Hybridon which uses gene technology to enhance immune responses. IR103 is in a Phase I trial.

- MDX010 is an artificial antibody product. Medarex is testing it against HIV in Phase II trials.

- Murabutide® is under study by Dr. Georges Bahr in France. It uses fragments of bacteria to stimulate the overall immune response. Murabutide is given by injection. Phase I results, published in 2003, were promising in terms of increases in CD4 cells and lower viral loads.

- Resveratrol is a chemical found in several plants and the skin of red grapes. It protects plants against pathogens and may have other immune-boosting properties. It is being studied in a Phase I trial in people with HIV.

- Reticulose® by Advanced Viral Research Corporation is a nucleic acid that stimulates the cell-killing arm of the immune system. It is administered as a subcutaneous (beneath the skin) injection. Early clinical trials showed that patients receiving Reticulose had increases in their CD4 and CD8 cells, weight increases, and fewer opportunistic infections than patients receiving placebo. No toxic side effects have been reported yet. Reticulose is in Phase III trials.

- SP-6310 by Samaritan Pharmaceuticals normalizes (reduces) levels of cortisol, a stress hormone. A Phase III study is being developed.

- Tesamorelin® (TH9507) by Theratechnologies is a growth hormone inducer. It is being studied in Phase III to treat visceral fat accumulation in lipodystrophy. Marketing rights for the United States have been sold to Serono.

- Tucaresol® by GlaxoSmithKline is an immune stimulator in Phase I trials.

- Zenapax® (daclizumab or anti-CD25) is being studied by the National Institutes of Health as a way to reduce viral load beyond what antiretroviral therapy (ART) can achieve.

Drugs No Longer in Development

The following drugs are no longer being developed for use against HIV:

- SP01A by Samaritan Pharmaceuticals has been replaced by SP-6310 (see above).

- WF10 by Dimethaid Research

Section 28.4

Therapeutic HIV Vaccines

Excerpted from "Therapeutic HIV Vaccines," AIDSinfo.gov, May 2006.
Reviewed by David A. Cooke, M.D., FACP, November 2010.

What is a vaccine?

A vaccine is a medical product designed to stimulate your body's immune system in order to prevent or control an infection. An effective vaccine trains your immune system to fight a particular microorganism so that it can't make you sick.

Although there are currently no vaccines to prevent or treat human immunodeficiency virus (HIV), researchers are developing and testing potential HIV vaccines. HIV vaccines designed to prevent HIV infection in HIV-negative people are called preventive vaccines. HIV vaccines designed to help control HIV infection in people who are already HIV-positive are called therapeutic vaccines. This section focuses on therapeutic HIV vaccines.

What is a therapeutic HIV vaccine?

A therapeutic HIV vaccine (also known as a treatment vaccine) is a vaccine used in the treatment of an HIV-infected person. Therapeutic HIV vaccines are designed to boost the body's immune response to HIV in order to better control the infection.

Currently, there are no therapeutic HIV vaccines approved by the Food and Drug Administration (FDA). However, therapeutic HIV vaccines are being tested in clinical trials to find out if they are safe and effective in treating people with HIV.

Researchers hope that if therapeutic vaccines are able to strengthen the body's natural anti-HIV immune response, people with HIV will not have to rely exclusively on the antiretroviral drugs now used to treat HIV infection. Currently, antiretroviral drugs must be taken for life, and some cause serious side effects.

All experimental therapeutic HIV vaccines are in very early stages of research, and no therapeutic vaccine is anticipated to be available to the general public for many years, if at all.

Will a therapeutic HIV vaccine be able to cure HIV?

Probably not. If therapeutic vaccines are effective, they may be able to help keep HIV infection under control. However, most researchers do not think therapeutic HIV vaccines will be able to completely eliminate HIV infection, because the virus hides in certain cells of the body where it can last for decades.

Will a therapeutic vaccine rule out the need for antiretroviral drugs?

Even an effective therapeutic HIV vaccine probably won't be able to replace antiretroviral drugs entirely. At best, a therapeutic HIV vaccine may help control HIV infection and keep people healthy while minimizing the need for antiretroviral drugs.

Who is eligible to receive a therapeutic vaccine?

Therapeutic vaccines are designed specifically for HIV-positive people who have healthy immune systems. Therapeutic vaccine recipients must have strong immune systems for the vaccine to generate an effective anti- HIV immune response. Clinical trials of therapeutic vaccines are recruiting volunteers with CD4 counts greater than 250 cells/mm^3, and most studies require a CD4 count greater than 350 cells/mm^3. People with weaker immune systems may be unable to produce a good immune response to a therapeutic HIV vaccine, and are therefore not eligible for these trials. Most trials require that therapeutic vaccine recipients continue taking antiretroviral drugs during the study.

What are the side effects of therapeutic vaccines?

Because testing is ongoing, not all of the side effects of therapeutic vaccines are known. However, side effects observed so far in clinical trials have been similar to the side effects that occur with FDA-approved vaccines. These side effects include the following:

- Soreness, swelling, redness, or pain at the site of injection

- Mild flu-like symptoms (fever, chills, muscle pain or weakness, nausea, headache, and dizziness)

Chapter 29

HIV/AIDS Clinical Trials

What Is an HIV/AIDS Clinical Trial?

Human immunodeficiency virus (HIV)/acquired immunodeficiency syndrome (AIDS) clinical trials are research studies in which new therapies and prevention strategies for HIV infection and AIDS are tested in humans. These studies are conducted by physicians and other healthcare professionals and can help determine the usefulness of experimental drugs and vaccines in treating or preventing HIV infection. Carefully conducted clinical trials are the fastest and safest way to help find treatments and prevention strategies that work.

New therapies are tested in humans only after laboratory and animal studies show promising results. In Phase I clinical trials, the experimental therapies are given to small numbers of people to help determine safe doses. Larger groups of patients may then receive the therapies in Phase II trials to help measure side effects and preliminary effectiveness. The treatments may then be used in even larger Phase III studies to compare the new treatment to ones already in use or to help estimate other effects of the drug.

What Is a Clinical Trial Protocol?

A clinical trial protocol is a detailed plan of how the trial will be conducted. Potential clinical trial participants learn details about the clinical trial protocol in a process called informed consent.

Excerpted from "What Is an HIV/AIDS Clinical Trial?" AIDSinfo.gov, September 2005. Reviewed by David A. Cooke, M.D., FACP, January 2011.

Informed consent is the process of learning key facts about a clinical trial before deciding whether or not to participate. To help someone decide whether or not to participate, study staff explain the details of the trial. Then the research team provides an informed consent document that includes details about the study, such as its purpose, duration, required procedures, and key contacts. Risks and potential benefits are also explained in the document. The participant then decides whether or not to sign the document. Informed consent is an ongoing process and the participant may withdraw from the trial at any time.

Benefits of Participating in an HIV/AIDS Clinical Trial

- Participants may gain access to new treatments not yet available to the public.

- Participants may receive expert medical care at leading health-care facilities.

- Participants have a chance to help others by contributing to medical research.

- Experimental drugs are often provided free of charge.

Risks of Participating in an HIV/AIDS Clinical Trial

- Experimental drugs may not have any benefits or may even be harmful.

- New drugs may have unanticipated side effects.

- Protocols may require a lot of the participant's time and frequent trips to the study site.

What Questions Should I Ask?

If you are interested in participating in a clinical trial, you may want to ask the following questions:

- What is the purpose of the study?

- What are the drug's side effects?

- What other treatment options do I have?

- Will I have to be in the hospital?

- How often will I have study visits?

- How long will the study last?

- Who will provide my medical care after the study is completed?
- What other drugs can I take if I participate in the study?
- What treatments must I avoid while participating in the study?
- Who will pay the costs of the study?
- How will my confidentiality be protected?

Chapter 30

HIV and AIDS Treatment for Children

How Serious Is Human Immunodeficiency Virus (HIV) for Children?

Where antiretroviral medications (ARVs) and good medical care for pregnant women are available, new infections of children are rare. There were about two million children around the world living with HIV in 2007.

Anyone age thirteen or younger is counted as a child in U.S. health statistics. In 1992, almost one thousand children were infected in the United States. By 2002, there were just ninety-two new infections. African American newborns are much more likely to be infected than children of other races.

Most children with HIV were born to mothers with HIV. Others got a transfusion of infected blood. In the developed world, blood for transfusions is screened and most pregnant women are taking ARVs.

Infected mothers can pass HIV to their newborns. This happens where mothers do not get good medical care while they are pregnant. It also happens where ARVs are not available, or where blood for transfusions is not always screened.

"Children and HIV," Fact Sheet #612, © 2009 AIDS InfoNet. Reprinted with permission. InfoNet fact sheets are updated frequently. Please visit the website at http://www.aidsinfonet.org for the newest version.

How Are Children Different?

Children's immune systems are still developing. They have a different response to HIV infection. CD4 cell counts and viral load counts are higher than in adults. An infant's viral load usually declines until age four or five. Then it stabilizes.

Children also respond differently to ARVs. They have larger increases in CD4 cell counts and more diverse CD4 cells. They seem to recover more of their immune response than adults.

Infants have more fat and water in their bodies. This affects the amount of medication available. Children have a very high rate of metabolism. This gradually slows as they mature.

The liver processes drugs and removes them from the body. It takes several years to mature. As it matures, drug levels in children can change a lot.

Bones develop quickly during the early years of life. ARVs can weaken bones in adults. This was also seen in children.

Research on Children

It is very difficult to recruit children into HIV clinical trials. In the United States, many children with HIV have already been in more than one research study. With falling infection rates, there are very few new cases of pediatric HIV. The United States has considered ending support for its pediatric trials network. Important research questions may be studied in adults.

A recent study found that children born to HIV-positive mothers have high rates of psychiatric disorders.

Treatment for Children

HIV-infected children should be treated by a pediatrician who knows about HIV.

Antiretroviral therapy (ART) works very well for children. The death rate of children with acquired immunodeficiency syndrome (AIDS) has dropped as much as for adults. However, manufacturers were not required to study their products in children until very recently in the United States. As a result, very few ARVs have been studied in children. Still, twelve ARVs are approved for use by children.

The correct doses are not always known. Children's doses are sometimes based on their weight. Another method is body surface area. This formula considers both height and weight. As mentioned above, several factors affect drug levels in children. Dosing may have to be adjusted several times as a child develops.

The doses of some medications for infants and very young children can be individualized. They come in liquid or powder form. Others come in a granular form. Some pills can be crushed and added to food or liquids. Some clinics teach children how to swallow pills. Children who can swallow pills have more medication options.

Doctors sometimes try to cut adult tablets into smaller pieces for children. However, this can result in doses that are too low. Some tablets are difficult to cut. Also, the medication may be unevenly distributed in the tablet

It is difficult to know when to start treatment for children. Immediate treatment might prevent immune system damage. Delayed treatment may provide better quality of life for several years. However, HIV-related diseases show up much faster in untreated children than in adults. Without treatment, about 20 percent of children die or develop AIDS within one year.

Children and Adherence

Adherence is a major challenge for children and infants. Both the child and the parents may need extra help. Many children do not understand why they should put up with medication side effects.

Their parents are usually HIV-positive. They may have their own difficulties with adherence. Their children may take different medications, on a different schedule. Many ARVs taste bad or have a strange texture. A feeding tube directly into the stomach may be necessary if an infant refuses to swallow medications.

The Bottom Line

Where ARVs and good medical care for pregnant women are available, new infections of children are rare.

Treatment of HIV-infected children is complicated. Not all ARVs are approved for use by children. The correct dosing is not always known. Children may have a difficult time tolerating medications and taking every dose as scheduled.

However, because children's immune systems are still developing, they might have a better chance of fully recovering from damage caused by HIV.

Children with HIV should be treated by a pediatrician with experience in HIV.

Chapter 31

HIV and AIDS Treatment for Pregnant Women

Human Immunodeficiency Virus (HIV) Testing and Pregnancy

I Am Pregnant, and I May Have HIV. Will I Be Tested for HIV When I Visit a Doctor?

In most cases, healthcare providers cannot test you for HIV without your permission. However, the U.S. Public Health Service recommends that all pregnant women be tested. If you are thinking about being tested, it is important to understand the different ways perinatal HIV testing is done. There are two main approaches to HIV testing in pregnant women: opt-in and opt-out testing.

In opt-in testing, a woman cannot be given an HIV test unless she specifically requests to be tested. Often, she must put this request in writing.

In opt-out testing, healthcare providers must inform pregnant women that an HIV test will be included in the standard group of tests pregnant women receive. A woman will receive that HIV test unless she specifically refuses. The Centers for Disease Control and Prevention (CDC) currently recommend that healthcare providers adopt an opt-out approach to perinatal HIV testing.

Excerpted from "HIV During Pregnancy, Labor and Delivery, and After Birth," AIDSinfo.gov, May 2009.

What Are the Benefits of Being Tested?

By knowing your HIV status, you and your doctor can decide on the best treatment for you and your baby and can take steps to prevent mother-to-child transmission of HIV. It is also important to know your HIV status so that you can take the appropriate steps to avoid infecting others.

What Happens If I Agree to Be Tested?

If you agree to be tested, your doctor should counsel you before the test about the way your life may change after you receive the test results. If the test indicates that you have HIV, you should be given a second test to confirm the results. If your second test is positive for HIV, you and your doctor will decide which treatment options are best for you and your baby. If the test indicates that you do not have HIV, you may receive counseling on HIV prevention.

What Happens If I Refuse to Be Tested?

If you decide that you do not want to be tested for HIV, your doctor may offer you counseling about the way HIV is transmitted and the importance of taking steps to prevent HIV transmission. He or she may also talk to you about the importance of finding out your HIV status so that you can take steps to prevent your baby from becoming infected.

Will My Baby Be Tested for HIV?

Healthcare providers recommend that all babies born to HIV-positive mothers be tested for HIV. However, states differ in the ways they approach HIV testing for babies:

- Some states require that babies receive a mandatory HIV test if the status of the mother is unknown.

- Some states require that healthcare providers test babies for HIV unless the mother refuses.

- Some states are required to offer an HIV test only to pregnant women (not their babies), which they can either accept or refuse.

- Some states have no specific requirements about testing pregnant women or their babies.

How Can I Find Out the Testing Policies of My State?

The U.S. Department of Health and Human Services (HHS) can provide you with HIV testing information for your state.

Treatment Regimens for HIV-Positive Pregnant Women

I Am HIV-Positive and Pregnant. Should I Take Anti-HIV Medications?

Yes. If you are HIV-positive and pregnant, it is recommended that you take anti-HIV medications to prevent your baby from becoming infected with HIV, and in some cases, for your own health. Anti-HIV medications are recommended for all pregnant women regardless of CD4 count and viral load. HIV treatment is an important part of preventing your baby from becoming infected with HIV and maintaining your health.

When Should I Consider Starting Anti-HIV Treatment?

When you start treatment will depend mostly on whether you need treatment only to prevent your baby from becoming infected with HIV or if you also need treatment for your own health. In general, it is recommended that pregnant women who are starting therapy for their own health be treated as soon as possible, including in the first trimester. For women who are beginning therapy only to prevent mother-to-child transmission, delaying anti-HIV medication until after the first trimester can be considered. You should discuss when to begin treatment with your doctor.

How Do I find Out Which HIV Treatment Regimen Is Best for Me?

Decisions about which HIV treatment regimen you will start should be based on many of the same factors that women who are not pregnant must consider. These factors include the following:

- Risk that the HIV infection may become worse
- Risks and benefits of delaying treatment
- Potential drug toxicities and interactions with other drugs you are taking
- The need to adhere to a treatment regimen closely
- The results of drug resistance testing

In addition to these factors, pregnant women must consider the following issues:

- Benefit of lowering viral load and reducing the risk of mother-to-child transmission of HIV

413

- Unknown long-term effects on your baby if you take anti-HIV medications during your pregnancy

- Information available about the use of anti-HIV medications during pregnancy

You should discuss your treatment options with your doctor so that together you can decide which treatment regimen is best for you and your baby.

What Treatment Regimen Should I Follow during My Pregnancy If I Have Never Taken Anti-HIV Medications?

Your best treatment options depend on when you were diagnosed with HIV, when you found out you were pregnant, at what point you sought medical treatment during your pregnancy, and whether you need treatment for your own health. Women who are in the first trimester of pregnancy and who do not have symptoms of HIV disease may consider delaying treatment until after ten to twelve weeks into their pregnancies. After the first trimester, pregnant women with HIV should receive at least azidothymidine (AZT: Retrovir® or zidovudine); your doctor may recommend additional medications depending on your CD4 count, viral load, and drug resistance testing.

I Am Currently Taking Anti-HIV Medications, and I Just Learned That I Am Pregnant. Should I Stop Taking My Medications?

Do not stop taking any of your medications without consulting your doctor first. Stopping HIV treatment could lead to problems for you and your baby. If you are taking anti-HIV medications and your pregnancy is identified during the first trimester, talk with your doctor about the risks and benefits of continuing your current regimen. Your doctor may recommend that you change the medications you take. If your pregnancy is identified after the first trimester, it is recommended that you continue with your current treatment. No matter what HIV treatment regimen you were on before your pregnancy, it is generally recommended that AZT become part of your regimen.

Will I Need Treatment during Labor and Delivery?

Most mother-to-child transmission of HIV occurs around the time of labor and delivery. Therefore, HIV treatment during this time is very important for protecting your baby from HIV infection. Several treatments can be used together to reduce the risk of transmission to your baby:

- Highly active antiretroviral therapy (HAART) is recommended even for HIV infected pregnant women who do not need treatment for their own health. If possible, HAART should include AZT (Retrovir® or zidovudine).

- During labor and delivery, you should receive intravenous (IV) AZT.

- Your baby should take AZT (in liquid form) every six hours for six weeks after birth.

If you have been taking any other anti-HIV medications during your pregnancy, your doctor will probably recommend that you continue to take them on schedule during labor.

Better understanding of HIV transmission has contributed to dramatically reduced rates of mother-to-child transmission of HIV. Discuss the benefits of HIV treatment during pregnancy with your doctor; these benefits should be weighed against the risks to you and to your baby.

Safety and Toxicity of Anti-HIV Medications during Pregnancy

I Am HIV-Positive and Pregnant. Are There Any Anti-HIV Medications That May Be Dangerous to Me or My Baby during My Pregnancy?

Yes. Although information on anti-HIV medications in pregnant women is limited, enough is known to make recommendations about medications for you and your baby. However, the long-term effects of babies' exposure to anti-HIV medications *in utero* are unknown. Talk to your doctor about which medications may be harmful during your pregnancy and what medication and dose changes are possible.

In general, protease inhibitors (PIs) are associated with increased levels of blood sugar (hyperglycemia), development of diabetes mellitus or worsening of diabetes mellitus symptoms, and diabetic ketoacidosis. Pregnancy is also a risk factor for hyperglycemia, but it is not known whether PI use increases the risk for pregnancy-associated hyperglycemia or gestational diabetes.

Two non-nucleoside reverse transcriptase inhibitors (NNRTIs), Rescriptor® (delavirdine) and Sustiva® (efavirenz), are not recommended for the treatment of HIV infected pregnant women. Use of these medications during pregnancy may lead to birth defects. Another NNRTI, Viramune® (nevirapine), may be part of your HIV treatment regimen. Long-term use of Viramune may cause negative side effects, such as exhaustion or weakness; nausea or lack of appetite; yellowing of eyes or skin; or signs of liver toxicity, such as severe skin rash, chills, fever, sore throat, or other flu-like symptoms, liver tenderness or enlargement, or elevated liver enzyme levels. These negative side effects are not normally seen with short-term use (one or two doses) of Viramune during pregnancy. However, because pregnancy and early symptoms of liver toxicity can be similar, your doctor should monitor you closely while you are taking Viramune. Also, Viramune should be used with caution in women who have never received HIV treatment and who have CD4 counts greater than 250 cells/mm³. Liver toxicity has occurred more frequently in these patients.

Nucleoside reverse transcriptase inhibitors (NRTIs) may cause mitochondrial toxicity, which may lead to a buildup of lactic acid in the blood. This buildup is known as hyperlactatemia or lactic acidosis. This toxicity may be of particular concern for pregnant women and babies exposed to NRTIs *in utero.*

There is very little known about the use of the entry inhibitors Fuzeon® (enfuvirtide) and Selzentry® (maraviroc) and the integrase inhibitor Isentress® (raltegravir) during pregnancy.

Delivery Options for HIV-Positive Pregnant Women

I Am HIV-Positive and Pregnant. What Delivery Options Are Available to Me When I Give Birth?

Depending on your health and treatment status, you may plan to have either a cesarean (also called c-section) or a vaginal delivery. The decision of whether to have a cesarean or a vaginal delivery is something that you should discuss with your doctor during your pregnancy.

How Do I Decide Which Delivery Option Is Best for My Baby and Me?

It is important that you discuss your delivery options with your doctor as early as possible in your pregnancy so that he or she can help you decide which delivery method is most appropriate for you.

Cesarean delivery is recommended for an HIV-positive mother when the following are true:

- Her viral load is unknown or is greater than 1,000 copies/mL at thirty-six weeks of pregnancy

- She has not taken any anti-HIV medications or has only taken AZT (Retrovir® or zidovudine) during her pregnancy

- She has not received prenatal care until thirty-six weeks into her pregnancy or later

To be most effective in preventing transmission, the cesarean should be scheduled at thirty-eight weeks or should be done before the rupture of membranes (also called water breaking).

Vaginal delivery is recommended for an HIV-positive mother when the following are true:

- She has been receiving prenatal care throughout her pregnancy

- She has a viral load less than 1,000 copies/mL at thirty-six weeks

Vaginal delivery may also be recommended if a mother has ruptured membranes and labor is progressing rapidly.

What Are the Risks Involved with These Delivery Options?

All deliveries have risks. The risk of mother-to-child transmission of HIV may be higher for vaginal delivery than for a scheduled cesarean. For the mother, cesarean delivery has an increased risk of infection, anesthesia-related problems, and other risks associated with any type of surgery. For the infant, cesarean delivery has an increased risk of infant respiratory distress.

Is There Anything Else I Should Know about Labor and Delivery?

Intravenous (IV) AZT should be started three hours before a scheduled cesarean delivery and should be continued until delivery. IV AZT should be given throughout labor and delivery for a vaginal delivery. It is also important to minimize the baby's exposure to the mother's blood. This can be done by avoiding any invasive monitoring and forceps- or vacuum-assisted delivery.

All babies born to HIV-positive mothers should receive anti-HIV medication to prevent mother-to-child transmission of HIV. The usual treatment for infants is six weeks of AZT; sometimes, additional medications are also given.

HIV-Positive Women and Their Babies After Birth

I Am an HIV-Positive Pregnant Woman, and I am currently on an HIV Regimen. Will My Regimen Change After I Give Birth?

Many women who are on an HIV treatment regimen during pregnancy decide to stop or change their regimens after they give birth. You and your doctor should discuss your postpartum treatment options during your pregnancy or shortly after delivery. Don't stop taking any of your medications without consulting your doctor first. Stopping HIV treatment could lead to problems.

How Will I Know If My Baby Is Infected with HIV?

Babies born to HIV-positive mothers are tested for HIV differently than adults. Adults are tested by looking for antibodies to HIV in their blood. A baby keeps antibodies from its mother, including antibodies to HIV, for many months after birth. Therefore, an antibody test given before the baby is eighteen months old may be positive even if the baby does *not* have HIV infection. For the first eighteen months, babies are tested for HIV directly, and not by looking for antibodies to HIV. When babies are more than eighteen months old, they no longer have their mother's antibodies and can be tested for HIV using the antibody test.

Preliminary HIV tests for babies are usually performed at three time points:

- Birth to fourteen days

- At one to two months of age

- At three to six months of age

If babies test negative on two of these preliminary tests, they should be given an HIV antibody test between twelve and eighteen months. Babies who test negative for HIV antibodies at this time are not HIV infected.

Babies are considered HIV-positive if they test positive on two of these preliminary HIV tests. Babies who test positive for HIV antibodies will need to be retested at fifteen to eighteen months. At eighteen months, babies should have an HIV antibody test to confirm HIV infection. A positive HIV antibody test given after eighteen months of age confirms HIV infection in children.

Are There Any Other Tests My Baby Will Receive After Birth?

Babies born to HIV-positive mothers should have a complete blood count (CBC) after birth. They should also be monitored for signs of anemia, which is the main negative side effect caused by the six-week AZT (Retrovir®, or zidovudine) regimen infants should take to reduce the risk of HIV infection. They may also undergo other routine blood tests and vaccinations for babies.

Will My Baby Receive anti-HIV Medication?

Yes. It is recommended that all babies born to HIV-positive mothers receive a six-week course of oral AZT to help prevent mother-to-child transmission of HIV. This oral AZT regimen should begin within six to twelve hours after your baby is born. Some doctors may recommend that AZT be given in combination with other anti-HIV medications. You and your doctor should discuss the options to decide which treatment is best for your baby.

In addition to HIV treatment, your baby should also receive treatment to prevent *P. carinii / jiroveci* pneumonia (PCP). The recommended treatment is a combination of the medications sulfamethoxazole and trimethoprim.[1] This treatment should be started when your baby is four to six weeks old and the six-week course of AZT is complete. The treatment should continue until your baby is confirmed to be HIV-negative. If your baby is HIV-positive, he or she will need to take this treatment indefinitely.

What Type of Medical Follow-Up Should I Consider for My Baby and Me After I Give Birth?

Seeking the right medical and supportive care services is important for you and your baby's health. These services may include the following:

- Routine medical care
- HIV specialty care
- Family planning services
- Mental health services
- Substance abuse treatment
- Case management

Talk to your doctor about these services and any others you may need. He or she should be able to help you locate appropriate resources.

What Else Should I Think about After I Give Birth?

The CDC recommends that women not breastfeed in areas where safe drinking water and infant formula are available (such as the United States). This is recommended to avoid transmission of HIV to infants through breast milk.

Physical and emotional changes during the postpartum period, along with the stresses and demands of caring for a new baby, can make it difficult to follow your HIV treatment regimen. Adherence to your regimen is important for you to stay healthy. Other issues you may want to discuss with your doctor include the following:

- Concerns you may have about your regimen and treatment adherence

- Feelings of depression (many women have these feelings after giving birth)

- Long-term plans for continuing medical care and HIV treatment for you and your baby

Notes

1. The combination of sulfamethoxazole and trimethoprim is known by other names.

Part Five

Common Co-Occurring Infections and Complications of HIV/AIDS

Chapter 32

Opportunistic Infections and Their Relationship to HIV/AIDS

People with healthy immune systems can be exposed to certain viruses, bacteria, or parasites and have no reaction to them—but people living with human immunodeficiency virus (HIV)/Acquired Immunodeficiency Syndrome (AIDS) can face serious health threats from what are known as "opportunistic" infections (OIs). These infections are called "opportunistic" because they take advantage of your weakened immune system, and they can cause devastating illnesses.

OIs are signs of a declining immune system. Most life-threatening OIs occur when your CD4 count is below 200 cells/mm^3. OIs are the most common cause of death for people with HIV/AIDS.

The Centers for Disease Control and Prevention (CDC) developed a list of more than twenty OIs that are considered AIDS-defining conditions—if you have HIV and one or more of these OIs, you will be diagnosed with AIDS, no matter what your CD4 count happens to be:

- Candidiasis of bronchi, trachea, esophagus, or lungs

- Invasive cervical cancer

- Coccidioidomycosis

- Cryptococcosis

- Cryptosporidiosis, chronic intestinal (greater than one month's duration)

- Cytomegalovirus disease (particularly CMV retinitis)

Excerpted from "Opportunistic Infections," AIDS.gov, October 2010.

- Encephalopathy, HIV-related
- Herpes simplex: chronic ulcer(s) (greater than one month's duration); or bronchitis, pneumonitis, or esophagitis
- Histoplasmosis
- Isosporiasis, chronic intestinal (greater than one month's duration)
- Kaposi sarcoma
- Lymphoma, multiple forms
- *Mycobacterium avium* complex
- Tuberculosis
- *Pneumocystis carinii* pneumonia
- Pneumonia, recurrent
- Progressive multifocal leukoencephalopathy
- Salmonella septicemia, recurrent
- Toxoplasmosis of brain
- Wasting syndrome due to HIV

Because they can be so dangerous to your health, it is essential that you understand the signs, symptoms, prevention, and management of OIs.

Can I Prevent Opportunistic Infections?

One of the goals of HIV treatment is to lower your risk of getting OIs. Antiretroviral therapy can help by increasing your number of CD4 cells, which will help protect you from OIs. You may also take medications used to prevent disease from occurring (this is known as prophylaxis).

The Basics of Opportunistic Infections

OIs can occur all over the body and be relatively localized (meaning they affect only one part of the body) or systemic or disseminated (meaning they spread to other parts of the body and other body systems). Whether and when you become susceptible to OIs is often related to your CD4 count.

CD4 Count Greater Than 500 Cells/mm³

In general, people with CD4 counts greater than 500 cells/mm³ are not at risk for opportunistic infections. For people with CD4 counts around 500, however, the daily fluctuations in CD4 cell levels can leave them vulnerable to minor infections, such as candidal vaginitis or yeast infections.

CD4 Count 500 Cells/mm³ to 200 Cells/mm³

At a CD4 count of 500 cells/mm³ to 200 cells/mm³, candidiasis (thrush) and Kaposi sarcoma are common OIs.

Candidiasis (thrush). This is a fungal infection that is normally seen in patients with CD4 counts in this range. It is treatable with antifungal medications. A trained provider can usually diagnose thrush with a visual examination.

Oral symptoms include: white patches on gums, tongue, or lining of the mouth; pain in the mouth or throat; difficulty swallowing; and loss of appetite.

Vaginal symptoms include: vaginal irritation; itching; burning; and thick, white discharge.

Kaposi sarcoma (KS). KS is caused by human herpes virus-8. Before the introduction of antiretroviral therapy, as many as one in five patients with AIDS had KS. It can cause lesions on the body and in the mouth. In addition, this virus can affect internal organs and disseminate to other parts of the body without any external signs. Treatment plans can include chemotherapy to shrink the lesions, as well as antiretroviral therapy to increase CD4 cell count. A diagnosis is typically made by inspecting a lesion and performing a direct biopsy on it.

Signs and symptoms of KS can include: appearance of a purplish lesion on skin; appearance of a purplish lesion in the mouth; occasionally gastrointestinal complaints with disseminated KS.

CD4 Count 200 Cells/mm³ to 100 Cells/mm³

At CD4 counts of 200 cells/mm³ to 100 cells/mm³, *Pneumocystis jiroveci (carinii)* pneumonia, histoplasmosis and coccidioidomycosis, and progressive multifocal leukoencephalopathy are common OIs.

***Pneumocystis jiroveci (carinii)* pneumonia (PCP).** PCP is a fungal infection and is the OI that most often causes death in patients with HIV. It is treatable with antibiotic therapy and close monitoring. If necessary, prophylaxis is available for patients who are at risk for

PCP, but who are not ready to start antiretroviral medication. Diagnosing PCP usually involves a hospital stay to ensure proper testing and treatment without complications.

Signs and symptoms of PCP can include shortness of breath, fever, dry cough, and chest pain.

Histoplasmosis and coccidioidomycosis. These are fungal infections that are found in many regions of the United States. They often present as severe, disseminated illnesses in patients with low CD4 counts. Diagnosis consists of blood tests and evaluation for possible exposures related to geographical areas.

Signs and symptoms of histoplasmosis and coccidioidomycosis can include fever, fatigue, weight loss, cough, chest pain, shortness of breath, and headache.

Progressive multifocal leukoencephalopathy (PML). PML is a severe neurological condition that is caused by the JC virus and typically occurs in patients with CD4 counts below 200. While there is no definitive treatment for this disease, it has been shown to be responsive to antiretroviral therapy. In some cases, the disease resolves without any treatment.

Signs and symptoms of PML can include dementia, seizures, difficulty speaking, confusion, and difficulty walking.

CD4 Count 100 Cells/mm^3 to 50 Cells/mm^3

At CD4 counts of 100 cells/mm3 to 50 cells/mm3, toxoplasmosis, cryptosporidiosis, cryptococcal infection or cryptococcosis, and cytomegalovirus are common OIs.

Toxoplasmosis. Toxoplasmosis is caused by the parasite *Toxoplasma gondii* that can cause encephalitis and neurological disease in patients with low CD4 counts. The parasite is carried by cats, birds, and other animals and is also found in soil contaminated by cat feces and in meat, particularly pork. Toxoplasmosis is treatable with aggressive therapy, and prophylaxis is recommended for patients with low CD4 counts (usually less than 200). Diagnosis of this condition often requires imaging studies (computed tomography [CT] or magnetic resonance imaging [MRI]) of the brain and a blood test.

Signs and symptoms of toxoplasmosis can include headache, confusion, motor weakness, fever, and seizures.

Cryptosporidiosis. Cryptosporidiosis is a diarrheal disease caused by the protozoa *Cryptosporidium*, and it can become chronic for people with low CD4 counts. Symptoms include abdominal cramps and severe chronic diarrhea. Infection with this parasite can occur through swallowing water that has been contaminated with fecal material (in swimming pools, lakes, or public water supplies); eating uncooked food (like oysters) that are infected; or by person-to-person transmission, including changing diapers or exposure to feces during sexual contact. Treatment and antiretroviral therapy are important.

Signs and symptoms of cryptosporidiosis can include chronic watery diarrhea, stomach cramps, weight loss, nausea, and vomiting.

Cryptococcal infection or cryptococcosis. Cryptococcal infection is caused by a fungus that typically enters the body through the lungs and can spread to the brain, causing cryptococcal meningitis. In some cases, it can also affect the skin, skeletal system, and urinary tract. This can be a very deadly infection if not caught and properly treated with antifungal medication. Although this infection is found primarily in the central nervous system, it can disseminate to other parts of the body, especially when a person has a CD4 count of less than 50.

Signs and symptoms of cryptococcal meningitis include fever, fatigue, headache, and neck stiffness. Some patients can have memory loss or mood changes.

Cytomegalovirus (CMV). CMV is an extremely common virus that is present in all parts of the world. It is estimated that a majority of the population have had CMV by the time they are forty years old. CMV can be transmitted by saliva, blood, semen, and other bodily fluids. It can cause mild illnesses when first contracted and many people may never have symptoms. However, it does not leave the body when someone is infected with CMV. In patients with HIV and low CD4 counts it can cause infections in the eye and gastrointestinal system.

Signs and symptoms of CMV include sore throat, swollen glands, fatigue, and fevers. In people with low CD4 counts it can cause blurred vision (if CMV infection is in the eye), painful swallowing, diarrhea, and abdominal pain.

CD4 Count Less than 50 Cells/mm³

At CD4 count less than 50 cells/mm^3, *Mycobacterium avium* complex is a common OI.

***Mycobacterium avium* complex (MAC).** MAC is a type of bacteria that can be found in soil, water, and many places in the environment. These bacteria can cause disease in people with HIV and CD4 counts less than 50. The bacteria can infect the lungs or the intestines, or in some cases, can become "disseminated." This means that it can spread to the bloodstream and other parts of the body. If this occurs, it can be a life-threatening infection. If a person's CD4 count is below 50, then medications are available to prevent this infection from occurring.

Signs and symptoms of MAC include fevers, night sweats, abdominal pain, fatigue, and diarrhea.

Chapter 33

Strategies for Managing Opportunistic Infections

Human immunodeficiency virus (HIV) infects the cells of your body's immune system. This, in turn, weakens the immune system, causing it to lose its ability to fight disease. This includes fairly common infections that may cause little or no harm in a healthy person, but take the opportunity of a weakened immune system to cause serious and even life-threatening disease. This is why they're called opportunistic infections, or OIs.

Regardless of where you are in your HIV disease, there are things that you can do to prevent and treat OIs. Preventing OIs applies to people at all stages of HIV disease. It includes:

- understanding what OIs are;
- learning how to prevent them;
- using preventive treatment when needed;
- treating them as they occur; and
- using maintenance therapy when needed.

A plan for treating OIs includes:

- Seeing your doctor regularly. This generally means every three months for most people or perhaps monthly for people dealing

Excerpted from "Strategies for Managing Opportunistic Infections," © 2010 Project Inform. Reprinted with permission. For more information, contact the National HIV/AIDS Treatment Hotline, 800-822-7422, or visit www.projectinform.org.

with complications. A doctor experienced in HIV disease who has treated people with HIV is better able to recognize and treat OIs and should be more familiar with preventive therapy.

- Noting and telling your doctor(s) about all the symptoms you have so they can diagnose problems early.

- Treating infections as they occur, completing treatment, and using maintenance therapy when needed. This may include the need for lifelong therapy.

Understanding OIs

The Centers for Disease Control (CDC) created a list of serious and life-threatening diseases. When these diseases occur in HIV-positive people, they're called AIDS-defining conditions. (AIDS is short for acquired immunodeficiency syndrome.) So when a person has an AIDS-defining condition, it results in an AIDS diagnosis for that person. An AIDS diagnosis can also occur if CD4 counts go below 200 or CD4 percentages fall below 14 percent.

OIs can be fairly common infections, like genital herpes. But that doesn't mean every HIV-positive person who has herpes also has AIDS. This is because herpes becomes an OI only when it uses a weakened immune system to become more aggressive, persistent, and harder to treat. So, if you have HIV and genital herpes you don't automatically have AIDS, but having a herpes outbreak that persists for a month despite its treatment is.

It's possible for people to get conditions that aren't on the CDC's list. Occasionally the CDC revises its list to include these new conditions. For example, hepatitis C is not currently an AIDS-defining OI. But more data show that people with HIV are at higher risk for more aggressive hepatitis C disease.

Learning How to Prevent OIs

Some OIs can be prevented. Others are more difficult to prevent because they're common and we're exposed to them often, like *Mycobacterium avium* complex (MAC). Or, we just don't know how they're spread, like *Pneumocystis jiroveci* pneumonia (PCP). But you can reduce your risk of some of these infections by practicing safer sex, washing food well, handling animals properly, and getting screened for them.

Several sexual infections can be found on the CDC's list. So if you've never been exposed to them, like herpes or human papillomavirus

(HPV)—which can cause cervical and anal cancers—then you can change your sexual behavior to reduce your risk for these infections.

If you like to cook, then thoroughly washing meats and peeling and washing fruits and vegetables can help reduce your risk for several dangerous infections. Boiling water, getting a good water filter, and avoiding raw and undercooked food can go a long way to protecting you. Ask questions about the food you want to order at restaurants.

Handling animals, whether they're pets in your home or on a farm or in the wild, can introduce several serious infections, including toxoplasmosis. You don't have to give up your pet. You can achieve this by making sure your cat or bird doesn't go outside, washing your hands well after handling every time, and avoiding their feces.

People with HIV should be screened for many OIs when they first find out they're HIV-positive, as part of their early lab screenings. In some cases, this allows people to know if they're already exposed to an organism and helps them learn how to prevent infections they don't already have. You can also consider getting vaccines for some infections like hepatitis A and B, which can cause more severe disease in HIV-positive people.

Other suggestions on preventing OIs:

- Wear gloves when gardening or changing a litter box.

- Learn about the infections you could get.

- Use a separate towel to wipe off gym equipment.

- Avoid being around people with known disease, such as pneumonia or tuberculosis (TB).

- Don't share syringes.

Treating OIs As They Occur

Because HIV replicates more as your immune system battles other infections, treating those infections as they occur is critical not only in clearing them, but also curbing further damage done by HIV.

The earlier something is diagnosed and treated, the more likely its treatment will be successful and result in full recovery. This means regular checkups by your doctor (every three months) and talking to him or her about your symptoms.

If you experience a new symptom and are between doctor visits, make an appointment. Don't wait to have something looked at. Keep a health journal or diary, or jot down when a symptom occurs and how long it remains. This may help your doctor figure out if a symptom is a drug side effect, a sign of an OI, or something else.

Many OIs have the same symptoms, and some infections can mask others. So, treatment may only deal with part of a problem.

Dealing with multiple infections may take diligence on your part when seeing many doctors and specialists. But it can easily become a full-time job juggling your appointments as your different doctors order many different lab tests. It's your primary doctor's job to manage all of this, even when s/he is busy. It can help to prepare for your appointments, write down your questions beforehand, and have someone like an advocate with you to record the answers.

Once an illness is diagnosed, completing your treatment is vital. Also, drugs that treat some OIs may interact with your HIV meds. Any time a new drug is added to your regimen, it's wise for you, your doctor, or pharmacist to assess whether it's safe to use with your other meds and adjust doses as needed.

Using Preventive Therapy

OIs are generally not a problem for people whose CD4 counts remain stable above 200. It's very rare for people with HIV to die of AIDS at this level. However, as your CD4s decline, your risk for getting OIs increases.

In general, if CD4 counts fall below 200, people are at higher risk for PCP. Preventive therapy is advised. For people with other symptoms of HIV infection, such as repeated fungal infections, PCP preventive therapy should be started sooner. If CD4 counts fall to 100–150, then preventive therapy for toxoplasmosis is recommended for people who test positive for it. If CD4 counts fall below 50, preventive therapy for MAC and cytomegalovirus (CMV) is advised. For people who suspect they've been exposed to TB, preventive therapy is also warranted.

Perhaps the best strategy for preventing OIs is to keep your CD4s above 200. This is reflected in the federal guidelines, which recommend people consider starting HIV therapy when their CD4 counts are 500 or below, and especially anyone with CD4 counts below 350. This is because HIV therapy stops HIV from destroying immune cells, preventing the further decline of the immune system.

Using Maintenance Therapy

After treating an OI, it's sometimes necessary to take medicines to prevent it from coming back. This is called maintenance therapy, and it could be taken for life. In some cases, it may be stopped if a person's immune system recovers by using potent HIV therapy.

Some people with repeated herpes outbreaks will take long-term therapy to prevent them from coming back. Similarly, some people troubled with repeated fungal infections will take long-term anti-fungal drugs. However, maintenance therapy is somewhat controversial. This is because these organisms can develop resistance to the drugs, leaving a person few options if or when a serious infection occurs.

When these types of infections continue to happen, it may come down to a quality of life issue. Maintenance therapy may be the only viable option for a person. So carefully weighing the risks and benefits is critical to making the right choice. Some will choose to risk losing viable treatments later to ease the problems of recurrent infections. Others will simply choose to treat these infections as they happen in hopes of preserving future treatment.

Chapter 34

HIV/AIDS and Co-Occurring Bacterial Infections

Chapter Contents

Section 34.1

Bacillary Angiomatosis

This information is reprinted with permission from DermNet, the website of the New Zealand Dermatological Society. Visit www.dermnetnz.org for patient information on numerous skin conditions and their treatment. © 2010 New Zealand Dermatological Society.

Bacillary angiomatosis is a systemic illness characterized by lesions similar to those of Kaposi sarcoma in the skin, mucosal surfaces, liver, spleen, and other organs. It is caused by bacterial infection with *Bartonella quintana* and *Bartonella henselae* (cause of catscratch disease). The disease is only rarely seen in healthy immunocompetent people. It mostly affects immunocompromised patients, particularly those with acquired immunodeficiency syndrome (AIDS) or human immunodeficiency virus (HIV).

How do you get bacillary angiomatosis?

Bacillary angiomatosis is caused equally by *Bartonella quintana* and *Bartonella henselae*. It is usually a result of exposure to flea-infested cats with *Bartonella henselae* and the human body louse for *Bartonella quintana* (cause of trench fever in soldiers during World War I). Nowadays, the disease occurs mainly in AIDS patients. It may also be a complication of catscratch disease in immunocompetent patients.

What are the signs and symptoms of bacillary angiomatosis?

The first sign is usually the appearance of numerous pinpoint purplish to bright red raised spots and nodules up to 10 cm on or just under the skin. These lesions resemble Kaposi sarcoma and often the disease is mistaken for this. There can be anywhere between one and one hundred lesions occurring on any part of the body, although they are rarely found on the palms, soles, or in the mouth. Lesions may be pinhead-sized spots or nodules up to 10 cm in diameter. Nodules are firm lumps and do not turn white with firm pressure. If injured, the lesions bleed profusely.

As the number of lesions increase, the patient may develop high fever, tender and swollen lymph nodes, nausea, vomiting, sweats, chills, and poor appetite.

The infection can also causes blood vessels to grow out of control and form tumor-like masses in other organs including the bone, liver, spleen, lymph nodes, heart, gastrointestinal tract, and respiratory tract, where airway obstruction may occur. The condition can become life threatening if not diagnosed and treated promptly.

What is the treatment of bacillary angiomatosis?

Bacillary angiomatosis is effectively treated with antibiotics. Erythromycin appears to be the antibiotic of choice and is given until lesions resolve, usually within three to four weeks of starting therapy. Other antibiotics used include doxycycline, cotrimoxazole, tetracycline, and rifampicin.

Large pus-filled lymph nodes or blisters may need to be drained. Supportive therapy includes hydration and analgesics for pain and fever. Warm moist compresses to affected nodes may decrease swelling and tenderness.

Section 34.2

Bacterial Pneumonia

What is it?

Bacterial pneumonia is a common problem for many human immunodeficiency virus (HIV)–positive people, even for those who have high CD4 cell counts or are responding well to HIV treatment. In one large study, HIV-positive adults were almost eight times more likely to experience bacterial pneumonia than HIV-negative adults—though the incidence of bacterial pneumonia has declined since the introduction of more potent combination antiretroviral (ARV) therapy in recent years.

Bacterial pneumonia and less severe airway (respiratory tract) infections can be caused by one of several bacteria. *Streptococcus pneumoniae* is the most common, followed by *Haemophilus influenzae*, *Pseudomonas aeruginosa*, and *Staphylococcus aureus*. Rarely, bacterial pneumonia can be caused by *Legionella pneumophila*, *Mycoplasma pneumoniae*, and *Chlamydia pneumoniae*.

Not only are HIV-positive people more likely to develop bacterial pneumonia as a result of one of these infections, they are also more likely to experience recurrent pneumonia. People with CD4 counts below 100, and those whose bacterial infection has spread beyond the lungs, are at increased risk of death from bacterial pneumonia.

HIV-positive people who smoke tobacco, use crack cocaine, are intravenous drug users, or suffer from alcoholism or liver disease are likely at a higher risk of developing bacterial pneumonia than HIV-positive people who don't have any of these cofactors.

What are the symptoms, and how is it diagnosed?

Symptoms of bacterial pneumonia include chills, shivering, and chest pain. Fever, rapid breathing, rapid heart rate, and wheezing are other signs of bacterial pneumonia.

A diagnosis of bacterial pneumonia depends mostly on the results of chest x-rays, blood tests (especially those looking for the bacteria and measuring white blood cell counts), and examination of sputum (phlegm) samples.

Because Pneumocystis pneumonia (PCP) is another common form of pneumonia, especially in HIV-positive people with suppressed immune systems, more advanced testing of sputum samples may be necessary. This is because bacterial pneumonia and pneumocystis pneumonia are treated very differently. In turn, it is important to rule out PCP in some HIV-positive people. Testing for PCP is recommended if the HIV-positive patient has fewer than 250 CD4 cells, other signs of immune deficiency (such as thrush), a history of PCP, or a history of another acquired immunodeficiency syndrome (AIDS)–related condition. Testing for tuberculosis, such as tuberculin skin testing (TST), may also be required.

Because of the increased risk of the infection spreading beyond the lungs in people with lower CD4 counts, and because drug-resistant *Staphylococcus aureus* requires different treatment, your provider may conduct a blood test to look for these conditions.

How is it treated?

Bacterial pneumonia is treated using drugs called antibiotics. There are typically three classes, or groups, of antibiotics healthcare providers will use when treating bacterial pneumonia:

- **Beta-lactams:** Recommended drugs in this class include high-dose amoxicillin (Amoxil®), amoxicillin-clavulanate (Augmentin®), cefpodoxime (Vantin®), and cefuroxime (Ceftin®).

- **Macrolides:** The two preferred macrolides are clarithromycin (Biaxin®) and azithromycin (Zithromax®). Macrolides are believed to effectively treat a large number of bacteria known to cause respiratory infections and pneumonia.

- **Tetracyclines:** The recommended drug in this class is doxycycline (Oracea®, Monodox®).

- **Fluoroquinolones:** Recommended drugs in this class include levofloxacin (Levaquin®), moxifloxacin (Avelox®), or gemifloxacin (Factive®).

Combining antibiotics is recommended, preferably a beta-lactam combined with a macrolide. Doxycycline may be used in place of a macrolide. For people who are allergic to penicillin or who have received a beta-lactam within the prior three months, a fluoroquinolone may be used.

In rarer cases, pneumonia may sometimes be caused by less common strains of bacteria. For people who are suspected to have infection with *Pseudomona aeruginosa*, a different combination of drugs is preferred. For the beta-lactam, the drugs piperacillin-tazobactam (Zosyn®), cefepime, imipenem, or meropenem are recommended, in combination with either ciprofloxacin (Cipro®) or levofloxacin (Levaquin®).

When methicillin-resistant *Staphylococcus aureus* (MRSA)—a potentially dangerous drug-resistant infection—is suspected as the cause of the pneumonia, experts recommend that vancomycin, possibly combined with clindamycin (Cleocin®) or linezolid (Zyvox®), be added to regular antibiotic therapy.

Pneumonia sometimes requires treatment in a hospital, where oxygen and other medications can be administered to ensure effectiveness and to make the patient more comfortable.

Patients usually start feeling better within two to three days after treatment is started. However, completing the full course of treatment is necessary, to ensure that the infection is controlled and to prevent the infection from becoming resistant to the medications being used.

A syndrome—called immune reconstitution inflammatory syndrome (IRIS)—where antiretroviral treatment can actually exacerbate the symptoms of an opportunistic infection due to a strengthened immune response, has not been reported with bacterial pneumonia.

How is it prevented?

According to the U.S. Department of Health and Human Services, maintaining the health of the immune system, using ARV therapy, is one of the best ways to reduce the risk of developing bacterial pneumonia.

HIV-positive people who have CD4 cell counts above 200 should talk with their doctors about receiving the twenty-three-valent polysaccharide pneumococcal vaccine (PPV) if they do not recall receiving one during the past five years. While the effectiveness of this vaccine has not been established in clinical trials involving HIV-positive people, it is believed to offer some benefit to HIV-positive people with relatively healthy immune systems. People with HIV should consider being revaccinated every five years. PPV may also be offered to people with CD4 counts below 200, however, there is no evidence of benefit in this group unless they also initiate ARV therapy.

Receiving a flu shot (influenza vaccination) every year may also be a good idea for HIV-positive people. Many people who experience the flu, a viral infection, can also develop bacterial infections that can lead to pneumonia. Reducing the risk of the flu may also reduce the risk of bacterial pneumonia.

For HIV-positive people who experience frequent recurrences of bacterial respiratory infections, including pneumonia, the regular use of antibiotics may be necessary. However, treatment guidelines recommend against taking antibiotics regularly unless they are also being used to prevent either PCP pneumonia or *Mycobacterium avium* complex (MAC). This is because there is an increased risk of side effects or bacterial drug resistance if these drugs are used on a regular basis.

Section 34.3

Mycobacterium Avium *Complex*

"You Can Prevent MAC (Disseminated Mycobacterium Avium Complex Disease)," Centers for Disease Control and Prevention, June 21, 2007.

- About 20 to 30 percent of people with acquired immunodeficiency syndrome (AIDS) get *Mycobacterium avium* complex (MAC) disease.

- Adults usually don't get MAC disease until their T-cell count drops below 50, but children can get it earlier.

- You can get MAC disease more than once.

- There are several drugs you can take to prevent MAC disease.

What is Mycobacterium avium *complex disease?*

Mycobacterium avium complex, also known as "MAC," is the name of a group of germs. These germs can infect people who are living with human immunodeficiency virus (HIV). Adults with HIV usually don't get MAC disease until their T-cell count drops below 50. Because MAC disease occurs later in the course of HIV infection, it usually is not the first sickness a person with HIV gets. Most people with HIV have

441

already been diagnosed with AIDS before they get MAC. About 20 to 30 percent of people with AIDS get MAC disease.

Can children get MAC disease?

Yes. The risk of MAC for children with HIV goes up as their T-cell count goes down, just as it does for adults. However, children who get MAC disease usually get it before their T-cell count falls to 50. Children with HIV usually have higher T-cell counts than adults with HIV.

What are the symptoms of MAC disease?

Although MAC usually infects persons through their lungs or intestines, it spreads quickly through the bloodstream, causing widespread or "disseminated" disease. People with disseminated MAC disease can have fever, night sweats, weight loss, abdominal pain, tiredness, and diarrhea.

How is MAC disease diagnosed?

MAC disease is diagnosed by laboratory tests that can identify the MAC germ in samples of blood, bone marrow, or tissue.

How do people get MAC disease?

People with AIDS probably get MAC disease through normal contact with air, food, and water. MAC disease has been found in many types of animals, including birds, chickens, pigs, cows, rabbits, and dogs. MAC germs can be found in most sources of drinking water, including treated water systems, and in dirt and household dust. MAC disease does not seem to be spread from one person to another.

How can I avoid MAC disease?

Because MAC germs are found in food, water, and soil, there is no easy way to avoid them. However, there are drugs that can prevent MAC germs from causing disease.

When should I get treatment to prevent MAC disease?

Because MAC disease occurs in people with very low T-cell counts, you should not get treatment to prevent MAC disease until your T-cell count is below 50. Your doctor will tell you when you or your child need to begin treatment for preventing MAC disease.

What drugs are used to prevent MAC?

Drugs which can reduce your chances of getting MAC disease include the following:

- clarithromycin [kla-REE-thro-MY-sin]
- azithromycin [a-ZEE-thro-MY-sin]
- rifabutin [rif-a-BU-tin]

Ask your doctor whether you should take one of these drugs.

Can the drugs used to prevent MAC disease cause side effects?

Yes. Rifabutin can cause eye irritation. If you are taking rifabutin or other drugs to prevent MAC, see your doctor regularly and report any side effects.

If I have already had MAC disease, can I get it again?

Yes. If you have had MAC disease, continue to take drugs to treat and prevent further MAC disease. MAC disease is most commonly treated with a combination of clarithromycin and ethambutol [eth-AM-bu-tol], with or without rifabutin.

Section 34.4

Tuberculosis

"Tuberculosis: A Guide for Adults and Adolescents with HIV,"
Centers for Disease Control and Prevention, June 21, 2007.

- Tuberculosis (TB) is caused by a germ called *Mycobacterium tuberculosis*.

- TB is spread through the air. You need to have close contact with a person who has TB to get it.

- Get tested for TB as soon as possible after learning you have human immunodeficiency virus (HIV). Go to your doctor or your health department for a skin test for TB.

- You can take medicines to prevent and to treat TB.

What is tuberculosis?

Tuberculosis (TB) is a disease caused by a germ called *Mycobacterium* (my-ko-bak-TEER-I-um) *tuberculosis*. TB most often affects the lungs, but TB germs can infect any part of the body. TB may be latent or active TB. "Latent" means that the germs are in the person's body but are not causing illness. If you have latent TB you will not have symptoms and cannot spread TB. However, if HIV has made your immune system too weak to stop the TB germs from growing, they can multiply and cause active TB (also called TB disease).

In people with HIV, TB in the lungs or anywhere else in the body is called an acquired immunodeficiency syndrome (AIDS)–defining condition. In other words, a person with both HIV and active TB has AIDS.

How is TB spread?

TB is spread from one person to another through the air. When a person who has TB disease of the lung or throat coughs, sneezes, or sings, TB germs may be sent into the air. A person who breathes air that contains these germs may get TB. People with TB disease are most likely to spread it to people they spend time with every day, such as family members, friends, or co-workers.

You can't get TB from shaking hands, sitting on a toilet seat, or sharing dishes or utensils.

How can I avoid TB?

Some activities and jobs may increase your chances of spending time with people who have TB and getting TB. These include working in a healthcare setting (a hospital, a clinic, a doctor's office), in jails and prisons, and in shelters for homeless people. You and your doctor should decide whether you should be working in such a place. If you do things that may increase your chances of getting TB, you and your doctor may decide that you need to be tested for TB more often than once a year.

If you can, avoid spending time with someone who has active TB but is not taking medicine or has just started taking medicine. A person who has been taking medicine for a few weeks can usually no longer spread TB to you. That person's doctor will say when it's safe for other people to spend time with him or her.

If you are exposed to a person with active TB, you should ask your doctor about getting treatment, even if your skin test was negative for TB.

How do I know if I might have active TB?

Your symptoms depend on where in your body the TB germs are growing. TB germs usually grow in the lungs. TB in the lungs may cause the following symptoms:

- A bad cough that lasts longer than three weeks

- Pain in the chest

- Coughing up blood or phlegm from deep inside the lungs

Other symptoms are as follows:

- Weakness or fatigue

- Weight loss

- No appetite

- Chills

- Fever

- Sweating at night

445

Does TB affect only the lungs?

No. Active TB most often affects the lungs. But it can also affect almost any other body organ, such as the kidneys or the spine. A person whose TB is not in the lungs or throat usually cannot give TB to other people.

Am I at greater risk of getting TB because I have HIV?

Yes. Latent TB is much more likely to become active TB in someone with HIV. This is because HIV weakens the immune system, which makes it harder for the body to fight off diseases like TB.

Since I have HIV, should I be tested for TB?

Yes. If you have not already had TB or a positive result from a skin test for TB in the past, get a tuberculin skin test, or TST at the health department or your doctor's office.

When you have the test, a healthcare worker will inject a small amount of testing fluid just under the skin on the lower part of your arm. After two or three days, the healthcare worker will check your arm to see whether you had a positive reaction to the test.

If you have a positive test result (which usually means you have latent TB), you may need other tests to see whether you have TB disease (active TB). These tests usually include a chest x-ray and a test of the phlegm you cough up. Because TB can grow somewhere else in your body, other tests may be done.

If you have a negative test result you should be tested again at least once a year, depending on your chances of getting TB. Discuss your chances of getting TB with your doctor.

If you are an HIV-infected mother whose baby was born after you got HIV, have your baby tested for TB when the baby is nine to twelve months old.

If I have latent TB, can drugs help prevent it from becoming active TB?

Yes. The drug isoniazid can help prevent latent TB from becoming active TB. People with HIV infection who need to take isoniazid are also given a vitamin called pyridoxine to prevent peripheral neuropathy (a disorder of the nervous system).

Get tested for latent TB, with a TST, as soon as possible after you learn you have HIV. If your skin test result is positive (but you do not have active TB), you will most likely be given nine months of treatment with isoniazid to prevent active TB. You need to take your medicine for the full nine months because TB germs die very slowly. Take your medicine exactly as your doctor or nurse tells you.

If you are a woman who is pregnant, you may still take isoniazid to fight TB. However, your doctor may tell you not to take the medicine until three months after delivery.

The germs that caused your latent TB might not be killed by isoniazid. In that case, you will be given another drug (probably rifampin) or a combination of drugs used to prevent TB.

If I have active TB, can it be cured?

Yes. The drugs that fight TB work as well in people with HIV as they do in people who do not have HIV.

Several drugs are used to treat active TB. You will need to take more than one drug for several months. Your symptoms may go away within a few weeks after you start taking the medicine. TB germs die very slowly, so you need to keep taking your medicine exactly as your doctor or nurse tells you (the right amount at the right time for the right length of time).

Can I give TB to other people?

Yes. If you have TB disease of the lungs or throat, you can probably spread TB to other people. You may need to stay home from work or school or other activities for a few weeks. After you've taken your medicine for a few weeks, you will probably no longer be able to spread TB to others, but you need to continue taking your medicine for six to nine months to be totally cured. Your doctor or nurse will tell you when you can return to work or school or other activities. The medicine should not affect your strength, your sexual function, or your ability to work. Taking the medicine as prescribed will keep you from again becoming sick with TB disease.

I am taking protease inhibitors to fight HIV infection. Can I also take medicine to cure TB?

Yes. But you should know that medicines for TB and the protease inhibitors affect each other. Your doctor will decide which combination of medicines will work best for you.

What is drug-resistant TB?

When TB germs are not killed by a certain drug, that TB is called "drug-resistant." TB germs may become resistant when patients do not take their medicine long enough or in the right amount at the right times. Follow your doctor's advice when taking medicines.

People who have drug-resistant TB can transmit it to others. Drug-resistant TB is found often in people who come from areas where TB is common (for example, Africa, Southeast Asia, Latin America) but it also occurs in parts of the United States.

When at least two of the best anti-TB drugs (isoniazid and rifampin) can't kill TB germs, the TB is called "multidrug-resistant" TB (MDR TB). A more serious form of MDR TB—"extensively drug resistant TB" (XDR TB)—is a relatively rare type of TB that is resistant to nearly all of the most effective medicines used to treat TB. A patient with MDR or XDR TB may need to see a doctor who is an expert on drug-resistant TB and who can recommend the best combination of drugs to fight the germs.

Chapter 35

HIV/AIDS and Co-Occurring Fungal Infections

Chapter Contents

Section 35.1

Candidiasis

What Is It?

Thrush, also called candidiasis, is a disease caused by a fungus (*Candida albicans*). Everyone has this fungus both on and inside their bodies. It can be found on the skin, in the stomach, the colon and rectum, the vagina, and in the mouth and throat. Most of the time, *Candida albicans* is harmless and actually helps keeps bacteria levels in check. Sometimes, however, there is an overgrowth of this fungus, which can lead to a variety of problems.

Both human immunodeficiency virus (HIV)–positive and HIV-negative people can develop candidiasis. Many women experience vaginal yeast infections, a type of candidiasis. Similarly, a person can experience an overgrowth of fungus in their mouth or the back of their throat. Stress, poor diet, or not getting enough rest can contribute to these problems. Also, a person who takes antibiotics for bacterial infections, especially for long periods of time, can develop thrush in their mouth or vagina. Candidiasis in the mouth (oral thrush) can also occur in people who use inhaled steroids, such as those used to treat asthma and other lung problems.

Poor oral hygiene and smoking can also play a role in fungal overgrowth in the mouth. Excessive alcohol and sugar consumption have also been linked to the development of candidiasis.

In HIV-positive people, oral thrush and vaginal yeast infections can occur at any time, regardless of their CD4 cell counts. The more the immune system becomes damaged, oral thrush and vaginal yeast infections are more likely to occur and recur more frequently. HIV-positive people with damaged immune systems, usually with a CD4 cell count less than 200, are also more likely to develop candidiasis deeper in their bodies, such as in their esophagus or their lungs. As with many opportunistic infections, candidiasis will usually improve or recur less often if antiretroviral therapy significantly increases CD4 cell counts.

What Are the Symptoms?

Symptoms of candidiasis depend on the part of the body affected. If you have any of the symptoms, you should contact your doctor.

Oral Candidiasis

Some of the general symptoms of oral thrush include burning pain in the mouth or throat, altered taste (especially when eating spicy or sweet foods), and difficulty swallowing. Oral candidiasis appears as white or pinkish-red blotches on the tongue, gums, the sides or roof of the mouth, and the back of the throat. Sometimes, oral candidiasis can cause the corners of the mouth to become chapped, cracked, and sore (angular cheilitis).

Vaginal Candidiasis

The most obvious symptom of vaginal yeast infections is a thick white discharge resembling cottage cheese. It can also cause itching and burning in or around the vagina, as well as a rash and tenderness of the outer lips of the vagina (the labia). HIV-positive women are more likely to experience recurrent vaginal yeast infections than HIV-negative women.

Esophageal Candidiasis

This is a type of candidiasis that occurs deep down in the throat and can't always be seen by looking into the mouth. It can cause chest pain, as well as pain and difficulty when swallowing. Esophageal candidiasis is much more common in HIV-positive people with suppressed immune systems.

How Is Candidiasis Diagnosed?

Most of the time, a doctor can diagnose candidiasis simply by looking in the mouth, at the back of the throat, or in the vagina. Sometimes it is necessary to scrape the overgrowth so that a sample can be sent to a lab.

X-rays and a special scope—called an endoscope—are used to look for candidiasis down the throat.

How Is Candidiasis Treated?

Just as there are three different types of candidiasis, there are three somewhat different ways to treat the disease.

Oral Candidiasis

The most common method of treating oral thrush is to use a medicated liquid that is swished around the mouth and swallowed, or a lozenge that is sucked, dissolved in the mouth, and swallowed. The treatment recommended by the U.S. Centers for Disease Control and Prevention (CDC) as the most effective and best tolerated is fluconazole (Diflucan® tablets). Diflucan is a tablet that must be swallowed. Studies have demonstrated that it is just as effective as clotrimazole and nystatin, but is more convenient and better tolerated. The dose is typically 100mg a day for seven to fourteen days.

Alternative treatments include:

- **Clotrimazole (Mycelex® troches):** These troches, or lozenges, are used either four or five times a day for one or two weeks. Lozenges should be dissolved in the mouth slowly and should not be chewed or swallowed whole. Clotrimazole can cause stomach upset.

- **Nystatin (Mycostatin® liquid or pastilles):** Nystatin is available in liquid and pastille (lozenge) form. The liquid dose is 5 milliliters four times a day for one or two weeks; it should be swished around the mouth slowly, for as long as possible (i.e., a few minutes), and then swallowed. One or two pastilles are taken four or five times a day for seven to fourteen days; they should be dissolved in the mouth slowly and should not be chewed or swallowed whole.

- **Itraconazole (Sporanox® liquid suspension):** This medication is a liquid that must be swallowed. While it is as effective as the three medications listed above, it is not as well tolerated as fluconazole tablets.

- **Ketoconazole (Nizoral®) or itraconazole (Sporanox®) capsules:** These capsules, which must be swallowed, are less effective that fluconazole. However, they are alternative options if the four medications listed above cannot be used.

Another possible treatment for oral candidiasis is gentian violet (Genapax®). This is a dye made from coal tar and can be purchased from some pharmacies, health food stores, and other places where complementary/alternative therapies are sold. Gentian violet is very messy and can stain clothing. It should be handled with care. For oral thrush, one of the best ways to apply the dye is by using a cotton swab.

Dip the swab in the dye and coat the Candida blotches in the mouth. It is best to avoid swallowing the drug, as it can cause stomach upset. Gentian violet can also stain the inside of the mouth, but this fades over time.

Vaginal Candidiasis

The most common method of treating vaginal yeast infections is to use a medicated cream or an insert (suppository) placed into the vagina. The most common treatments for vaginal candidiasis are available over-the-counter and can be purchased in many pharmacies. Many vaginal creams and suppositories can weaken condoms and diaphragms, which can increase the risk of pregnancy and HIV transmission:

- **Clotrimazole (Gyne-Lotrimin® cream):** Five grams of this cream are applied every day, using a special applicator, for seven to fourteen days.

- **Clotrimazole (Mycelex® vaginal suppositories):** Available in 100 mg and 500 mg strength suppositories and are available by prescription. The 100 mg suppositories are used every day for seven days. Alternatively, two 100 mg suppositories can be used every day for a total of three days. The 500 mg suppository is much more powerful than the 100 mg inserts and only needs to be inserted once.

- **Miconazole (Monistat® vaginal cream):** Five grams of this cream are applied every day, using a special applicator, for seven days.

- **Miconazole (Monistat® vaginal suppositories):** Available in 100 mg, 200 mg, and 500 mg strengths. The 100 mg and 200 mg suppositories are available over the counter and the 500 mg suppositories are available by prescription. The 100 mg suppositories are used once a day for seven days and the 200 mg suppositories are used once a day for three days. The 500 mg suppository only needs to be inserted once.

- **Terconazole (Terazol 3® and Terazol 7® creams):** Terazol 3 contains a higher dose of terconazole than Terazol 7. Terazol 7 is applied every day, using a special applicator, for seven days. Terazol 3 is applied every day for three days.

- **Terconazole (Terazol 3® suppositories):** These suppositories contain 80 mg terconazole and are inserted every day for three days.

- **Tioconazole (Vagistat® ointment):** This ointment contains 300 mg tioconazole and is inserted, using a special applicator, only once.

- **Butoconazole (Femstat® cream):** Five grams of this cream are applied every day, using a special applicator, for three days.

As with oral candidiasis, if vaginal yeast infections do not go away while using these creams or suppositories, or if the infection returns soon after treatment is stopped, more potent drugs such as nystatin (Mycostatin®) liquid, itraconazole (Sporanox®) liquid, or fluconazole (Diflucan®) tablets can be prescribed by a doctor. Women who are pregnant should not use these oral drugs. They may harm the developing fetus.

Another possible treatment for vaginal yeast infections is gentian violet (Genapax®). This is a dye made from coal tar and can be purchased from some pharmacies, health food stores, and other places where complementary/alternative therapies are sold. Genapax can be purchased in a tampon formulation; each tampon contains 5 mg of gentian violet. Gentian violet tampons can be messy and can stain clothing and undergarments. They should be handled and inserted with care. To treat vaginal yeast infections, gentian violet tampons are inserted once or twice a day for one to two weeks.

Esophageal Candidiasis

Because esophageal candidiasis is considered to be more severe, deeper in the body, and harder to treat than either oral thrush or vaginal yeast infections, more powerful drugs—using higher doses than those used to treat oral of vaginal candidiasis—are usually needed to treat it. These drugs can cause liver enzymes to increase. They can also interact with other medications, including protease inhibitors, nonnucleoside reverse transcriptase inhibitors, as well as certain antihistamines and sedatives. Be sure to check with your doctor about other drugs you are taking before taking these antifungal treatments:

- **Fluconazole (Diflucan®):** To treat esophageal candidiasis, an intravenous solution or 200 mg tablet of fluconazole is taken once a day for two or three weeks. Fluconazole is considered the first choice for treating esophageal candidiasis, because blood levels of fluconazole fluctuate less than either itraconazole or ketoconazole.

- **Itraconazole (Sporanox®):** This drug is frequently used to treat esophageal candidiasis. Many doctors are now recommending that the liquid formula (itraconazole cyclodextrin solution) be used. If the itraconazole tablets are used, they are often taken with another drug, flucytosine (Ancobon®), to increase effectiveness. For oral candidiasis, the dose of itraconazole used is usually 100 mg a day for one or two weeks. For esophageal candidiasis, the dose is usually 200 mg a day for two or three weeks. Itraconazole tablets should be taken with food; itraconazole liquid should be taken on an empty stomach.

- **Ketoconazole (Nizoral®):** 400 mg of Nizoral is taken every day for three or four weeks. This drug interacts with many antiretroviral drugs. It can increase indinavir (Crixivan®), saquinavir (Invirase®), and amprenavir (Agenerase®) levels in the blood. Ritonavir (Norvir®) can increase the amount of ketoconazole in the blood and, as a result, the daily ketoconazole dose should not exceed 200 mg.

Severe or Drug-Resistant Candidiasis

Sometimes, candidiasis can become resistant to the "azole" drugs (all of those listed above) or is so severe that it cannot be adequately treated using any of these treatments. As a result, a drug called amphotericin B is often used. It is usually administered in a hospital through an intravenous (IV) line. The two types of amphotericin B are standard amphotericin B (Fungizone®) and liposomal amphotericin B (Abelcet®, AmBisome®, Amphotec®).

Amphotericin B can cause serious side effects, including kidney damage, allergic reactions (e.g., fever, chills, altered blood pressure), bone marrow damage, nausea, vomiting, and headache. The risk of kidney damage is increased if amphotericin B is combined with cidofovir (Vistide®) or ganciclovir (Cytovene®), two drugs used to treat cytomegalovirus (CMV), and pentamidine (NebuPent®), a drug used to treat *Pneumocystis carinii* pneumonia (PCP). The risk of bone marrow damage is increased if amphotericin B is taken at the same time as AZT (Retrovir®), flucytosine (Ancobon®), or ganciclovir.

Generally speaking, the liposomal amphotericin B brands are less toxic than standard amphotericin B. However, standard amphotericin B is faster acting than any of the liposomal drugs and is usually the drug of choice when candidiasis or other fungal infections are severe and an immediate threat to life.

How Should Pregnant Women Be Treated for Candidiasis?

Because many of the drugs used to treat fungal infections can be toxic to the developing fetus, the Centers for Disease Control and Prevention (CDC) recommend that topical treatments—such as vaginal creams or suppositories for vaginal candidiasis—be used whenever possible.

Can Candidiasis Be Prevented?

There is no guaranteed way to prevent oral thrush, vaginal yeast infections, or the more serious forms of candidiasis from occurring. These infections are more likely to occur in HIV-positive people with compromised immune systems (less than 200 CD4 cells). Thus, one way to help prevent candidiasis from occurring is to keep the immune system healthy, such as by using antiretroviral drugs, reducing stress, eating right, and getting plenty of rest.

There is still some debate regarding the use of antifungal drugs to prevent candidiasis. There have been a few studies showing that fluconazole (Diflucan®) can reduce the number of oral or vaginal fungal infections experienced by HIV-positive people with compromised immune systems. However, it may be possible that prolonged use of fluconazole—or any of the "azole" drugs—may lead to the development of drug-resistant *Candida albicans*. This can prevent the drugs from working correctly when they are most needed. Because of this, many doctors do not recommend that these drugs be used continuously to prevent candidiasis. However, the prolonged or continual use of antifungals may be the best option for people with a history of frequent outbreaks of oral thrush or vaginal yeast infections.

There are a number of health tips all HIV-positive people should consider to help prevent candidiasis:

- **Watch your diet:** It may be helpful to avoid foods high in sugar, dairy, yeast, wheat, and caffeine. These types of ingredients are believed to promote fungal overgrowth.

- **Eat yogurt:** Many experts also recommend eating lots of yogurt that contains *Lactobacillus acidophilus*, a "good" bacteria believed to keep *Candida albicans* in check. Not all yogurt brands contain this bacteria, so be sure the packaging says "contains *Lactobacillus acidophilus*."

- **Practice good oral hygiene:** This includes brushing regularly, flossing, using an antiseptic mouthwash (e.g., Listerine®), and reducing or eliminating the use of tobacco products such as chewing tobacco and cigarettes.

- **For vaginal yeast infections:** To help reduce the risk of vaginal infections, wear loose, natural-fiber clothing and undergarments with a cotton crotch. Also, stay away from deodorant tampons and feminine deodorant sprays.

Are There Any Experimental Treatments?

Candidiasis is a problem for many people, regardless of whether or not they are infected with HIV. This is especially true for people who have strains of Candida that are resistant to currently available drugs. Thus, new drugs are always being developed for candidiasis and other fungal infections.

Section 35.2

Cryptococcal Meningitis

What is it?

Cryptococcal meningitis is a serious infection of the brain and spinal column that can occur in people living with human immunodeficiency virus (HIV). It is caused by a fungus—*Cryptococcus neoformans*.

Cryptococcus neoformans is very common in the environment and can be found in soil and in bird droppings. If soil containing *Cryptococcus neoformans* is kicked up into the air, it can be inhaled and deposited in the lungs. From there, the fungus can travel through the blood to the spinal column and brain, where it can cause disease.

While most adults and children have been exposed to this fungus at some point during their lives, they generally have immune systems that are healthy enough to prevent *Cryptococcus neoformans* from causing disease. At one time, between 5 and 8 percent of people with HIV developed cryptococcal meningitis. Since the introduction of potent combination antiretroviral (ARV) therapy, however, that number has dropped significantly. People with compromised immune systems, particularly HIV-positive people with CD4 cell counts below 50, are more likely to experience cryptococcal meningitis.

Cryptococcal meningitis results in inflammation and swelling of the brain. This can be extremely debilitating and/or painful and can cause damage to the brain. *Cryptococcus neoformans* can also cause disease in the lungs and, less commonly, in the kidneys, skin, urinary tract, and lymph nodes.

If it is not treated correctly, cryptococcal meningitis can be fatal. Thus, it is very important for HIV-positive people with compromised immune systems to monitor their health closely and report any symptoms to their healthcare provider.

What are the symptoms, and how is it diagnosed?

Many of the symptoms of cryptococcal meningitis are similar to those seen in other diseases. These include: fever, fatigue, stiff neck, body aches, headaches (often severe), nausea/vomiting, and skin lesions. Other important symptoms include confusion, muddled thinking, vision problems, and possibly seizures.

People diagnosed with cryptococcal meningitis often have symptoms of infection outside the brain. This includes coughing and shortness of breath, from infection in the lungs, and skin lesions that can look like another infection called molluscum contagiosum. It is always advisable for HIV-positive people to report any symptoms, now matter how mild, to their healthcare provider.

There are two ways to diagnose cryptococcal meningitis. The first involves looking for the fungus in the bloodstream. This is nothing more than a simple blood test. The second, most common way to diagnose cryptococcal meningitis involves the liquid—the cerebrospinal fluid (CSF)—that surrounds the brain and the spine. To collect this fluid, a doctor or a technician must perform a lumbar puncture, also called a spinal tap. Once a small amount of CSF has been removed from the spine, a laboratory can look for *Cryptococcus neoformans* in the fluid. A spinal tap is also done to check the amount of pressure in the brain. Because cryptococcal meningitis can cause the brain to swell, the pressure of the CSF can increase. Knowing the CSF pressure can help determine how severe the disease is. If the pressure is extremely high, additional CSF might be drained to ease symptoms and prevent damage to the brain.

This is what is involved in a spinal tap:

1. Your lower spine, just above your hips, will be punctured with a hollow needle. Your lower back will be cleaned and a local anesthetic (e.g., Novocain®) will be injected near the site of the puncture.

2. You will lie on your side with your back to the person performing the test. You will be asked to bring your knees up to your abdomen and to bend your forehead toward your knees. Alternatively, you will be asked to sit up, with your knees tucked under your chin and your head dropped into your chest.

3. The needle is inserted through your lower back into the spinal column. You may feel a "pop" but, generally speaking, it is not painful. It is very important that you take deep breaths to keep yourself relaxed and that you remain perfectly still.

4. It takes approximately five minutes to remove enough CSF for analysis.

5. To check the pressure of the CSF, the person conducting the spinal tap will attach a machine called a manometer to the needle.

6. If you experience discomfort, you should communicate this to the person performing the test—without moving—so that he or she can reposition the needle.

7. After the spinal tap is completed, you will be asked to lie on your back for fifteen to thirty minutes. Less than 1 percent of people experience a severe headache due to the movement of the CSF during a spinal tap.

Some doctors also request brain scans using magnetic resonance imagining (MRI). This is usually done before a spinal tap to check for other diseases than can cause symptoms similar to cryptococcal meningitis.

How is it treated?

The standard recommended treatment for all forms of cryptococcal meningitis involves two drugs. The first, amphotericin B (Fungizone®), is given every day through an IV line. The second, flucytosine (Ancobon®), is taken orally.

Amphotericin B can cause side effects, some of them serious. Side effects include nausea, fever, chills, muscle pain, low potassium levels, damage to the bone marrow and its ability to produce red blood cells and white blood cells, and kidney damage. Tip: Take a regular dose of acetaminophen (e.g., Tylenol®), ibuprofen (e.g., Advil®), naproxen (e.g., Aleve®), or diphenhydramine (e.g., Benadryl®) approximately half an hour before receiving amphotericin B—this can help prevent or reduce some side effects during and after receiving the infusion.

Liposomal amphotericin B—a drug involving microscopic spheres of lipids (fats) that contain amphotericin B—may be prescribed for patients who become very ill while taking Fungizone or develop kidney problems. If liposomal amphotericin B is used, experts recommend a dose between 4 and 6 milligrams per kilogram of body weight per day.

After two weeks of taking amphotericin B and flucytosine, you will need to have another blood test and/or spinal tap to check for *Cryptococcus neoformans*. If the test is positive, combination treatment will be continued. If the tests are negative, both drugs are stopped and another drug, fluconazole (Diflucan®), is immediately started. This is necessary to help prevent the cryptococcal meningitis from recurring. Fluconazole is taken by mouth, every day, at a dose of 400 mg.

Fluconazole treatment may be stopped if the patient sees his or her CD4 cell count increase to levels above 200 for at least six months in response to ARV drug treatment. However, some specialists recommend a spinal tap before discontinuing fluconazole treatment, to make sure that there is no detectable *Cryptococcus neoformans* infection in the CSF. Fluconazole treatment should be restarted if the CD4 cell count falls below 200 again.

Because cryptococcal meningitis can cause the brain to swell, which can lead to debilitating symptoms and brain damage, it is often necessary to drain CSF from the spinal column to reduce the amount of pressure in the brain. These spinal taps may need to be repeated daily during the first few weeks of treatment to keep CSF pressure low.

A syndrome—called immune reconstitution inflammatory syndrome (IRIS)—where initiating antiretroviral treatment can actually exacerbate the symptoms of an opportunistic infection due to a strengthened immune response, has been reported in up to 30 percent of people diagnosed with cryptococcal meningitis. For this reason, some experts recommend waiting to start ARV therapy until people have been on treatment for cryptococcal meningitis for two weeks.

How is it prevented?

Because *Cryptococcus neoformans* can be found in many parts of the environment, it is very difficult to prevent coming into contact with the fungus. Moreover, *Cryptococcus neoformans* can live in a person's body for many months or possibly years before it causes disease, depending on the health of the person's immune system.

Since *Cryptococcus neoformans* will most likely lead to cryptococcal meningitis in people with damaged immune systems, the best possible way to prevent this disease is to keep the immune system healthy. This includes starting ARV therapy before the immune system becomes impaired.

For people who do have compromised immune systems (less than 50 CD4 cells), it is possible to take fluconazole (Diflucan®), an oral pill (200 mg) taken once a day, to help prevent cryptococcal meningitis and other serious fungal infections. However, most experts don't recommend using fluconazole to prevent this disease. This is because cryptococcal meningitis is quite rare. As explained in the first part of this section, only 5 to 8 percent of HIV-positive people with severely suppressed immune systems experience this disease. Because fluconazole can cause side effects and may cause *Cryptococcus neoformans* or other fungi to become resistant to the drug—which would prevent fluconazole from being effective when it is most needed—many experts are concerned that the risks of using this drug on a long-term basis might outweigh the its potential benefits.

Section 35.3

Pneumocystis Carinii *Pneumonia*

"You Can Prevent PCP," Centers for Disease Control and Prevention, June 21, 2007.

- *Pneumocystis carinii* pneumonia (PCP) is the most common serious infection among persons with human immunodeficiency virus (HIV). It can be fatal.

- PCP can be prevented and treated.

- Trimethoprim-sulfamethoxazole (TMP-SMX), also known as Bactrim®, Septra®, or Cotrim®, is the best medicine for preventing and treating PCP.

- You should take all medicines as prescribed by your doctor.

What is PCP?

Pneumocystis carinii (NEW-mo-SIS-tis CA-RIN- nee-eye) pneumonia, or PCP, is a severe illness found in people with HIV. It is caused by a germ called *Pneumocystis carinii*. Most people infected with this germ don't get pneumonia because their immune systems are normal. People whose immune systems are badly damaged by HIV can get PCP. People with HIV are less likely to get PCP today than in earlier years. However, PCP is still the most common serious infection among people with acquired immunodeficiency syndrome (AIDS) in the United States.

How do I know if I have PCP?

If you have PCP, you probably will have fever, cough, or trouble breathing. People with PCP may die if the infection is not treated quickly. See your doctor immediately if you have these symptoms. PCP can be diagnosed only by laboratory tests of fluid or tissue from the lungs.

How do you catch PCP?

Most scientists believe PCP is spread in the air, but they don't know if it lives in the soil or someplace else. The PCP germ is very common. Since it is difficult to prevent exposure to PCP, you should get medical care to prevent PCP.

How can I protect myself from PCP?

PCP can be prevented. The best drug for preventing PCP is trimethoprim-sulfamethoxazole (try- METH-o-prim - sul-fa- meth-OX-uh-sole), or TMP-SMX. TMP-SMX is a combination of two medicines. It has many different brand names, such as Bactrim®, Septra®, and Cotrim®. Adults and older children can take TMP-SMX as a tablet. You can also get TMP- SMX as a liquid.

I was vaccinated for pneumonia. Won't that protect me against PCP?

No. The pneumonia vaccine protects you against another kind of pneumonia, but not against PCP. There is no vaccine for PCP.

When should I start treatment to prevent PCP?

You should have your blood tested regularly to check the strength of your immune system. Your doctor should prescribe TMP-SMX to prevent PCP if your CD4 cell count falls below 200. Your doctor may also put you on TMP-SMX if you show certain symptoms, such as having a temperature above 100°F that lasts for two weeks or longer, or if you get a fungal infection in the mouth or throat (commonly called "thrush"). Having thrush is believed to raise your risk for getting PCP.

What are the side effects of TMP-SMX?

TMP-SMX can make some people have a rash or feel sick. If the drug reaction is not severe, TMP-SMX should be continued because it works so much better than any other medicine to prevent PCP.

Are there other medicines to prevent PCP?

Yes. Check with your doctor about the possibility of other treatments. Take all of your medicines as prescribed by your doctor. Don't change how many pills you are taking without speaking with your doctor.

Can I get PCP more than once?

Yes. If you have already had PCP you can get it again. TMP-SMX can prevent second infections with PCP. Therefore, you should take TMP-SMX even after you have had PCP to prevent getting it again.

Can children get PCP?

Yes. Children with HIV or AIDS can also get PCP.

Is PCP sexually transmitted?

No. PCP is not sexually transmitted.

Chapter 36

HIV/AIDS and Co-Occurring Parasitic Infections

Chapter Contents

Section 36.1

Cryptosporidiosis

"You Can Prevent Cryptosporidiosis," Centers for Disease
Control and Prevention, November 27, 2007.

- Crypto (full name is cryptosporidiosis) is a disease caused by a microscopic parasite (a type of germ). It causes diarrhea, stomach cramps, and fever.

- You get crypto by putting anything in your mouth that has been in contact with the feces (solid waste, bowel movement) of a person or animal infected with crypto.

- You can help keep crypto out of your mouth by washing your hands, practicing safer sex, not swallowing water when you swim, washing and cooking your food, and drinking only safe water.

What is cryptosporidiosis?

Cryptosporidiosis (krip-toe-spo-rid-e-O-sis) is a disease caused by a microscopic parasite, or germ, called *Cryptosporidium parvum*. Both the disease and the germ are often called "crypto."

What are the symptoms of crypto?

Most people who get crypto have watery diarrhea, stomach cramps, an upset stomach, or a slight fever. In some people, the diarrhea can be so severe that they lose weight. Other people with crypto have no symptoms.

How does crypto affect someone with acquired immunodeficiency syndrome (AIDS) or human immunodeficiency virus (HIV)?

Crypto can cause severe illness for a long time in people infected with HIV. You can die from crypto. If your CD4 (sometimes called T helper) cell count is below 200/mm³, crypto may give you symptoms for a long time. If your CD4 cell count is above 200, your symptoms may last only one to three weeks. But even after your symptoms go away, you may still be carrying crypto. If you are carrying crypto, even without symptoms, you can give it to someone else. Also, your own symptoms may come back if your CD4 cell count later drops below 200.

How is crypto spread?

Crypto is spread in the feces (bowel movements). Crypto is *not* spread by contact with blood. You can get crypto by putting anything in your mouth that has touched the feces of a person or animal infected with crypto. You can't tell by looking whether something has been in contact with feces, so you need to be aware of what these things may be. Things likely to be contaminated with feces include the following:

- Skin around a person's anus (especially important with sex partners)
- Animals (skin or fur of farm animals and household pets)
- Cat litter boxes
- Children in diapers
- Clothing, bedding, toilets, or bedpans used by someone with diarrhea
- Dirt (in gardens, yards, parks, etc.)
- Uncooked or unwashed food
- Water (for bathing, swimming, or drinking)

Can crypto be treated?

Yes. Antiretroviral medicines (HIV medicines) will decrease or get rid of crypto symptoms. However, crypto may come back if the immune system gets weaker. Some drugs may reduce or eliminate the symptoms of crypto. If you suspect you may have crypto, talk with your healthcare provider to determine which treatment is right for you. If you have diarrhea, you might become dehydrated. Drink plenty of fluids to prevent dehydration. Oral rehydration drinks work well.

How can I protect myself from crypto?

Wash your hands. Wash your hands often with soap and water. Always wash your hands well after you touch anything that might have had contact with even the smallest amounts of human or animal feces (see previous list). Even if you wear gloves when you handle these things, you should still wash your hands well when you finish.

Practice safer sex. People with crypto may have it on their skin in the anal and genital areas, thighs, and buttocks. You can't tell by looking if someone has crypto, so you may want to protect yourself in these ways with any sex partner:

- Avoid "rimming" (kissing or licking the anus). Rimming is likely to spread crypto even if you and your partner wash well before.

- Always wash your hands well with soap and water after touching your partner's anus or rectal area.

Be careful around animals. If you visit a farm, try to avoid touching the animals, especially young animals (calves and lambs). Be sure not to directly touch the feces from any animal. After the visit, wash your hands well with soap and water before you prepare food or put anything in your mouth. Have someone who does not have HIV clean your shoes. If you must clean your shoes yourself, wear disposable gloves and wash your hands well after taking off the gloves.

Most domestic animals (dogs, cats, birds) are safe as household pets. However, avoid contact with pets that may have crypto. Pets most likely to have crypto include puppies or kittens younger than six months, dogs or cats with diarrhea, and stray pets. Have someone who does not have HIV clean litter boxes or cages. If you must do the cleaning yourself, wear disposable gloves and wash your hands well with soap and water after taking off the gloves. Have any new puppy or kitten younger than six months or any pet with diarrhea tested for crypto.

Be careful when swimming or using hot tubs. Do not swallow water when you swim or use a hot tub. Crypto may be present in fresh water, saltwater, or even swimming pool water. Protect yourself and others—do not swim or use public hot tubs if you have diarrhea. Crypto is not killed by the amount of chlorine used in swimming pools, hot tubs, and at water parks.

Wash and/or cook your food. The outsides of vegetables and fruits may have crypto on them. Washing removes crypto from the surface, and cooking kills crypto. Wash all vegetables or fruit you will eat raw. If you can, peel fruit before eating. Cook food whenever possible. Cooked food and processed or packaged foods should be safe if, after cooking or processing, the food is not handled by someone with crypto.

Drink safe water. Do not drink water straight from lakes, ponds, rivers, streams, or springs. Do not drink tap water without boiling it if the public health department announces that tap water may not be safe for drinking. You may choose to take extra steps to lower the risk of getting crypto from tap water (see below). These steps may take time and may cost money, so you may want to talk about these with your doctor. If you take these extra steps, you should do so all the time, not just at home. Also, remember that water and ice from a refrigerator ice maker and drinks made at a fountain are often made with tap water.

Ways to be sure your water is safe:

- *Boil the water:* Boiling is the best way to kill crypto. Heat the water at a rolling boil for at least one minute or at least three minutes if living at higher altitudes (>6,500 feet or 2,000 meters). After it cools, put it in a clean container, seal it with a lid, and store it in the refrigerator. Use this water for drinking, cooking, or making ice. Clean containers and ice trays with soap and water before use. Do not touch the inside of them after cleaning.

- *Distill the water:* You can also remove crypto from your water by using a home distiller. These devices use heat to remove crypto. Store distilled water the same way you would store boiled water.

- *Filter the water:* Filters trap crypto from the water flowing through them. You must replace filter cartridges regularly and properly or the filter will fail. Have someone who does not have HIV change the filter cartridges for you. If you change the cartridge yourself, wear gloves and wash your hands well with soap and water when done. Filters may not remove crypto as well as boiling does because even good filters may let some crypto through.

Not all home water filters remove crypto.
The following filters are most effective for removing crypto:

- Filters that work by reverse osmosis

- Filters that have "absolute" one-micron pores

- Filters that meet National Sanitation Foundation (NSF) Standard #53 and #58.

Drink bottled water. Bottled water from a protected well or protected spring is less likely to contain crypto than bottled water from a river, stream, or lake; but you cannot be sure it is safe. Any bottled water that has been distilled or treated by one or more of the methods listed under "Filter the water" should be safe.

Drinks that are safe: Carbonated (bubbly) drinks in cans or bottles, fruit drinks in cans or bottles, steaming hot tea or coffee, pasteurized dairy products, pasteurized juices.

Drinks that may not be safe: Water fountains and beverages prepared at soda fountains, drinks made by mixing frozen concentrate with tap water, iced tea or coffee, unpasteurized dairy products or juices, fresh fruit juices.

Take extra care when traveling. Poor water treatment and food sanitation in developing countries may increase your risk for getting crypto. Take even greater precautions than you would at home. Avoid especially food and drink from street vendors, uncooked foods, tap water, and unpasteurized drinks. Talk with your healthcare provider about other advice on travel abroad.

Section 36.2

Toxoplasmosis

"You Can Prevent Toxo," Centers for Disease Control
and Prevention, June 21, 2007.

- Toxo can be prevented.

- People with human immunodeficiency virus (HIV) infection should be tested for toxo.

- Toxo usually causes illness in people whose CD4 count is below 100.

- Trimethoprim-sulfamethoxazole (TMP-SMX), also known as Bactrim®, Septra®, or Cotrim®, is the best drug for preventing toxo.

What is toxo?

Toxoplasmosis [tox-o-plaz-MO-sis], or "toxo," is a common infection among people with HIV and acquired immunodeficiency syndrome

(AIDS). It usually affects the central nervous system, including the brain. Many people infected with toxo have no symptoms. However, people with HIV or AIDS often get ill from toxo infection.

What are the symptoms of toxo-related illness?

The most common symptoms of toxo-related illness are headache, confusion, and fever. Other symptoms include seizures, poor coordination, and nausea.

How is toxo spread (or transmitted)?

Toxo can be spread in two ways: (1) by eating undercooked meat; and (2) through contact with infected cat stool.

How can I protect myself from toxo infection?

- Don't eat undercooked or raw red meat. Cook meat until its inside temperature reaches 150°F. If you don't have a meat thermometer, cook meat until it is no longer pink in the center. Red meat is also safe from toxo if it has been frozen for at least twenty-four hours, smoked, or cured. Chicken, other fowl, and eggs almost never contain toxo. However, you should still cook these foods until well done because of the risk for other diseases.

- Take special care if you have a cat. You do not need to give up your cat.

- Ask someone who is not infected with HIV and is not pregnant to change the litter box daily. This will help get rid of any toxo germs before they can infect you. If you must clean the box yourself, wear gloves and wash your hands well with soap and water right after changing the litter.

- Keep your cat indoors to prevent it from hunting.

- Feed your cat only cat food or cook all meat thoroughly before giving it to your cat.

- Do not give your cat raw or undercooked meat.

- If you adopt or buy a cat, get one that is healthy and at least one year old. Avoid stray cats and kittens. They are more likely than other cats to be infected with toxo.

- Wash your hands well after touching raw meat and after gardening, yard work, and other outdoor activities.

- Wash all fruits and vegetables well before eating them raw.

What happens when someone with HIV has toxo infection?

When someone is infected with toxo, it hides in inactive tissue eggs (or cysts), usually in the brain or muscles. These infections stay inactive as long as the infected person's immune system is strong. However, when HIV weakens the immune system, toxo can cause illness.

In the United States, from 15 percent to 40 percent of people with HIV infection have been infected with toxo and probably have tissue cysts. Up to half of all persons with AIDS who have toxo infection and a CD4 count under 100 get toxo-related illness.

What should I do to prevent an inactive toxo infection from becoming active?

The most important thing you can do is to get the best care you can for your HIV infection. Take your antiretroviral medicine just the way your doctor tells you to. If you get sick from your medicine, call your doctor for advice. Toxo most affects HIV-infected people whose CD4 counts are below 100. If you were not tested for toxo when you were tested for HIV, ask your doctor to test you for toxo at your next appointment.

If you have toxo infection and your CD4 count falls below 100, your doctor will prescribe TMP-SMX to prevent illness. TMP-SMX is also used to prevent *Pneumocystis carinii* pneumonia (PCP). If you can't take TMP-SMX, other drugs are available for toxo and PCP.

If I have had toxo-related illness, can I get it again?

Yes. If you have had toxo-related illness, you will need to take drugs for the rest of your life to prevent getting it again.

Chapter 37

HIV/AIDS and Co-Occurring Viral Infections

Chapter Contents

Section 37.1

Cytomegalovirus

"You Can Prevent CMV," Centers for Disease
Control and Prevention, June 21, 2007.

- Cytomegalovirus (CMV) infection is very common; between 50
  and 85 percent of all Americans have CMV by age forty.
- In people with human immunodeficiency virus (HIV), CMV can
  cause retinitis (ret-in-I-tis), which can cause blindness.
- You can take steps to reduce your chance of infection with CMV
  and to protect yourself from CMV-related diseases.

What is CMV?

CMV, or cytomegalovirus (si-to-MEG-a-lo-vi-rus), is a virus that is
found in all parts of the world. For someone with HIV or acquired immunodeficiency syndrome (AIDS), CMV can cause retinitis (blurred
vision and blindness), painful swallowing, diarrhea, and pain, weakness, and numbness in the legs.

How is CMV spread?

CMV spreads from one person to another in saliva (spit), semen,
vaginal secretions, blood, urine, and breast milk. You can get CMV
when you touch these fluids with your hands, then touch your nose or
mouth. People can also get CMV through sexual contact, breastfeeding,
blood transfusions, and organ transplants.

How can I protect myself from CMV?

You may already have CMV. However, you can take steps to avoid
CMV, such as the following:

- Washing your hands frequently and thoroughly.
- Using condoms. (However, no protective method is 100 percent
  effective, and condom use cannot guarantee absolute protection
  against any sexually transmitted disease.)

- Talking to your doctor if you expect to receive a blood transfusion. Most blood banks don't screen blood for CMV.

If you work in a daycare center, you should take these special precautions:

- Wash your hands thoroughly after contact with urine or saliva.

- Avoid oral contact with saliva or objects covered with saliva (such as cups, pacifiers, toys, etc.).

- Talk with your doctor about whether you should continue to work in a daycare center.

How do I know if I have CMV?

A blood test can tell you if you have CMV, but this test is not commonly performed. CMV doesn't always cause symptoms. Some people have fatigue, swollen glands, fever, and sore throat when they first get CMV. But these are also symptoms of other illnesses, so most people don't know it when they get CMV.

How is CMV different for someone with HIV?

Once CMV enters a person's body, it stays there. Most people with CMV never get CMV-related diseases. However, in people with HIV or AIDS, the virus can cause severe disease.

How can I prevent CMV disease?

The most important thing you can do is to get the best care you can for your HIV infection. Take your antiretroviral medicine just the way your doctor tells you to. If you get sick from your medicine, call your doctor for advice. CMV disease mostly affects HIV-infected people whose CD4 cell counts are below 100. Oral (taken by mouth) ganciclovir (gan-CY-clo- veer) may be used to prevent CMV disease, but it is expensive, has side effects, and may not work for all people. Normally, ganciclovir is not recommended, but you may want to talk with your doctor about it.

Section 37.2

Herpes Simplex Virus

Excerpted from "Herpes Simplex Virus (Oral and Genital
Herpes)," from AIDSmeds.com. Reprinted with permission.
Copyright © 2010 CDM Publishing, L.L.C.

What is it?

Herpes is a general term for two different diseases: one that affects
the area around the mouth (oral herpes, also known as cold sores) and
another that affects the area around the genitals (genital herpes). Viruses cause both of these diseases. The herpes simplex virus-1 (HSV-1)
causes oral herpes; both HSV-1 and herpes simplex virus-2 (HSV-2)
cause genital herpes. While HSV-1 and HSV-2 are different viruses,
they look very much the same and are treated similarly.

Herpes cannot be cured. Once someone is infected with either virus,
it cannot be cleared from the human body.

Both HSV-1 and HSV-2 live in nerve cells, usually under the skin.
Neither virus is always active. They often remain silent or inactive in
these cells, sometimes for many years or even a lifetime. This is called
"latency." For reasons not entirely understood by researchers, the viruses
can become active and cause symptoms, which include sores around the
mouth or near the genitals. This is called "reactivation." These symptoms
can come and go in what is known as outbreaks, or "flare-ups."

During a flare-up, the virus becomes active and causes a chain of
events leading to a cluster of small bumps to form. The bumps may
rupture, heal, and then disappear for an indefinite period of time.

Anyone infected with either virus, regardless of their human immunodeficiency virus (HIV) status, can experience oral or genital herpes
flare-ups. Approximately 70 percent of all adults living in the United
States are infected with one—or both—viruses. HSV-1 is spread via
direct contact with an infected area, usually during a flare-up of the
disease. Kissing and oral-genital sex can spread HSV-1. More serious
sexual activity, including penile-vaginal or penile-anal intercourse,
is the main route by which HSV-2 is spread. Both types of HSV can
actively reproduce without causing symptoms; this is known as viral

"shedding." A person with HSV can infect another person when they are shedding, even if they do not currently have any sores.

Anybody infected with either virus can experience flare-ups. In people who have healthy immune systems, a herpes flare-up usually lasts a few weeks. In people with compromised immune systems, including people with HIV and acquired immunodeficiency syndrome (AIDS), the herpes sores can last longer than a month. Severe herpes flare-ups can be incredibly painful. In a very small number of cases, herpes can spread to other organs, including the eyes, the throat, the lungs, and the brain.

What are the symptoms, and how is it diagnosed?

The symptoms of herpes depends on the site of disease:

- **Oral herpes (cold sores):** Sores around the mouth and nostrils. They may itch or be painful.

- **Genital herpes:** Sores on the penis in males or near or in the vagina in women. Genital herpes can also cause sores near the anus, including the area between the anus and the genitals (the perineum). Sometimes, genital herpes can cause pain when urinating or defecating.

How is herpes diagnosed?

Oral and genital herpes are well-known diseases. Most doctors and other healthcare providers know herpes when they see it. In turn, both types of herpes can often be diagnosed—and treatment recommended— simply by examining the sores. However, guidelines published by the Centers for Disease Control and Prevention (CDC) recommend that mouth sores in particular be confirmed by laboratory testing, as oral herpes can sometimes be more difficult to diagnose in people with HIV.

When in doubt, a small sample of the sore is sent to a lab for testing. If the virus is found in the sample, a confirmed diagnosis can be made.

Because a large number of people are infected with HSV-1 and/or HSV-2, there is no value in having blood samples tested for the presence of antibodies to either virus. Being infected with the virus does not necessarily mean that herpes sores will occur.

How is herpes treated?

Herpes cannot be cured. Once either virus is inside the body and settles itself into the nerve cells, it cannot be eliminated. However, herpes sores can be treated. Treatment can speed up healing time, reduce pain, and delay or prevent additional flare-ups. Typically, treatment is used only during a flare up. This is called "episodic therapy." In people with compromised immune systems, flare-ups can be frequent and may require long-term therapy to prevent recurrences. This is called "suppressive therapy." Some people can tell when they are about to have a flare-up, usually because of tingling at the site where a sore will appear. This is called the "prodrome" stage.

There are four treatments available for the treatment of herpes:

- **Acyclovir (Zovirax®):** Acyclovir has been studied and used for many years as a treatment for oral and genital herpes. It has been studied specifically in people with HIV and herpes and has been shown to be safe and effective. Acyclovir is available in a topical cream, pills, and an intravenous formulation. Most experts agree that the cream is not very effective and that pills are best for mild to moderate flare-ups or long-term suppressive therapy. Intravenous acyclovir is used to treat serious flare-ups or outbreaks that affect internal organs (especially HSV infection of the central nervous system). The oral dose used to treat flare-ups is 400 mg taken either three or four times a day, usually for five to ten days. Treatment will work best if it is started within twenty-four hours of the first sign of symptoms or the prodrome stage. For this reason, people with more frequent outbreaks not on suppressive therapy may wish to keep acyclovir on hand in case of a flare-up. The dose can be doubled if the herpes sores fail to respond. Taking 400 mg of the drug three times daily or 800 mg of the drug twice a day for a prolonged period of time can help prevent flare-ups from recurring. However, this is usually recommended only for patients who have a history of frequent recurrences.

- **Valacyclovir (Valtrex®):** Valacyclovir is a "pro-drug" of acyclovir and has been approved specifically for the treatment of herpes in HIV-positive people. Unlike acyclovir, valacyclovir needs to be broken down by the body before its active ingredient— acyclovir—can begin controlling the disease. This allows for higher amounts of acyclovir to remain in the body, thus requiring a lower dose of the drug to be taken by mouth. For mild to moderate herpes flare-ups the dose of valacyclovir in people with HIV is 500 mg twice daily. For episodic therapy, valacyclovir is taken for five to ten days. However, the drug can be taken every day for a prolonged period of time using half the dose needed to treat flare-ups (500 mg every day). Treatment will work best if it is started within twenty-four hours of the first sign of symptoms or the prodrome stage. For this reason, people with more frequent outbreaks not on suppressive therapy may wish to keep valacyclovir on hand in case of a flare-up. Like acyclovir, valacyclovir rarely causes side effects.

- **Famciclovir (Famvir®):** Famciclovir is the pill form of a topical cream called penciclovir (Denavir®). Usually, 500 mg of the drug is taken by mouth, twice daily, for five to ten days. Treatment will work best if it is started within twenty-four hours of the first sign of symptoms or the prodrome stage. A dose of 500 mg twice daily, taken for a prolonged period of time, is considered to be a safe and effective preventative therapy for recurrent herpes flare-ups.

- **Trifluridine (Viroptic®):** Trifluridine drops are used to treat HSV infection of the eye(s). One drop is placed in the affected eye every two hours, for up to twenty-one days. It cannot be used to treat or prevent HSV disease of other parts of the body.

In some cases, herpes flare-ups do not respond to acyclovir, valacyclovir, or famciclovir, probably due to the emergence of drug-resistant forms of HSV-1 and HSV-2. HIV-positive patients with suppressed immune systems—usually a CD4 cell count less that 100—who have been receiving long-term acyclovir for the treatment and prevention of recurrent herpes flare-ups have been known to develop drug-resistant herpes. Because acyclovir is similar to both valacyclovir and famciclovir, simply switching to these two drugs is not usually effective.

At the present time, foscarnet (Foscavir®) is the most common treatment for acyclovir-resistant herpes. The drug must be administered via an intravenous (IV) line, usually three times a day, often in a hospital or under the close supervision of an in-home nurse.

Some healthy tips:

- During a flare-up, it is important to keep the sores and the area around the sores as clean and dry as possible. This will help your natural healing processes. Some doctors recommend warm showers in order to cleanse the infected area. Afterward, towel dry gently, or dry the area with a hair dryer on a low or cool setting. To prevent chafing, some people also find it helpful to avoid tight-fitting undergarments. Most creams and lotions do no good and may even irritate the area.

- The amino acids lysine and arginine have been shown to play a role in herpes flare-ups. According to some new research, lysine can help control herpes flare-ups. Arginine, on the other hand, can actually make flare-ups worse. In turn, foods that are rich in lysine—but low in arginine—can help control both oral and genital herpes. Fish, chicken, beef, lamb, milk, cheese, beans, brewer's yeast, mung bean sprouts, and most fruits and vegetables have more lysine than arginine, except for peas. Gelatin, chocolate, carob, coconut, oats, whole wheat and white flour, peanuts, soybeans, and wheat germ have more arginine than lysine.

Can herpes be prevented?

Vaccines to prevent herpes virus infections are currently being studied and it is felt that an effective vaccine may be available in three to five years. Vaccines will only function to prevent the infection from occurring in the first place—they won't likely help control flare-ups in patients who are already infected.

People who are infected with herpes can transmit the virus during periods where the virus is shedding, but there are no symptoms. Because of this, the Centers for Disease Control and Prevention (CDC) recommends that people with herpes who have a regular sex partner who is not infected with herpes may want to take suppressive treatment as an added precaution, in addition to consistent and correct condom use.

Are there any experimental treatments?

Some researchers are studying new therapies for the treatment of herpes, including a topical foscarnet cream and a topical gel of the anti-CMV drug cidofovir. Another topical drug being studied for oral and genital herpes is trifluridine, a drug already approved for the treatment of herpes infection of the eye.

Section 37.3

Herpes Zoster Virus

What is it?

Shingles is an infection caused by the same virus that causes chickenpox (the varicella-zoster virus, which is a type of herpes virus). You cannot develop shingles unless you have had a previous infection of chickenpox (usually as a child). Shingles can occur in people with suppressed immune systems, which includes people with human immunodeficiency virus (HIV) and people over sixty years of age (especially those with diabetes, cancer, or other diseases that can suppress immunity).

Up to 95 percent of people in the United States have antibodies against the varicella-zoster virus and many develop chickenpox at some point in their lives, usually when they are school-aged children. Even though the pox lesions heal, the virus does not die—it continues to live quietly in nerve roots near the spinal cord. While the immune system cannot kill the virus completely, it can prevent the virus from becoming active again, usually for the rest of an infected person's life. However, if the immune system becomes suppressed, the virus can escape the nerve roots and become active. Instead of coming back as chickenpox (varicella), it comes back as shingles (zoster).

When shingles occurs, it only affects one side of the body, usually in the form of a belt-like streak along a single line of nerves. The most common site is the back, upper abdomen, or face. It can also affect the eyes and more rarely the inner ear. Shingles can be very painful, but it can be treated.

You cannot transmit shingles to someone who has had chickenpox in the past or has been vaccinated against the varicella-zoster virus. However, the rash that occurs with shingles can "shed" the varicella-zoster virus. Someone who has not had chickenpox or has not been vaccinated against this virus can develop chickenpox if they come into contact with a shingles rash.

Approximately 3 to 5 percent of people infected with the varicella-zoster virus will experience shingles at some point in their lives, most of them after the age of fifty. Shingles is fifteen to twenty-five times more likely to occur in HIV-positive people, regardless of the CD4 cell count. In other words, the CD4 cell count doesn't need to be low for shingles to be a risk; it can develop even when the immune system appears relatively healthy. In HIV-positive people with significant immune suppression (CD4 cell count below 50), there is an increased risk of zoster infection of other parts of the body, including the retina at the back of the eye. This can result in rapid blindness.

What are the symptoms?

The first signs of shingles are often fever, chills, fatigue, headache, and an upset stomach, which can lead people to mistakenly believe they have the flu. These symptoms are often followed by sensations of numbness, tingling, or pain on one side of the body or face. Many people describe the pain as burning, throbbing, and stinging, with intermittent sharp stabs of severe pain. Some people experience severe itching or aching rather than pain.

After several days of these symptoms, a belt-like rash that extends from the midline of the body outward will develop. The rash will be made up of grape-like clusters of small, clear, fluid-filled blisters on reddened skin. Within three days after the rash appears, the fluid-filled blisters will turn yellow, dry up, and crust over. Shingles rash can sometimes take longer to crust over in HIV-positive people with severely suppressed immune systems.

After the rash crusts over, it can take two weeks or longer for the shingles to heal completely, sometimes leaving pitted scars.

In about 10 to 25 percent of cases, shingles can occur in the eye, which is known as "ophthalmicus" shingles. The symptoms range from pain and redness of the eye to impaired vision and chronic twitching of the eyelid. In the worst cases, this can lead to permanent damage and blindness. Also, rarely, shingles can spread to the nerves in the inner ear, which can lead to hearing loss, vertigo, and loss of balance.

It can take up to six weeks for shingles pain to go away completely. Sometimes, shingles can do long-lasting damage to a nerve, which may result in pain, numbness, or tingling for months or years after the rash has healed completely (this is called "post-herpetic neuralgia").

How is shingles diagnosed?

Initial flu-like symptoms can be mistaken for other diseases. As soon as the rash develops, however, shingles is relatively easy to diagnose, as the rash is fairly unique. In turn, your doctor may be able to tell you what it is—and have you start treatment immediately—simply by looking at the rash. To be sure, or if your doctor has doubts, he or she can take a small sample of the rash and send it to a lab to look for the varicella-zoster virus.

How is shingles treated?

Like most herpes viruses, varicella-zoster cannot be cured. However, shingles can be treated. Treatment can speed up healing time, reduce pain, and delay or prevent shingles from recurring. Most of the time, pills taken by mouth can be used to treat shingles. Sometimes, if the infection is severe or doesn't respond effectively to the pills, it might be necessary to be admitted to the hospital to receive intravenous (IV) treatment.

There are three treatments available for the treatment of shingles:

- **Acyclovir (Zovirax®):** Acyclovir has been studied and used for many years as a treatment for shingles. It has been studied specifically in people with HIV and has been shown to be safe and effective. Treatment is most effective if it is initiated within forty-eight to seventy-two hours after the first symptoms appear. Intravenous acyclovir is used to treat more serious outbreaks of shingles. The oral dose used to treat shingles is 800 mg taken five times a day for seven to ten days (until the rash has crusted over). Taking lower doses of the drug for a prolonged period of time can help prevent shingles from recurring. However, this is usually recommended only for patients who have a history of frequent recurrences.

- **Valacyclovir (Valtrex®):** Valacyclovir is a "pro-drug" of acyclovir. Unlike acyclovir, valacyclovir needs to be broken down by the body before its active ingredient—acyclovir—can begin controlling the disease. This allows for higher amounts of acyclovir to remain in the body, thus requiring a lower dose of the drug to be taken by mouth. For the treatment of shingles, 1,000 mg of valacyclovir is taken three times a day for seven days or until the rash has completely crusted over. Treatment is most effective if it is initiated within forty-eight to seventy-two hours after the first symptoms appear. Like acyclovir, valacyclovir rarely causes side effects. Valacyclovir is actually the preferred form of acyclovir to use for the treatment of shingles (IV acyclovir is still the preferred choice for the treatment of severe shingles).

- **Famciclovir (Famvir®):** Famciclovir is the pill form of a topical cream called penciclovir (Denavir®). The dose of famciclovir is 500 mg three times a day for seven days or until the rash has completely crusted over. Treatment is most effective if it is initiated within forty-eight to seventy-two hours after the first symptoms appear.

Oral drugs to treat shingles work best if they are started within three days of the start of symptoms. Thus, it's always best to contact your healthcare provider immediately if you notice burning, sharp pain, tingling, or numbness in or under your skin on one side of your body or face.

In some cases, shingles does not respond to acyclovir, valacyclovir, or famciclovir, probably due to the emergence of drug-resistant forms of the virus. Fortunately, this has occurred in only a few HIV-positive people. Because acyclovir is similar to both valacyclovir and famciclovir, simply switching to these two drugs is not usually effective. At the present time, foscarnet (Foscavir®) is the most common treatment for acyclovir-resistant shingles. The drug must be administered via an intravenous (IV) line, usually three times a day, often in a hospital or under the close supervision of an in-home nurse.

Painkillers can also be used to manage the discomfort of shingles. Most of the time, mild painkillers (e.g., Tylenol® and Advil®) are helpful. Stronger painkillers, including some that can be taken by mouth or applied directly to the skin (e.g., Lidoderm® brand lidocaine patches), are also available and can be obtained with a doctor's prescription. In some cases a doctor may use a corticosteroid, like prednisone, to relieve pain and possibly speed healing time. There are no data on the use of immune suppressing drugs like prednisone to treat shingles in people with HIV, however.

During an episode of shingles, it is important to keep the sores and the area around the sores as clean and dry as possible. This will help your natural healing processes. Keeping the sores clean can also prevent them from becoming infected with bacteria, which can sometimes occur. Some doctors recommend warm showers in order to cleanse the affected area. Afterward, towel dry gently, or dry the area with a hair dryer on a low or cool setting. To prevent chafing, some people also find it helpful to avoid tight-fitting undergarments. Most creams and lotions do no good and may even irritate the area.

Can shingles be prevented?

There are two kinds of live vaccines against the varicella-zoster virus. One vaccine, called Varivax®, is typically recommended for children and guards against initial infection and chickenpox. The other vaccine, called Zostavax®, is used to protect a person from developing shingles.

The Varivax vaccine is recommended for HIV-positive children who've never had chicken pox, are at least eight years old, and have a CD4 count of at least 200. While there haven't been any studies testing the safety and effectiveness of Varivax in HIV-positive adolescents and adults who've never had chicken pox, many expert groups recommend it for older HIV-positive people, provided that their CD4 count is at least 200. If the vaccine ends up causing disease—a possibility when live vaccines are used—treatment with acyclovir is recommended.

Zostavax, the vaccine to prevent shingles in people who have already had chickenpox, is not currently recommended for HIV-positive adults. This is because it is more potent than Varivax and may cause more extensive side effects, including severe rash and disseminated disease, in people with compromised immune systems. Zostavax has not yet been fully evaluated in people with compromised immune systems, including people with HIV. It is probably best that the vaccine be avoided by all HIV-positive people, regardless of their immune system status, until necessary clinical trials are completed.

At the present time, keeping the immune system healthy is the best way to prevent shingles. This means keeping your viral load low and your CD4 cells high using anti-HIV drug treatment and by adopting a healthy lifestyle.

Section 37.4

Human Papillomavirus

Excerpted from "Human Papillomavirus and HIV Disease," © 2010 Project Inform. Reprinted with permission. For more information, contact the National HIV/AIDS Treatment Hotline, 800-822-7422, or visit www.projectinform.org.

The human papillomavirus (HPV) is the most common sexually transmitted infection in the United States. About twenty million people are infected at any one time. Nearly half of all sexually active people have had HPV at some point in their lives. Since it often doesn't cause symptoms, many never know they've had it.

Though most types of HPV do not cause serious disease, some can lead to cancerous conditions. Left untreated, these high-risk types can cause cervical and anal cancers and other cancers much less often in the vulva, penis, and scrotum. HPV has become a growing concern for people living with human immunodeficiency virus (HIV) since they're at higher risk for both HPV infection and disease.

What Is HPV?

HPV is a virus that lives in the flat, thin cells on the surface of your skin, called epithelial cells. These cells are also found on the surface of the vagina, vulva, cervix, anus, penis head, mouth, and throat, which is why having sex can easily pass the virus on to others. Most people who get HPV clear the infection on their own, often within six months to a year.

More than two hundred types of HPV exist. Some do not appear to cause health problems while others cause the common wart. (Most of these are caused by types 1, 2, and 4.) About forty types are responsible for genital warts, while about a dozen high-risk types can cause dysplasia, which are abnormal cells that can lead to cancer. HPV types 6 and 11 cause about 90 percent of genital warts. Types 16 and 18 cause about 70 percent of cervical and anal cancers. Other high-risk types include 31, 35, 39, 45, 51, 52, and 58.

Some people fear that having genital warts can lead to cancer. The HPV types that cause genital warts are not linked to cancer. However, if you have one type of HPV you may also have others, which could be ones that cause cancer. This is especially true for people with HIV.

What Are the Symptoms?

Symptoms often don't appear when you have HPV, for both high- and low-risk types. This makes it difficult to know if you have HPV; but it also means that considering HPV may be en essential part of your routine healthcare. Some doctors may not consider it an important issue, which may leave you to bring up the topic during your visits.

For genital warts, symptoms include small bumps or growths on the skin. They can appear as one or several bumps, or even in groups. They can be round and flat or differ in size. Other times they're shaped like the surface of a cauliflower. Genital warts can appear on the vagina, vulva, cervix, penis, scrotum, anus, and the areas around the sex organs like the groin or inner thighs. Rarely, genital warts appear in the mouth or throat. When they're present, genital warts are usually painless, though some itching or discomfort may occur.

For dysplasia, since symptoms are often not present, it's important to get regular Pap smears to diagnose dysplasia as early as possible. Pap smears can be used to check the cervix as well as the anus. Routine Pap tests in women have greatly decreased the number of cervical cancers in the United States since the 1960s to about eleven thousand each year.

How Is HPV Spread?

HPV is passed through skin-to-skin contact. It is very easily passed during oral, vaginal, and anal sex through mucous membranes, body fluids, and small breaks in the skin. This includes surfaces of skin that you can see, like the surface of the vulva, and on what you can't see, such as the surface of the cervix or anus.

Who Is at Risk for HPV?

You are more at risk for HPV infection and disease if you're sexually active, especially at an early age. The more sex partners you have and having a sex partner who has had many partners also puts you at higher risk. HPV occurs more often in people seventeen to thirty-three years of age, though anyone can get HPV. Also, if you smoke, you are at an increased risk for getting HPV.

People living with HIV are more at risk for getting HPV and for having more stubborn symptoms. This includes genital warts that persist or reappear after treatment and higher rates of cervical and anal dysplasia. Sexually active gay and bisexual men have about a seventeen times higher risk of anal dysplasia and cancer. All people living with HIV are also at a higher risk for anal dysplasia, whether or not they've had anal sex.

How Do You Prevent HPV?

The only way to prevent getting HPV is by not having sex. Since this is not an option for many people, there are other ways to reduce your risk of getting HPV. Limiting the number of partners and choosing partners who've had few or no sexual partners can reduce your risk.

Using a condom can help you prevent getting HPV, but it doesn't fully protect you. This is because HPV can live in skin areas that are not covered by a condom. However, studies show a noticeable drop in HPV cases when condoms are used. Also, stopping smoking will help reduce your risk of getting HPV.

Lastly, for women, getting an HPV vaccine can greatly reduce their risk of getting certain types of HPV. Currently, the vaccine called Gardasil® protects against low-risk HPV types 6 and 11 and high-risk types 16 and 18. For those who haven't already had these types of HPV, Gardasil is nearly 100 percent effective. Federal guidelines recommend Gardasil for girls eleven to twelve years of age before they become sexually active, though girls as young as nine and women up to age twenty-six are also recommended.

A second vaccine, Cervarix®, is now in large study and should be available soon. It protects against high-risk HPV types 16, 18, 31, and 45. It also is nearly 100 percent effective in those who haven't already had those four types. Cervarix will not prevent genital warts.

Getting a vaccine does not substitute for getting regular Pap tests. Women who get vaccinated should still stay on regular Pap schedules. Since higher rates of anal dysplasia occur in people with HIV, these individuals may want to discuss with their doctors about getting anal Paps done. Neither vaccine is used in boys or men, though some studies are now looking at its safety and effectiveness.

How Is HPV Diagnosed?

Genital warts are diagnosed by a visual exam by your doctor. The areas can include the outside of the body in and around the genital area and inside the body in the vagina, cervix, anus, or rectum.

Dysplasia is diagnosed through a cervical or anal Pap test done by your doctor. An HPV deoxyribonucleic acid (DNA) test may also be done. If it hasn't been done and the Pap results come back showing dysplasia, your doctor may do the DNA test to see what types of HPV are present. DNA tests are currently done in women only.

Other types of exams may also be done depending upon the results from or in addition to a Pap test. To further examine the cervix, your doctor may use a colposcope, which is a special microscope that looks at the cells of the cervix, vagina, and vulva. To examine the anus, you may have a DRE (digital rectal examination) done, which is when your doctor inserts a finger into the anus to check for bumps or other abnormal tissue. An HRA (high-resolution anoscopy) may also be done, which is when your doctor inserts a special microscope into the anus to more closely check the tissue.

A biopsy of cervical or anal tissue may also be done. This is done during a Pap test and removes a small piece of tissue to be screened for abnormal cells. The procedure can be painful.

HPV and Cervical Dysplasia

Standards of care for screening cervical dysplasia have been in place since the 1960s. All women should start getting routine Pap smears within three years of becoming sexually active and no later than twenty-one years. Routine most often means every three years if Pap results come back normal and more frequently if the results show dysplasia.

HPV and Anal Dysplasia

Infection with HPV in the anus is rather common. It most often happens due to anal intercourse; however, it can occur from other areas having been infected. Only a fraction of people with anal HPV infection will develop a lasting case of anal intraepithelial neoplasia (AIN). Although even fewer will go on to develop anal cancer, the rate of anal cancer continues to rise, especially in HIV-positive people.

How Is HPV Treated?

Treating HPV focuses on treating its symptoms, like genital warts and dysplasia. Since most people's immune systems are able to rid their bodies of HPV on their own within six to twelve months, treatments have not been developed to get rid of the virus. Many treatments for HPV disease exist, and they may depend upon the level of disease you have. You can discuss the options with your health provider to find one that best suits you. Even after treatment, both genital warts and dysplasia can return, so treatment may take several months. It's wise to continue checking and report symptoms, should they reappear.

Treating genital warts may be done by you or by your doctor. Treating dysplasia must be done by your doctor. Some treatments cause more discomfort than others, and some require recovery time. People living with HIV more often need more aggressive treatment to treat their HPV disease.

Special Concerns for People Living with HIV

HPV infection and disease are more common and persistent in people living with HIV. HIV-positive women are at a higher risk for cervical dysplasia. HIV-positive men and women are both at increased risk for anal dysplasia, whether or not they've engage in anal sex. A much higher rate of anal dysplasia occurs in gay and bisexual men living with HIV. Nearly all HIV-positive men who have had receptive anal intercourse have anal HPV infection.

Treating HPV disease is an emerging issue for people with HIV. Standards of care are not in place to screen and treat anal dysplasia. Expanding research over the past two years has helped bring this concern closer to the forefront for both people with HIV and their doctors. However, this still may lead to gaps in medical attention, especially for people living with HIV. Those with CD4 cell counts below 100 are more likely to have more persistent HPV disease and may not respond to HPV treatments as well as others do.

Therefore, it's wise to engage with your health provider in more routine screening for cervical and especially anal dysplasia. Though an anal Pap smear is similar to a cervical Pap, some doctors may not know how to do one or are comfortable with doing one.

Special Concerns for Pregnant Women, Children, and People over Fifty

The risk of passing HPV on to a baby during pregnancy or birth is very low. However, treating HPV can affect a pregnancy. Make sure to tell your doctor if you're pregnant or considering pregnancy when discussing your treatment options. Some treatments, like Condylox®, should not be used because of possible birth defects. Since the HPV that causes genital warts and dysplasia is sexually transmitted, few concerns apply to children. The HPV vaccine Gardasil is recommended for girls starting at age nine, before sexual activity starts. There is currently no vaccine to protect boys from HPV.

Since cases of HPV more often occur in people aged seventeen to thirty-three, people over fifty are generally less at risk for getting the infection. However, it's still possible for an adult to get HPV at any age. If your immune system is weakened or if you smoke, then you are more at risk for HPV disease. HPV infection and disease is not well studied in people over fifty.

What May Help to Ask about at a Doctor's Visit?

• Do you have enough information about me and my risks for HPV?

• What is my risk for getting HPV and developing HPV disease?

• What tests should I get done to screen for possible HPV?

• How often do you recommend I get a cervical and/or anal Pap smear done?

Section 37.5

Progressive Multifocal Leukoencephalopathy

"Progressive Multifocal Leukoencephalopathy Information Page,"
National Institute of Neurological Disorders and Stroke,
National Institutes of Health, May 14, 2010.

What is progressive multifocal leukoencephalopathy?

Progressive multifocal leukoencephalopathy (PML) is caused by the reactivation of a common virus in the central nervous system of immune-compromised individuals. Polyomavirus JC (often called JC virus) is carried by a majority of people and is harmless except among those with lowered immune defenses. The disease occurs, rarely, in organ transplant patients; people undergoing chronic corticosteroid or immunosuppressive therapy; and individuals with cancer, such as Hodgkin disease, lymphoma, and sarcoidosis. PML is most common among individuals with acquired immune deficiency syndrome (AIDS). Studies estimate that prior to effective antiretroviral therapy, as many as 5 percent of people with AIDS eventually developed PML. For them, the disease was most often rapidly fatal.

With current human immunodeficiency virus (HIV) therapy, which effectively restores immune system function, as many as half of all HIV-PML patients survive, although they sometimes have an inflammatory reaction in the regions affected by PML. The symptoms of PML are the result of an infection that causes the loss of white matter (which is made up of myelin, a substance that surrounds and protects nerve fibers) in multiple areas of the brain. Without the protection of myelin, nerve signals can't travel successfully from the brain to the rest of the body. Typical symptoms associated with PML are diverse, since they are related to the location and amount of damage in the brain, and evolve over the course of several days to several weeks. The most prominent symptoms are clumsiness; progressive weakness; and visual, speech, and sometimes personality changes. The progression of deficits leads to life-threatening disability and death over weeks to months. A positive diagnosis of PML can be made on brain biopsy, or by combining observation of a progressive course of the disease, consistent white matter lesions visible on a magnetic resonance image (MRI) scan, and the detection of the JC virus in spinal fluid.

Is there any treatment?

Currently, the best available therapy is reversal of the immune-deficient state. This can sometimes be accomplished by alteration of chemotherapy or immunosuppression (even if it means losing non-vital transplanted organs). In the case of HIV-associated PML, immediately beginning anti-retroviral therapy will benefit most individuals.

What is the prognosis?

The mortality rates for those with HIV-PML have fallen dramatically from approximately 90 percent to around 50 percent, according to most reports. For non-AIDS individuals with PML, the prognosis remains grim; the disease usually lasts for months and 80 percent die within the first six months, although spontaneous improvement has been reported. Those who survive PML can be left with severe neurological disabilities.

What research is being done?

The National Institute of Neurological Disorders and Stroke (NINDS) and other institutes of the National Institutes of Health (NIH) conduct research related to PML in laboratories at the NIH, and support additional research through grants to major medical institutions across the country. Much of this research focuses on finding better ways to prevent, treat, and ultimately cure disorders such as PML.

Section 37.6

Viral Hepatitis

Excerpted from "Hepatitis," AIDS.gov, October 2010.

Hepatitis is a broad term referring to inflammation of the liver. Hepatitis can be caused by a variety of things, including toxins, certain drugs, heavy alcohol use, and bacterial infections—but most hepatitis infections are caused by viruses. Viral hepatitis is the leading cause of liver cancer and the most common reason for liver transplantation.

Different types of hepatitis are labeled with letters from the alphabet. These include hepatitis A, B, C, D, and E. The most common types in the United States are A, B, and C.

Hepatitis and Human Immunodeficiency Virus (HIV)

You can get some forms of viral hepatitis the same way you get HIV—through unprotected sexual contact and injection drug use. Hepatitis B and Hepatitis C are common forms of hepatitis among people who are at risk for, or living with, HIV/AIDS (acquired immunodeficiency syndrome). When someone is infected with both HIV and hepatitis B or C, we say that they are co-infected.

Another common form of hepatitis—hepatitis A (HAV)—is an acute liver disease, which is spread through contact with the feces of an infected person. HAV does not lead to chronic infection in the way that hepatitis B and C do, but it can cause serious illness that can last for months.

There is a vaccine that can prevent hepatitis A infection. The Centers for Disease Control and Prevention (CDC) encourage people at high risk for HIV infection—including men who have sex with men and injection drug users—to be vaccinated.

Hepatitis B and Co-Infection

Hepatitis B is caused by the hepatitis B Virus (HBV). HBV is the world's leading cause of chronic liver disease. It is typically transmitted through sexual intercourse, injection drug use, and from mother to baby during pregnancy. You can have HBV without having any symptoms, and sometimes it will clear up naturally without progressing to a chronic infection. People who have chronic HBV infection, however, can develop hepatitis or even liver cancer.

There is a vaccine that will protect you from HBV. The CDC recommends universal HBV vaccination of susceptible patients with HIV/AIDS.

Treatment for HBV infection involves using medications similar to those that treat HIV. HBV treatment is complex—if you have HBV, a properly trained healthcare provider will need to monitor your treatment closely.

If you are co-infected with HIV and HBV, you have a higher risk for developing chronic hepatitis B infection. In addition, HIV infection can increase the amount of HBV virus that is circulated in your body. For these reasons, if you have HIV/HBV co-infection, you should be evaluated for liver disease and talk with your healthcare provider about treatment options.

Hepatitis C and Co-Infection

Hepatitis C (HCV) is one of the most common co-infections associated with HIV. According to CDC, about 25 percent of HIV-infected persons in the United States are also infected with HCV.

If you have HCV, you may not have any symptoms. In order to diagnose HCV, you will need to have tests to check the amount of HCV in your blood. In addition, you may need to have imaging studies and a liver biopsy to determine whether you have liver damage and how serious it is.

HIV infection can increase the amount of HCV virus that is circulated in your body, so if you are co-infected, you will be at higher risk for progressing to liver disease, cirrhosis, and liver cancer. You will also have an increased risk of hepatotoxicity, or general liver damage, which can be caused by your HIV medications.

There is no vaccine for HCV, but treatment is available. Not everyone is a good candidate for this treatment, so you will need to talk with your healthcare provider to find out whether you will benefit. HCV treatment has significant side effects, so it's important to learn about them before you consent to therapy.

If you have HIV/HCV co-infection, you should also ask your healthcare provider if you need to be immunized against Hepatitis A (which causes acute, but not chronic, infection) and hepatitis B to prevent further infections and liver damage.

Chapter 38

HIV/AIDS and Co-Occurring Cancer

Chapter Contents

Section 38.1

HIV Infection and Cancer Risk

Excerpted from National Cancer Institute, January 29, 2010

Do people infected with human immunodeficiency virus (HIV) have an increased risk of cancer?

Yes. People infected with HIV have a substantially higher risk of some types of cancer than uninfected people of the same age.[1-4] Three of these cancers are known as "acquired immunodeficiency syndrome (AIDS)–defining cancers" or "AIDS-defining malignancies": Kaposi sarcoma, non-Hodgkin lymphoma, and cervical cancer. A diagnosis of any one of these cancers marks the point at which HIV infection has progressed to AIDS.

People infected with HIV are about eight hundred times more likely than uninfected people to be diagnosed with Kaposi sarcoma, at least seven times more likely to be diagnosed with non-Hodgkin lymphoma, and, among women, at least three times more likely to be diagnosed with cervical cancer.[1, 3]

In addition, people infected with HIV are also at higher risk of several other types of cancer.[1, 3, 4] These "non-AIDS-defining cancers" include anal cancer, Hodgkin lymphoma, liver cancer, and lung cancer.

People infected with HIV are at least nine times more likely to be diagnosed with anal cancer than uninfected people, at least ten times more likely to be diagnosed with Hodgkin lymphoma, and three to four times as likely to be diagnosed with liver and lung cancers.[1, 3]

People infected with HIV do not have increased risks of breast, colorectal, prostate, or many other common types of cancer.[1, 3] Screening for these cancers in HIV-infected people should follow current guidelines.

Why do people infected with HIV have a higher risk of cancer?

Infection with HIV weakens the immune system and reduces the body's ability to destroy cancer cells and fight infections that may lead to cancer.[2, 5]

Many people infected with HIV are also infected with other viruses that increase the risk of certain cancers.[1-7] The following are the most important of these cancer-causing viruses:

- Human herpesvirus 8 (HHV8), also known as Kaposi sarcoma–associated herpesvirus (KSHV), is the cause of Kaposi sarcoma.

- Epstein Barr virus (EBV) causes some subtypes of non-Hodgkin and Hodgkin lymphoma.

- Human papillomavirus (HPV) causes cervical cancer and some types of anal, penile, vaginal, vulvar, and head and neck cancer.

- Hepatitis B virus (HBV) and hepatitis C virus (HCV) both can cause liver cancer.

Infection with most of these viruses is more common among people infected with HIV than among uninfected people.

In addition, the prevalence of some traditional risk factors for cancer, especially smoking (a known cause of lung cancer) and heavy alcohol use (which can increase the risk of liver cancer), is higher among people infected with HIV.[1, 4]

Has the introduction of antiretroviral therapy changed the cancer risk of people infected with HIV?

The introduction of highly active antiretroviral therapy (HAART) in the mid-1990s greatly reduced the incidence of Kaposi sarcoma and non-Hodgkin lymphoma among people infected with HIV.[1-4, 6, 7] HAART lowers the amount of HIV circulating in the blood, thereby allowing partial restoration of immune system function. Although lower than before, the risk of these two cancers is still much higher among people infected with HIV than among people in the general population. This persistently high risk may be due, at least in part, to the fact that immune system function remains substantially impaired in people treated with HAART. In addition, over time, HIV can develop resistance to the drugs used in HAART, and many people infected with HIV have had difficulty in accessing medical care or taking their medication as prescribed.[3]

Although the introduction of HAART has led to reductions in the incidence of Kaposi sarcoma and non-Hodgkin lymphoma among HIV-infected individuals, it has not reduced the incidence of cervical cancer, which has essentially remained unchanged.[1-4, 7, 8] Moreover, the incidence of several non-AIDS-defining cancers, particularly Hodgkin lymphoma and anal cancer, may have been increasing among HIV-infected individuals since the introduction of HAART.*1, 3, 4, 7, 9* The influence of HAART on the risk of these other cancer types is not well understood.

What can people infected with HIV do to reduce their risk of cancer or to find cancer early?

Taking HAART as indicated based on current HIV treatment guidelines lowers the risk of the major AIDS-defining cancers and increases overall survival.

The risk of lung cancer can be reduced by quitting smoking. Because HIV-infected people have a higher risk of lung cancer, it is especially important that they do not smoke.

The higher incidence of liver cancer among HIV-infected people appears to be related to more frequent co-infection with hepatitis virus (particularly HCV) and alcohol abuse/dependence than among uninfected people.[4, 9] Therefore, HIV-infected individuals should know their hepatitis status. If blood tests show that they have previously been infected with HBV or HCV, they should consider reducing their alcohol consumption. In addition, if they currently have viral hepatitis, they should discuss with their healthcare provider whether HBV- or HCV-suppressing therapy is an option for them.[9, 10] Some drugs may be used for both HBV-suppressing therapy and HAART.[9]

Because HIV-infected women have a higher risk of cervical cancer, it is important that they be screened regularly for this disease. Studies have suggested that Pap test abnormalities are more common among HIV-infected women and that HPV deoxyribonucleic acid (DNA) tests may not be as effective as Pap tests in screening these women for cervical cancer.[8, 11]

Some researchers recommend anal Pap smear screening to detect and treat early lesions before they progress to anal cancer.[12] This type of screening may be most beneficial for men who have had sexual intercourse with other men. HIV-infected patients should discuss such screening with their medical providers.

Selected References

1. Engels EA, Biggar RJ, Hall HI, et al. Cancer risk in people infected with human immunodeficiency virus in the United States. *International Journal of Cancer* 2008; 123(1):187–94.

2. Angeletti PC, Zhang L, Wood C. The viral etiology of AIDS-associated malignancies. *Advances in Pharmacology* 2008; 56:509–57.

3. Engels EA, Pfeiffer RM, Goedert JJ, et al. Trends in cancer risk among people with AIDS in the United States 1980–2002. *AIDS* 2006; 20(12):1645–54.

4. Silverberg MJ, Abrams DI. AIDS-defining and non-AIDS-defining malignancies: Cancer occurrence in the antiretroviral therapy era. *Current Opinion in Oncology* 2007; 19(5):446–51.

5. Grogg KL, Miller RF, Dogan A. HIV infection and lymphoma. *Journal of Clinical Pathology* 2007; 60(12):1365–72.

6. Powles T, Macdonald D, Nelson M, Stebbing J. Hepatocellular cancer in HIV-infected individuals: Tomorrow's problem? *Expert Review of Anticancer Therapy* 2006; 6(11):1553–58.

7. Spano JP, Costagliola D, Katlama C, Mounier N, Oksenhendler E, Khayat D. AIDS-related malignancies: State of the art and therapeutic challenges. *Journal of Clinical Oncology* 2008; 26(29):4834–42.

8. Heard I. Prevention of cervical cancer in women with HIV. *Current Opinion in HIV and AIDS* 2009; 4(1):68–73.

9. Macdonald DC, Nelson M, Bower M, Powles T. Hepatocellular carcinoma, human immunodeficiency virus and viral hepatitis in the HAART era. *World Journal of Gastroenterology* 2008; 14(11):1657–63.

10. McGinnis KA, Fultz SL, Skanderson M, et al. Hepatocellular carcinoma and non-Hodgkin's lymphoma: The roles of HIV, hepatitis C infection, and alcohol abuse. *Journal of Clinical Oncology* 2006: 24(31):5005–9.

11. Massad LS, Seaberg EC, Wright RL, et al. Squamous cervical lesions in women with human immunodeficiency virus: Long-term follow-up. *Obstetrics and Gynecology* 2008; 111(6):1388–93.

12. Goldie SJ, Kuntz KM, Weinstein MC, et al. The clinical effectiveness and cost-effectiveness of screening for anal squamous intraepithelial lesions in homosexual and bisexual HIV-positive men. *Journal of the American Medical Association* 1999; 281(19):1822–29.

Section 38.2

Kaposi Sarcoma

Kaposi sarcoma is a disease of blood vessels that was considered very rare before the start of the acquired immunodeficiency syndrome (AIDS) pandemic. AIDS is due to infection with human immuno-deficiency virus (HIV).

There are four types of Kaposi sarcoma:

- The classic type of Kaposi sarcoma affects elderly men of Mediterranean and Middle European descent and in men in Sub-Saharan Africa.

- HIV-associated Kaposi sarcoma mainly affects men who have sex with men.

- Endemic or African Kaposi sarcoma arises in some parts of Africa in children and young adults.

- Iatrogenic Kaposi sarcoma is due to drug treatment causing immune suppression.

Classic Kaposi sarcoma is rare and unassociated with HIV infection. It most often arises in middle-aged to elderly men of Mediterranean or Jewish descent (less than 10 percent are women), particularly if they come from a rural environment. They have a higher than expected rate of diabetes mellitus.

In the United States, Kaposi sarcoma was particularly common in the 1980s especially among HIV-positive men who had sex with men. It occurs less frequently in intravenous drug users and is rare in women, hemophiliacs, or their sexual partners. HIV-associated Kaposi sarcoma is more common in women in some parts of Africa. It has become less common in the United States and Europe because of effective highly active antiretroviral therapy (HAART) treatment for HIV disease.

African Kaposi sarcoma is becoming more prevalent with the rise in HIV infection. It is one of the most common forms of cancer, especially in children, in Uganda and Zambia.

Iatrogenic Kaposi sarcoma is a particular concern for organ transplant patients, especially in geographic areas associated with high levels of infection with Kaposi sarcoma herpes virus (KSHV). Most have the virus prior to transplantation, but the drugs cause it to reactivate.

What Is Kaposi Sarcoma Due To?

Kaposi sarcoma is associated with:

- infection with Kaposi sarcoma herpes virus (KSHV). This virus is also called human herpes virus 8. It is most often found in men who have sex with men but it can also occur in heterosexuals. Data is emerging that nonsexual modes of transmission can occur, possibly via saliva or arthropod bites.

- production of certain cytokines or cell signaling proteins.

- genetic factors.

- hormonal factors.

Researchers sometimes classify Kaposi sarcoma as a reactive hyperplasia and sometimes as a neoplasm (cancer); at times they may consider it multicentric and other times metastatic.

KSHV may lie dormant, or replicate and cause disease. As well as causing Kaposi sarcoma, it may also be the cause of some forms of non-Hodgkin lymphoma and Castleman disease.

How Does It Present?

Kaposi sarcoma presents as red to purplish spots (macules) and raised bumps (papules and nodules) anywhere on the skin or mucous membranes. Initially, the lesions are small and painless but they can ulcerate and become painful. There are various forms:

- Localized nodular
- Locally aggressive
- Generalized lymphadenopathic
- Patch stage
- Localized plaques

- Exophytic lesions

- Infiltrative plaques

- Disseminated cutaneous and visceral disease

- Telangiectatic

- Keloidal

- Ecchymotic

- Lymphangioma-like/cavernous disease

Kaposi sarcoma often starts as flat patches on one or both lower legs, often in association with lymphedema. The patches evolve into plaques, nodules, or scaly tumors.

Kaposi sarcoma in association with HIV infection may develop at any time during the course of illness. Generally, the greater the immunosuppression (e.g., with CD4 cell counts less than 200/mm^3) the more extensive and aggressive the Kaposi sarcoma will be.

Kaposi sarcoma lesions can also occur internally; in the gut, lungs, genitals, lymphatic system, and elsewhere. These internal lesions may cause symptoms (e.g., discomfort with swallowing, bleeding, shortness of breath, swollen legs, etc.)

Diagnosis

The appearance of Kaposi sarcoma lesions is often typical but a skin biopsy of a lesion allows a definite diagnosis. The tumor is made up of spindle cells and vascular structures with a characteristic pattern of clefting (vascular slits).

Blood tests may show no abnormality, depending whether there are associated disorders such as AIDS. Anemia may arise if there is bleeding. KSHV assays or antibody titers to KSHV are difficult to interpret.

Staging and Prognosis

There have been various attempts to classify Kaposi sarcoma, depending on whether it is localized or disseminated in the skin, and if there is lymph node or internal organ involvement. The degree of immunosuppression present may also be used in staging systems.

Kaposi sarcoma has a variable course. Some patients develop only a few minor skin lesions while others have much more extensive external and internal disease. The latter lesions may result in fatal complications (e.g., from bleeding, obstruction, or perforation of an organ). Kaposi sarcoma is not curable, but it can be treated and its symptoms controlled.

Treatment

In HIV disease, if the lesions are not widespread or troublesome, often the best approach is simply to treat the underlying HIV infection with highly active antiretroviral drug combinations that suppress HIV replication (HAART). These drugs reduce the frequency of Kaposi sarcoma and may also prevent its progression or the development of new lesions. It is not yet clear why this approach works; one opinion is that the improvement in immune function results in reduced levels of tumor growth-promoting proteins.

Iatrogenic Kaposi sarcoma may improve or clear if it is possible to stop immune suppressive medication.

The choice of more specific treatment depends largely on the extent of the disease.

Treating Localized Lesions

Small, localized lesions are generally only treated if they are painful or they are causing cosmetic problems. It should be noted that lesions tend to recur after local treatments. Treatments include:

- Cryotherapy with liquid nitrogen.

- Radiotherapy. This is most useful for classic Kaposi sarcoma and is less effective for HIV-associated disease.

- Surgical excision of individual nodules.

- Laser therapy, using pulsed dye laser or pulsed carbon dioxide laser.

- Injection with anti-cancer drugs such as vinblastine.

- Topical application of alitretinoin gel (Panretin®).

Treating Extensive or Internal Lesions with Systemic Therapy

A combination of anti-cancer drugs are given, but at lower than usual dosages if there is immunosuppression.

Other chemotherapy treatments that are used in some international centers include bleomycin, etoposide, paclitaxel, docetaxel, and liposomal forms of the standard anti-cancer drugs, doxorubicin or daunorubicin. "Liposomal" means that the drugs are coated in small fat bubbles, or liposomes, which allows better absorption, hopefully resulting in fewer side effects.

Immunotherapy includes the use of interferon-alpha and imiquimod, sirolimus and thalidomide.

Clinical trials into a wide range of other therapies are ongoing. Some examples of these are:

- Photodynamic therapy (a combination of a photosensitizer and light energy).

- Isotretinoin (a vitamin-A derivative).

- Cytokine inhibitors.

- The pregnancy hormone human chorionic gonadotropin (HCG); Kaposi sarcoma lesions disappear in some women when they become pregnant.

- Ganciclovir, cidofovir, and foscarnet (antiviral medications) have been recently reported to result in lower rates of Kaposi sarcoma among those being treated for cytomegalovirus (CMV) retinitis (inflammation of the retina caused by cytomegalovirus) and are currently being studied. Acyclovir, another antiviral, has been tried, but does not appear to work.

Section 38.3

AIDS-Related Lymphoma

Excerpted from PDQ® Cancer Information Summary. National Cancer Institute; Bethesda, MD. "AIDS-Related Lymphoma Treatment (PDQ®): Patient Version." Updated September 2009. Available at http://cancer.gov. Accessed May 20, 2010.

General Information about AIDS-Related Lymphoma

AIDS-related lymphoma is a disease in which malignant (cancer) cells form in the lymph system of patients who have acquired immunodeficiency syndrome (AIDS).

AIDS is caused by the human immunodeficiency virus (HIV), which attacks and weakens the body's immune system. The immune system is then unable to fight infection and diseases that invade the body. People with HIV disease have an increased risk of developing infections, lymphoma, and other types of cancer. A person with HIV disease who develops certain types of infections or cancer is then diagnosed with AIDS. Sometimes, people are diagnosed with AIDS and AIDS-related lymphoma at the same time.

Lymphomas are cancers that affect the white blood cells of the lymph system, part of the body's immune system.

Types of Lymphoma

Lymphomas are divided into two general types: Hodgkin lymphoma and non-Hodgkin lymphoma. Both Hodgkin lymphoma and non-Hodgkin lymphoma may occur in AIDS patients, but non-Hodgkin lymphoma is more common. When a person with AIDS has non-Hodgkin lymphoma, it is called an AIDS-related lymphoma.

Non-Hodgkin lymphomas are grouped by the way their cells look under a microscope. They may be indolent (slow-growing) or aggressive (fast-growing). AIDS-related lymphoma is usually aggressive. There are three main types of AIDS-related lymphoma:

- Diffuse large B-cell lymphoma
- B-cell immunoblastic lymphoma

507

- Small non-cleaved cell lymphoma

Symptoms of AIDS-Related Lymphoma

Possible signs of AIDS-related lymphoma include weight loss, fever, and night sweats.

These and other symptoms may be caused by AIDS-related lymphoma. Other conditions may cause the same symptoms. A doctor should be consulted if any of the following problems occur:

- Weight loss or fever for no known reason

- Night sweats

- Painless, swollen lymph nodes in the neck, chest, underarm, or groin

- A feeling of fullness below the ribs

Diagnosing AIDS-Related Lymphoma

Tests that examine the body and lymph system are used to help detect (find) and diagnose AIDS-related lymphoma.

The following tests and procedures may be used:

- **Physical exam and history:** An exam of the body to check general signs of health, including checking for signs of disease, such as lumps or anything else that seems unusual. A history of the patient's health habits and past illnesses and treatments will also be taken.

- **Complete blood count (CBC):** A procedure in which a sample of blood is drawn and checked for the following:

  - The number of red blood cells, white blood cells, and platelets

  - The amount of hemoglobin (the protein that carries oxygen) in the red blood cells

  - The portion of the sample made up of red blood cells

- **Lymph node biopsy:** The removal of all or part of a lymph node. A pathologist views the tissue under a microscope to look for cancer cells. One of the following types of biopsies may be done:

  - *Excisional biopsy:* The removal of an entire lymph node.

  - *Incisional biopsy:* The removal of part of a lymph node.

- *Core biopsy:* The removal of tissue from a lymph node using a wide needle.

- *Fine-needle aspiration (FNA) biopsy:* The removal of tissue from a lymph node using a thin needle.

- **Bone marrow aspiration and biopsy:** The removal of bone marrow, blood, and a small piece of bone by inserting a hollow needle into the hipbone or breastbone. A pathologist views the bone marrow, blood, and bone under a microscope to look for abnormal cells.

- **HIV test:** A test to measure the level of HIV antibodies in a sample of blood. Antibodies are made by the body when it is invaded by a foreign substance. A high level of HIV antibodies may mean the body has been infected with HIV.

- **Epstein-Barr virus (EBV) test:** A test to measure the level of EBV antibodies in a sample of blood, tissue, or cerebrospinal fluid (CSF). Antibodies are made by the body when it is invaded by a foreign substance. A high level of EBV antibodies may mean the body has been infected with EBV.

- **Chest x-ray:** An x-ray of the organs and bones inside the chest. An x-ray is a type of energy beam that can go through the body and onto film, making a picture of areas inside the body.

Prognosis

Certain factors affect prognosis (chance of recovery) and treatment options.

The prognosis (chance of recovery) and treatment options depend on the following:

- The stage of the cancer

- The number of CD4 lymphocytes (a type of white blood cell) in the blood

- Whether the patient has ever had AIDS-related infections

- The patient's ability to carry out regular daily activities

Stages of AIDS-Related Lymphoma

After AIDS-related lymphoma has been diagnosed, tests are done to find out if cancer cells have spread within the lymph system or to other parts of the body.

The process used to find out if cancer cells have spread within the lymph system or to other parts of the body is called staging. The information gathered from the staging process determines the stage of the disease. It is important to know the stage in order to plan treatment, but AIDS-related lymphoma is usually advanced when it is diagnosed.

There are three ways that cancer spreads in the body.

The three ways that cancer spreads in the body are:

- **Through tissue:** Cancer invades the surrounding normal tissue.

- **Through the lymph system:** Cancer invades the lymph system and travels through the lymph vessels to other places in the body.

- **Through the blood:** Cancer invades the veins and capillaries and travels through the blood to other places in the body.

When cancer cells break away from the primary (original) tumor and travel through the lymph or blood to other places in the body, another (secondary) tumor may form. This process is called metastasis. The secondary (metastatic) tumor is the same type of cancer as the primary tumor. For example, if breast cancer spreads to the bones, the cancer cells in the bones are actually breast cancer cells. The disease is metastatic breast cancer, not bone cancer.

Stages of AIDS-related lymphoma may include E and S:

- **E:** "E" stands for extranodal and means the cancer is found in an area or organ other than the lymph nodes or has spread to tissues beyond, but near, the major lymphatic areas.

- **S:** "S" stands for spleen and means the cancer is found in the spleen.

The following stages are used for AIDS-related lymphoma:

- Stage I
- Stage II
- Stage III
- Stage IV

Stage I

Stage I AIDS-related lymphoma is divided into stage I and stage IE:

- **Stage I:** Stage I cancer is found in one lymph node group.

- **Stage1E:** Stage IE cancer is found in an area or organ other than the lymph nodes.

Stage II

Stage II AIDS-related lymphoma is divided into stage II and stage IIE:

- **Stage II:** Cancer is found in two or more lymph node groups on the same side of the diaphragm (the thin muscle below the lungs that helps breathing and separates the chest from the abdomen).

- **Stage IIE:** Cancer is found in an area or organ other than the lymph nodes and in lymph nodes near that area or organ, and may have spread to other lymph node groups on the same side of the diaphragm.

Stage III

Stage III AIDS-related lymphoma is divided into stage III, stage IIIE, stage IIIS, and stage IIIS+E:

- **Stage III:** Cancer is found in lymph node groups on both sides of the diaphragm (the thin muscle below the lungs that helps breathing and separates the chest from the abdomen).

- **Stage IIIE:** Cancer is found in lymph node groups on both sides of the diaphragm and in an area or organ other than the lymph nodes.

- **Stage IIIS:** Cancer is found in lymph node groups on both sides of the diaphragm and in the spleen.

- **Stage IIIS+E:** Cancer is found in lymph node groups on both sides of the diaphragm, in an area or organ other than the lymph nodes, and in the spleen.

Stage IV

In stage IV AIDS-related lymphoma, the cancer either:

- is found throughout one or more organs other than the lymph nodes and may be in lymph nodes near those organs; or

- is found in one organ other than the lymph nodes and has spread to lymph nodes far away from that organ.

Patients who are infected with the Epstein-Barr virus or whose AIDS-related lymphoma affects the bone marrow have an increased risk of the cancer spreading to the central nervous system (CNS).

For treatment, AIDS-related lymphomas are grouped based on where they started in the body, as follows:

- **Peripheral/systemic lymphoma:** Lymphoma that starts in lymph nodes or other organs of the lymph system is called peripheral/systemic lymphoma. The lymphoma may spread throughout the body, including to the brain or bone marrow.

- **Primary CNS lymphoma:** Primary CNS lymphoma starts in the central nervous system (brain and spinal cord). Lymphoma that starts somewhere else in the body and spreads to the central nervous system is not primary CNS lymphoma.

Treatment Option Overview

There are different types of treatment for patients with AIDS-related lymphoma. Some treatments are standard (the currently used treatment), and some are being tested in clinical trials. A treatment clinical trial is a research study meant to help improve current treatments or obtain information on new treatments for patients with cancer. When clinical trials show that a new treatment is better than the standard treatment, the new treatment may become the standard treatment. Patients may want to think about taking part in a clinical trial. Some clinical trials are open only to patients who have not started treatment.

Treatment of AIDS-related lymphoma combines treatment of the lymphoma with treatment for AIDS.

Patients with AIDS have weakened immune systems and treatment can cause further damage. For this reason, patients who have AIDS-related lymphoma are usually treated with lower doses of drugs than lymphoma patients who do not have AIDS.

Highly active antiretroviral therapy (HAART) is used to slow progression of HIV (which is a retrovirus). Treatment with HAART may allow some patients to safely receive anticancer drugs in standard or higher doses. Medicine to prevent and treat infections, which can be serious, is also used.

AIDS-related lymphoma usually grows faster than lymphoma that is not AIDS-related and it is more likely to spread to other parts of the body. In general, AIDS-related lymphoma is harder to treat.

Three types of standard treatment are used:

- Chemotherapy

- Radiation therapy

- High-dose chemotherapy with stem cell transplant

Chemotherapy

Chemotherapy is a cancer treatment that uses drugs to stop the growth of cancer cells, either by killing the cells or by stopping them from dividing. When chemotherapy is taken by mouth or injected into a vein or muscle, the drugs enter the bloodstream and can reach cancer cells throughout the body (systemic chemotherapy). When chemotherapy is placed directly into the spinal column (intrathecal chemotherapy), an organ, or a body cavity such as the abdomen, the drugs mainly affect cancer cells in those areas (regional chemotherapy). Combination chemotherapy is treatment using more than one anticancer drug. The way the chemotherapy is given depends on the type and stage of the cancer being treated.

Intrathecal chemotherapy may be used in patients who are more likely to have lymphoma in the central nervous system (CNS).

Colony-stimulating factors are sometimes given together with chemotherapy. This helps lessen the side effects chemotherapy may have on the bone marrow.

Radiation Therapy

Radiation therapy is a cancer treatment that uses high-energy x-rays or other types of radiation to kill cancer cells or keep them from growing. There are two types of radiation therapy. External radiation therapy uses a machine outside the body to send radiation toward the cancer. Internal radiation therapy uses a radioactive substance sealed in needles, seeds, wires, or catheters that are placed directly into or near the cancer. The way the radiation therapy is given depends on the type and stage of the cancer being treated.

High-Dose Chemotherapy with Stem Cell Transplant

High-dose chemotherapy with stem cell transplant is a method of giving high doses of chemotherapy and replacing blood-forming cells destroyed by the cancer treatment. Stem cells (immature blood cells) are removed from the blood or bone marrow of the patient or a donor and are frozen and stored. After the chemotherapy is completed, the stored stem cells are thawed and given back to the patient through an infusion. These reinfused stem cells grow into (and restore) the body's blood cells.

New Treatments

This summary describes treatments that are being studied in clinical trials. It may not mention every new treatment being studied.

Targeted therapy. Targeted therapy is a type of treatment that uses drugs or other substances to identify and attack specific cancer cells without harming normal cells. Monoclonal antibody therapy is one type of targeted therapy being studied in the treatment of AIDS-related lymphoma.

Monoclonal antibody therapy is a cancer treatment that uses antibodies made in the laboratory from a single type of immune system cell. These antibodies can identify substances on cancer cells or normal substances that may help cancer cells grow. The antibodies attach to the substances and kill the cancer cells, block their growth, or keep them from spreading. Monoclonal antibodies are given by infusion. These may be used alone or to carry drugs, toxins, or radioactive material directly to cancer cells.

Clinical Trials

For some patients, taking part in a clinical trial may be the best treatment choice. Clinical trials are part of the cancer research process. Clinical trials are done to find out if new cancer treatments are safe and effective or better than the standard treatment.

Many of today's standard treatments for cancer are based on earlier clinical trials. Patients who take part in a clinical trial may receive the standard treatment or be among the first to receive a new treatment.

Patients who take part in clinical trials also help improve the way cancer will be treated in the future. Even when clinical trials do not lead to effective new treatments, they often answer important questions and help move research forward.

Patients can enter clinical trials before, during, or after starting their cancer treatment.

Some clinical trials only include patients who have not yet received treatment. Other trials test treatments for patients whose cancer has not gotten better. There are also clinical trials that test new ways to stop cancer from recurring (coming back) or reduce the side effects of cancer treatment.

Follow-Up

Some of the tests that were done to diagnose the cancer or to find out the stage of the cancer may be repeated. Some tests will be repeated in order to see how well the treatment is working. Decisions about whether to continue, change, or stop treatment may be based on the results of these tests. This is sometimes called re-staging.

Some of the tests will continue to be done from time to time after treatment has ended. The results of these tests can show if your condition has changed or if the cancer has recurred (come back). These tests are sometimes called follow-up tests or check-ups.

Treatment Options for AIDS-Related Lymphoma

AIDS-Related Peripheral/Systemic Lymphoma

There is no standard treatment plan for AIDS-related peripheral/systemic lymphoma. Treatment is adjusted for each patient and is usually one or more of the following:

- Combination chemotherapy
- High-dose chemotherapy and stem cell transplant
- A clinical trial of monoclonal antibodies
- A clinical trial of different treatment combinations

AIDS-Related Primary Central Nervous System Lymphoma

Treatment of AIDS-related primary central nervous system lymphoma is usually radiation therapy.

Chapter 39

Other AIDS-Related Health Concerns

Chapter Contents

Section 39.1

AIDS Dementia Complex

Dementia is a brain disorder that affects a person's ability to think clearly and can impact his or her daily activities. Acquired immunodeficiency syndrome (AIDS) dementia complex (ADC)—dementia caused by human immunodeficiency virus (HIV) infection—is a complicated syndrome of different nervous system and mental symptoms. These are somewhat common in people with HIV disease.

The frequency of ADC increases with advancing HIV disease and as CD4 counts decline. It's fairly uncommon in people with early HIV disease, and more common in people with severely weakened immune systems. Severe ADC is almost exclusively seen in advanced HIV disease.

ADC consists of many conditions. These can easily be mistaken for symptoms of other common problems including depression, drug side effects, or infections like toxoplasmosis or lymphoma. Because ADC varies so much from person to person, it's poorly understood and there's no way to tell how a person will progress with ADC.

What Is ADC?

ADC is characterized by severe changes in four areas: a person's ability to understand and remember information (cognition); behavior; ability to move their bodies (motor coordination); or emotions (mood). These changes are called ADC when they're believed to be related to HIV itself rather than other factors.

Cognitive impairment often appears as memory loss, speech problems, inability to concentrate, and poor judgment. These are often the first symptoms a person will notice. They include the need to make lists in order to remember routine tasks or forgetting, in mid-sentence, what one was talking about.

Behavioral changes are the least understood. They can be described as impairments in one's ability to perform common tasks and activities of daily living. These changes are found in 30 to 40 percent of people with early ADC.

Motor impairment is often characterized by a loss of control of the bladder; loss of feeling in and loss of control of the legs; and stiff, awkward, or obviously slowed movements. It's not common in early ADC. A change in handwriting may be an early sign.

Mood impairments are defined as changes in emotional responses. In ADC, this is associated with several conditions, such as severe depression, severe personality changes (psychosis), and, less commonly, intense excitability (mania).

The Symptoms of ADC

Diagnosing ADC is heavily dependent on the keen judgment of doctors, often together with psychiatric, brain, or neurology experts. It's difficult to determine impairments in mood and behavior since there's no standard course of ADC. In one person it may be very mild with periods of varying severity of symptoms. In another it can be abrupt, severe, and progressive.

Sometimes symptoms are overlooked or dismissed by caregivers, who may believe the symptoms are due to advanced HIV disease or depression. ADC symptoms may include poor concentration, forgetfulness, loss of short- or long-term memory, social withdrawal, slowed thinking, short attention span, irritability, apathy (lack of caring or concern for oneself or others), weakness, poor coordination, impaired judgment, vision problems, and personality change.

ADC occurs more commonly in children with HIV than adults. It presents similarly and is often more severe and progressive.

Possible Early Stage Symptoms

- Difficulty concentrating
- Difficulty remembering phone numbers or appointments
- Slowed thinking
- Longer time needed to complete tasks
- Reliance on keeping lists
- Mental status tests and other mental capabilities may be normal
- Irritability
- Unsteady gait (walk) or difficulty keeping balance

- Poor hand coordination or writing
- Depression

Possible Middle Stage Symptoms

- Symptoms of muscle weakness
- Poor performance on regular tasks
- More concentration and attention required
- Slow responses and frequently dropping objects
- Feelings of indifference or apathy
- Slowness in normal activities, like eating and writing
- Walking, balance, and coordination require a great deal of effort

Possible Late Stage Symptoms

- Loss of bladder or bowel control
- Difficulty walking
- Loss of initiative or interest
- Withdrawing from life
- Psychosis or mania
- Confinement to bed

How Does HIV Cause ADC?

While it is clear that HIV can cause serious disease in the nervous system, how it causes ADC is unclear. In general, nervous system and mental disorders are caused by the death of nerve cells. While HIV does not directly infect nerve cells, it's thought it can somehow kill them indirectly.

Macrophages—white blood cells that are common in the brain and act as large reservoirs for HIV—appear to be HIV's first target in the central nervous system. Infected macrophages can carry HIV into the brain from the bloodstream. From there, these cells likely cause damage in many different ways.

What If You Think You Have ADC?

- Don't be afraid to tell your doctor or any other providers that you suspect something is wrong. Find a second opinion if you need one.

- Keep a notepad with you and write down your symptoms whenever they occur. This will greatly help your doctor to help you.

- Build as much support as possible, including friends, family, and professionals. Although it's possible to treat ADC, it may take a while for some symptoms to go away.

Incidence

Anecdotal reports indicate that there are fewer people with ADC since HIV therapy became standard. People who develop ADC today tend to be "sicker" than those before the use of HIV therapy. The rate of ADC dropped from 53 percent in 1987 to 3 percent in 1988 (after the first HIV drug was approved).

Early in the epidemic, many new AIDS cases were attributed to ADC. Many doctors now report that they're no longer seeing people who have just ADC. It has increasingly become a disease of late-stage AIDS when people suffer from multiple infections.

Diagnosing ADC

Three tests are required to diagnose ADC accurately: a mental status exam, one of the standard scans (computed tomography [CT] and/or magnetic resonance imaging [MRI]), and a spinal tap. These may also help tell ADC apart from other brain diseases like toxoplasmosis, progressive multifocal leukoencephalopathy (PML), or lymphoma. However, ADC can occur along with these other brain diseases, so diagnosing multiple conditions can be more difficult.

A mental status exam helps reveal problems like short- or long-term memory loss, difficulty concentrating, and abstract thinking as well as swings in mood. Imaging scans of the brain are also used. Certain lab tests can examine cerebrospinal fluid (CSF) that's been obtained by a spinal tap.

CT scans are x-rays that can show signs of destroyed brain tissue. MRI, or magnetic resonance imaging, is a more sensitive scan. Results from both tests can help rule out other causes for the symptoms.

Testing CSF may help determine ADC, but they're not conclusive. Mostly they're used to rule out other causes of the symptoms. Many people with ADC have higher levels of certain proteins or white blood cells in their CSF. However, not everyone with these levels turn out to have ADC. Also, people with advanced ADC are more likely to have higher HIV levels in their CSF, though this is also not conclusive.

Treating ADC

The best therapies to treat ADC appear to be HIV drugs, and high-dose Retrovir® (zidovudine, AZT) is the most studied drug for it. However, many specialists contend that how well a potent regimen controls HIV overall is more important than the actual drugs used. This may or may not include using standard, or even high-dose, Retrovir as part of the regimen.

Generally speaking, creating an HIV regimen to treat ADC follows three principals: (1) Start a potent regimen (usually three drugs) to decrease viral load to undetectable levels; (2) In people on HIV therapy, consider their drug history and resistance test results; and (3) If possible, use HIV drugs that cross the blood-brain barrier as part of the new regimen.

It's believed that an HIV drug that crosses the blood-brain barrier might help prevent or treat ADC. Findings from earlier in the epidemic show that high-dose Retrovir (1,000–1,200mg/day) can cross the blood-brain barrier and effectively treat it. Several researchers have reported improvements in symptoms. However, many with HIV are often unable to tolerate its side effects.

While Retrovir may be the most researched drug, other HIV drugs that cross the blood-brain barrier may be equally useful. These include Zerit®, Ziagen®, Viramune®, Agenerase®, and to a lesser degree Crixivan® and Epivir®. Sustiva® does not cross it to a significant degree, but some experts speculate it may be useful in treating ADC.

Treating the Symptoms

Psychoactive drugs are often used to treat ADC symptoms: antipsychotics, anti-depressants, anxiolytics, psycho-stimulants, anti-manics, and anti-convulsants. These drugs do not treat the underlying cause of ADC, or even stop its progression. However, they may ease some of its symptoms. Haldol® (haloperidol) is often used though it has many side effects, so smaller doses of 5–10mg daily should be used.

Ritalin® (methylphenidate) has been used successfully in people with ADC to ease apathy and to increase energy, concentration, and appetite. Daily doses of 5–10mg are often enough.

In cases of severe behavior disorders, drugs like Thorazine® and Mellaril® can be used to control agitation. Ativan® (lorazepam) and Valium® (diazepam) may also be used for sedation and controlling anxiety. Others include Trilafon® (perphenazine), Navane® (thiothixene), Moban® (molindone), and Prozac® (fluoxetine) with Wellbutrin® (bupropion).

Section 39.2

Oral Health Issues

Excerpted from "Oral Health Issues," AIDS.gov, October 2010.

Your Mouth, Your Health

When you are focused on your overall health and wellbeing—and especially when you are dealing with illness—it can be easy to overlook dental issues and oral healthcare.

But good dental hygiene is an important part of managing your human immunodeficiency virus (HIV) disease. If you wait until you are having problems with your teeth and gums to see a dentist, you can end up dealing with infection, pain, and tooth loss.

Poor oral health can even lead to malnutrition. If you can't chew or swallow because your mouth hurts, you may not eat enough to keep yourself healthy.

HIV and Oral Health

Your mouth may be the first part of your body to show signs of HIV infection. Oral opportunistic infections, such as candidiasis (thrush), are sometimes the first indicator that your immune system is not working properly—and oral health can be an important indicator of how HIV is affecting your body.

Anyone can have oral health problems, but HIV disease can make you more susceptible to the following:

- Oral warts

- Fever blisters

- Oral hairy leukoplakia

- Thrush

- Canker sores

- Cavities

- Gum disease (periodontitis and gingivitis)

523

People with HIV/acquired immunodeficiency syndrome (AIDS) may also experience dry mouth, which increases the risk of tooth decay and can make chewing, eating, swallowing, and even talking difficult. Some HIV medications can cause dry mouth.

The best ways to avoid these problems include the following:

- See your dentist regularly and ask about the best way to care for your mouth and teeth.

- Brush your teeth at least twice a day. (After every meal is better!)

- Floss every day. Flossing cleans parts of your teeth that your toothbrush can't reach.

- Take all your HIV medications on schedule—this will protect your immune system and prevent oral opportunistic infections.

- Let your doctor know if your HIV meds are causing you to have dry mouth. There are remedies.

- Examine your mouth often and tell your primary care provider if you notice any unusual changes in the way your mouth looks or feels.

- If you do not have a dentist, ask your regular clinic or provider to refer you to one.

Section 39.3

HIV-Related Pain

Pain is common in people living with human immunodeficiency virus (HIV)—HIV-positive people. One study of HIV-positive people found that more than 50 percent had pain. Pain can occur at all stages of HIV disease and can affect many parts of the body. Usually pain occurs more often and becomes more severe as HIV disease progresses. But each individual is different. Some people may experience a lot of pain, while others have little or none.

What Causes Pain?

HIV-related pain can have many causes:

- A symptom of HIV itself
- A symptom of other illnesses or infections
- A side effect of HIV drugs

Regardless of the reason, pain should be evaluated and treated to help HIV-positive people have a good quality of life.

Common Types of Pain

The first step in managing HIV-related pain is identifying the type, and if possible, the cause of pain. Some common types of pain include the following:

Peripheral Neuropathy

Pain due to nerve damage, mostly in the feet and hands. It may be described as numbness, tingling, or burning. Nerve damage can be caused by HIV drugs or other medical conditions such as diabetes. The older HIV drugs that caused the most peripheral neuropathy are not commonly used today.

Abdominal Pain

There are many possible causes of abdominal pain:

- A side effect of some HIV drugs (for example cramps)

- Infections caused by bacteria or parasites

- Problems of the intestinal tract such as irritable bowels

- Inflammation of the pancreas (pancreatitis) caused by some HIV drugs or by drinking alcohol

- Bladder or urinary tract infections (especially in women)

- Menstrual cramps or conditions of the uterus, cervix, or ovaries

Headache

Head pain can be mild to severe, and may be described as pressure, throbbing, or a dull ache. The most common causes of mild headaches include muscle tension, flu-like illness, and HIV drug side effects. Moderate or severe headaches can be caused by sinus pressure, tooth infections, brain infections, brain tumors, bleeding in the brain, migraines, or strokes. Sometimes the cause cannot be determined.

Joint, Muscle, and Bone Pain

This pain can also be mild to severe. It may be related to conditions such as arthritis, bone disease, injury, or just aging. It can also be a side effect of some HIV drugs and medications for other conditions like hepatitis or high cholesterol.

Herpes Pain

Herpes is a family of viruses common in HIV-positive people. Herpes viruses stay in the body for life, going into hiding and flaring up later. The varicella-zoster herpes virus first causes chickenpox and later can cause shingles, a painful rash along nerve pathways. Herpes simplex virus types 1 and 2 cause painful blisters around the mouth ("cold sores") or genital area. Even after a herpes sore heals, a person may still have persistent pain.

Other Types

- Painful skin rashes due to infections or HIV drug side effects

- Chest pain caused by lung infections such as tuberculosis (TB), bacterial pneumonia or *Pneumocystis carinii* pneumonia (PCP)

- Mouth pain caused by ulcers ("canker sores") or fungal infections like thrush

- Fibromyalgia or related chronic pain conditions

- Pain due to cancer anywhere in the body

Assessing Pain

Once the type of pain is identified, the next step is to evaluate its characteristics. The goals of pain assessment are to:

- **Define the severity of pain (how much it hurts):** Your healthcare provider may ask you to assign a number to your pain, from one (very mild pain) to ten (the worst possible pain). Pictures can also describe pain. A smiling face represents little or no pain, while a crying face represents severe pain.

- **Describe details of your pain:** Your healthcare provider may ask you to describe how your pain feels, for example sharp, dull, throbbing, or burning. Is it new (acute) or have you had it for a while (chronic)? Where is it located? Is it constant or does it come and go?

You may be having pain but do not want to complain. Talking about pain to your healthcare provider is not the same thing as complaining! Telling your healthcare provider exactly how you feel is the best thing you can do to find out what is wrong and get the right treatment.

Pain Management

Once the type and characteristics of pain are identified, you and your healthcare provider will decide how to manage or treat it. The following factors will play a role in selecting the right type of treatment for you:

- Cause, type, and severity of pain

- Whether it is short-term or long-term

- History of substance abuse

If your pain is being caused by a medication you are taking or another illness, your healthcare provider will want to take care of that first. If you are still experiencing pain, there are many options for pain relief.

Non-Medicinal Therapies

Pain relief without medications such as:

- Massage
- Relaxation techniques
- Physical therapy
- Acupuncture
- Heat and cold therapy
- Hypnosis
- Mental imagery or visualization

While these may be enough to relieve pain, they are often used along with pain medications.

Non-Opioid Medications

Pain relief medicines that do not contain narcotics (opiates). They are available over the counter or by prescription. These medicines relieve mild to moderate pain related to inflammation or swelling. Some people with a history of drug addiction prefer non-opioid pain medicines such as:

- Tylenol® (acetaminophen).
- Non-steroidal anti-inflammatory drugs (NSAIDs) such as aspirin or ibuprofen (for example, Advil®).
- Cyclooxygenase-2 (COX-2) inhibitors, a type of NSAID that is less likely to cause stomach problems, for example Celebrex® (celecoxib).
- Steroids, natural or manufactured hormones that reduce inflammation. Examples include prednisone and hydrocortisone.

Non-opioid pain medicines can cause side effects including liver damage (Tylenol), easy bleeding (aspirin), stomach pain or damage (aspirin and other NSAIDs), and heart problems (COX-2 inhibitors).

Opioids/Narcotics

Narcotics and related drugs known as opioids are the strongest pain relievers, available only by prescription. They are used to treat moderate to severe pain.

Opioids are classified by how fast and how long they work:

- **Immediate-release opioids:** Act rapidly but pain relief lasts for a shorter period of time

- **Sustained-released opioids:** Take longer to start working but pain relief lasts longer

Opioids are also classified by their strength:

- Mild to moderate pain relievers (they are often mixed with non-opioid medicines to improve their action):
  - Hydrocodone
  - Vicodin® (hydrocodone plus acetaminophen)
  - Codeine
  - Tylenol with codeine (acetaminophen plus codeine)
  - Ultram® (tramadol)
- Severe pain relievers:
  - Morphine
  - Fentanyl
  - OxyContin® (oxycodone)
  - Methadone or buprenorphine (not commonly prescribed in first-line pain reliever treatment)

Opioids can cause side effects including drowsiness, nausea, and constipation. Overdoses can slow down breathing and cause death. Opiates can lead to dependence or addiction and may be a problem for people with a history of substance use.

Topical or Local Therapies

These are medications that are injected or applied to the skin around a painful area. Examples include the local anesthetic Xylocaine® (lidocaine) and capsaicin, which comes from chili peppers.

Other Therapies

There are medicines prescribed for other purposes that also have pain-relieving properties:

- **Anti-depressants:** Relieve neuropathic pain such as peripheral neuropathy. An example is Cymbalta® (duloxetine).

- **Anti-convulsants:** Usually used to treat seizures, some of these drugs work for peripheral neuropathy. An example is Neurontin® (gabapentin).

Determine If the Pain Treatment Works

Once you start medication or other pain treatment, your healthcare provider should assess your pain regularly to see if treatment is working. Sometimes pain medications can stop working over time.

What to Do If You Have Pain

When you experience pain, it is important to know how to get fast, safe relief.

Do not ignore your pain. Pain is the body's way of telling us something is wrong. Ignoring pain often makes matters worse and can cause more damage in the long run.

Assess your pain. When pain occurs ask yourself the following questions:

- How long have I had the pain?

- Did it happen suddenly or over time?

- Is the pain sharp or dull?

- What makes the pain worse?

- Does anything ease the pain?

- Is the pain limited to one place or does it spread out to other areas?

- Are there other symptoms (for example numbness, cough, or fever)?

Notify your healthcare provider. Report pain to your provider without delay. Describing your pain will help find the cause and how best to treat it.

Take your pain medicine as directed. If you need pain medications, make sure you take them exactly as prescribed. Pain medications work best if they are taken at the first sign of pain. Breaking the cycle of pain means taking medications before your pain is at its worst.

Be responsible. Pain medications are very effective when taken as prescribed. Taking them incorrectly can be dangerous. Opioids are addictive, meaning you can develop physical and emotional dependence on a drug. High doses can cause breathing problems. In the worst cases, incorrect use of opioids can be fatal.

Tell your healthcare provider if treatment does not work. If your pain medicine is not relieving your pain, talk to your providers. You may be taking a medication that will not work for you, or you may have built a tolerance to the drugs over time. You may need to change doses or switch to a new medication.

Pain is common among HIV-positive people. But it can be managed using a variety of methods. Talk to your healthcare provider if you are having pain. He or she can work with you to find the cause, manage the pain, and improve your quality of life.

Section 39.4

Wasting Syndrome

"Wasting Syndrome," Fact Sheet #519, © 2010 AIDS InfoNet. Reprinted with permission. InfoNet fact sheets are updated frequently. Please visit the website at http://www.aidsinfonet.org for the newest version.

What Is AIDS Wasting?

Acquired immunodeficiency syndrome (AIDS) wasting is the involuntary loss of more than 10 percent of body weight, plus more than thirty days of either diarrhea or weakness and fever. Wasting is linked to disease progression and death. Losing just 5 percent of body weight can have the same negative effects. Wasting is still a problem for people with AIDS, even people whose human immunodeficiency virus (HIV) is controlled by medications.

Part of the weight lost during wasting is fat. More important is the loss of muscle mass. This is also called "lean body mass," or "body cell mass." Lean body mass can be measured by bioelectrical impedance analysis (BIA) or by a full body x-ray (dual energy x-ray absorptiometry; DEXA) scan. These are simple, painless office procedures.

AIDS wasting and lipodystrophy can both cause some body shape changes. Wasting is the loss of muscle. Lipodystrophy can cause a loss of fat under the skin. Wasting is not the same as fat loss caused by lipodystrophy. However, wasting in women can start with a loss of fat.

What Causes AIDS Wasting?

Several factors contribute to AIDS wasting.

Low food intake. Low appetite is common with HIV. Also, some AIDS drugs have to be taken with an empty stomach, or with a meal. It can be difficult for some people with AIDS to eat when they're hungry. Drug side effects such as nausea, changes in the sense of taste, or tingling around the mouth also decrease appetite. Opportunistic infections in the mouth or throat can make it painful to eat. Infections in the gut can make people feel full after eating just a little food. Finally, lack of money or energy may make it difficult to shop for food or prepare meals.

Poor nutrient absorption. Healthy people absorb nutrients through the small intestine. In HIV disease, several infections (including parasites) can interfere with this process. HIV may directly affect the intestinal lining and reduce nutrient absorption. Diarrhea causes loss of calories and nutrients.

Altered metabolism. Food processing and protein building are affected by HIV disease. Even before any symptoms show up, you need more energy. This might be caused by the increased activity of the immune system. People with HIV need more calories just to maintain their body weight.

Hormone levels can affect the metabolism. HIV seems to change some hormone levels. Also, cytokines play a role in wasting. Cytokines are proteins that produce inflammation to help the body fight infections. People with HIV have very high levels of cytokines. This makes the body produce more fats and sugars, but less protein.

Unfortunately, these factors can work together to create a "downward spiral." For example, infections may increase the body's energy requirements. At the same time, they can interfere with nutrient absorption and cause fatigue. This can reduce appetite and make people less able to shop for or cook their meals. They eat less, which accelerates the process.

How Is Wasting Treated?

There is no standard treatment for AIDS wasting. However, successful antiretroviral treatment usually leads to healthy weight gain. Treatments for wasting deal with each of the causes mentioned above.

Reducing nausea and vomiting helps increase food intake. Also, appetite stimulants including Megace® and Marinol® have been used.

Megace, unfortunately, is associated with increases in body fat. Marinol (dronabinol) is sometimes used to increase appetite. It is a synthetic form of a substance found in marijuana. Medications that fight nausea can also help. AIDS activists have long urged the legalization of marijuana. It reduces nausea and stimulates the appetite. In the late 1990s, several states legalized the medical use of marijuana.

Treating diarrhea and opportunistic infections in the intestines helps alleviate poor nutrient absorption. There has been a lot of progress in this area. However, two parasitic infections—cryptosporidiosis and microsporidiosis—are still extremely difficult to treat. Another approach is the use of nutritional supplements like Ensure® and Advera®. These have been specifically designed to provide easy-to-absorb nutrients. However, they have not been carefully studied and contain a lot of sugar. Nutritional supplements like Juven® or whey protein may also help increase weight. Consult with your healthcare provider before using nutritional supplements. Supplements should be used in addition to a balanced diet.

Treating changes in metabolism. Hormone treatments are being examined. Human growth hormone (Serostim®) increases weight and lean body mass, while decreasing fat mass. However, it is extremely expensive, can cause serious side effects, and can cost over $40,000 per year. Some nutritional experts believe it can be effective at doses lower than the U.S. Food and Drug Administration (FDA)–approved dose. Testosterone and anabolic (muscle building) agents like oxandrolone or nandrolone might also help treat wasting. They have been studied alone and in combination with exercise.

Progressive resistance training (PRT) is a form of exercise using small weights. A recent study found that PRT gave results like oxandrolone (an anabolic steroid) in increasing lean body mass. PRT was also more effective than oxandrolone in increasing physical functioning. It is also less expensive.

The Bottom Line

AIDS wasting is not well understood. However, it is clear that people with HIV disease need to avoid the loss of lean body mass. Various treatments for wasting are being studied.

Be sure to monitor your weight. Maintain your intake of nutritious foods even if your appetite is low. Get treatment right away for serious diarrhea or any infection of your digestive system. These might cause problems with the absorption of nutrients.

Part Six

Living with HIV Infection

Chapter 40

Coping with an HIV/AIDS Diagnosis

Chapter Contents

Section 40.1

How to Cope: Things to Keep in Mind

Excerpted from "Mental Health,"
U.S. Department of Veterans Affairs, December 2009.

Many people are surprised when they learn that they have been diagnosed with HIV. Some people feel overwhelmed by the changes that they will need to make in their lives. It is normal to have strong reactions when you find out you are HIV-positive, including feelings such as fear, anger, and a sense of being overwhelmed. Often people feel helpless, sad, and anxious about the illness.

Some things to keep in mind about your feelings:

- No matter what you are feeling, you have a right to feel that way.

- There are no "wrong" or "right" feelings—feelings just are.

- Feelings come and go.

- You have choices about how you respond to your feelings.

There are many things you can do to deal with the emotional aspects of having HIV/AIDS. What follows are some of the most common feelings associated with a diagnosis of HIV/AIDS and suggestions on how to cope with these feelings. You may experience some, all, or none of these feelings, and you may experience them at different times.

Denial

People who find out that they are HIV-positive often deal with the news by denying that it is true. You may believe that the HIV test came out wrong or that there was a mix-up of test results. This is a natural and normal first reaction.

At first, this denial may even be helpful, because it can give you time to get used to the idea of infection. However, if not dealt with, denial can be dangerous—you may fail to take certain precautions or reach out for the necessary help and medical support.

It is important that you talk out your feelings with your health care provider or someone you trust. It is important to do this so that you can begin to receive the care and support you need.

Anger

Anger is another common and natural feeling related to being diagnosed with HIV. Many people are upset about how they got the virus or angry that they didn't know they had the virus.

Ways to deal with feelings of anger include the following:

- Talk about your feelings with others, such as people in a support group, or with a counselor, friend, or social worker.

- Try to get some exercise—like gardening, walking, or dancing— to relieve some of the tension and angry feelings you may be experiencing.

- Avoid situations—involving certain people, places, and events— that cause you to feel angry or stressed out.

Sadness or Depression

It is also normal to feel sad when you learn you have HIV/AIDS. If, over time, you find that the sadness doesn't go away or is getting worse, talk with your doctor or someone else you trust. You may be depressed.

Finding the right treatment for depression takes time—so does recovery. If you think you may be depressed, don't lose hope. Instead, talk to your healthcare provider and seek help for depression.

Fear and Anxiety

Fear and anxiety may be caused by not knowing what to expect now that you've been diagnosed with HIV, or not knowing how others will treat you after they find out you have HIV. You also may be afraid of telling people—friends, family members, and others—that you are HIV-positive.

Ways to control your feelings of fear and anxiety include the following:

- Learn as much as you can about HIV/AIDS.

- Get your questions answered by your healthcare provider.

- Talk with your friends, family members, and healthcare providers.

- Join a support group.

- Help others who are in the same situation, such as by volunteering at an HIV/AIDS service organization. This may empower you and lessen your feelings of fear.

- Talk to your doctor about medicines for anxiety if the feelings don't lessen with time or if they get worse.

Section 40.2

Things You Can Do to Enhance Your Emotional Well-Being

Excerpted from "Mental Health,"
U.S. Department of Veterans Affairs, December 2009.

It is completely normal to have an emotional reaction upon learning that you have human immunodeficiency virus (HIV), such as anxiety, anger, or depression. These feelings do not last forever. There are many things that you can do to help take care of your emotional needs. Here are just a few ideas:

- Talk about your feelings with your doctor, friends, family members, or other supportive people.

- Try to find activities that relieve your stress, such as exercise or hobbies.

- Try to get enough sleep each night to help you feel rested.

- Learn relaxation methods like meditation, yoga, or deep breathing.

- Limit the amount of caffeine and nicotine you use.

- Eat small, healthy meals throughout the day.

- Join a support group.

There are many kinds of support groups that provide a place where you can talk about your feelings, help others, and get the latest information about HIV and acquired immunodeficiency syndrome (AIDS). Check with your healthcare provider for a listing of local support groups.

More specific ways to care for your emotional well being include various forms of therapy and medication. Used by themselves or in combination, these may be helpful in dealing with the feelings you are experiencing. Therapy can help you better express your feelings and find ways to cope with your emotions. Medicines that may be able to help with anxiety and depression are also available.

The most important thing to remember is that you are not alone; there are support systems in place to help you, including doctors, psychiatrists, family members, friends, support groups, and other services.

Section 40.3

Connecting with Others

You're not alone. It's one of the most important things to keep in mind as you adjust to the fact that you're living with human immunodeficiency virus (HIV). And thanks to the internet, it's more true today than it's ever been.

Nobody should face an HIV diagnosis all by themselves. So, whatever your reservations, make sure you connect with a community of HIV-positive people. It's a key step toward solving both the emotional and practical problems of living with HIV.

Finding Support in Person

In the United States, every state has a number of local HIV/AIDS organizations. An HIV/AIDS organization can be a true lifeline in many ways. Most organizations offer most, if not all, of these critical services:

- Support groups, in which you regularly meet and talk with other HIVers in the area (some organizations even offer specific

support groups for drug users, gay men, women, recently diagnosed people, and so on)

- Counseling for mental health issues or substance abuse

- Case managers, who can help coordinate the mental and physical care you need, and get you connected with government assistance (such as Medicaid, disability insurance, and help paying
for medications)

- Classes or workshops on topics such as learning more about HIV,
taking your HIV meds properly, nutrition, fitness, and other important issues

- HIV prevention counseling, including free condoms and discussions about how to protect yourself from other sexually transmitted diseases while also ensuring you don't pass HIV to others

Go on a retreat! Connecting with other HIV-positive people can be
a challenge, especially if you live in remote areas or work full time.
One little known option is to go on an HIV retreat. There are an as-
sortment of retreats across the country where you can meet and get
to know other positive people. Some are even free or low cost, others
have scholarships. They range from carefree holidays to educational
weekends. There are retreats beach side, in the mountains, and in the
middle of the biggest U.S. cities. These retreats are geared for the newly
positive as well as people who have long ago processed their diagnosis
and are just looking for a chance to unwind.

Finding Support Online

There are many ways for you to connect with others on the internet
to get the support you need, including the following:

- Bulletin boards

- Ask the experts

- Personal stories

Chapter 41

Staying Healthy with Diet and Exercise When You Have HIV/AIDS

Chapter Contents

Section 41.1

HIV and Nutrition

"Diet and Nutrition," U.S.
Department of Veterans Affairs, December 10, 2009.

Why Is Nutrition Important?

Nutrition is important for everyone because food gives our bodies the nutrients they need to stay healthy, grow, and work properly. Foods are made up of six classes of nutrients, each with its own special role in the body:

- Protein builds muscles and a strong immune system.

- Carbohydrates (including starches and sugars) give you energy.

- Fat gives you extra energy.

- Vitamins regulate body processes.

- Minerals regulate body processes and also make up body tissues.

- Water gives cells shape and acts as a medium where body processes can occur.

Having good nutrition means eating the right types of foods in the right amounts so you get these important nutrients.

Do I Need a Special Diet?

There are no special diets, or particular foods, that will boost your immune system. But there are things you can do to keep your immunity up.

When you are infected with human immunodeficiency virus (HIV), your immune system has to work very hard to fight off infections—and this takes energy (measured in calories). This means you may need to eat more food than you used to.

If you are underweight—or you have advanced HIV disease, high viral loads, or opportunistic infections—you should include more protein as well as extra calories (in the form of carbohydrates and fats). You'll find tips for doing this below.

If you are overweight, you should follow a well-balanced meal plan such as the U.S. government's Food Pyramid guide. Keep in mind, you may need to eat more food to meet your extra needs.

How Do I Keep from Losing Weight?

Weight loss is a common problem for people infected with HIV, and it should be taken very seriously. Losing weight can be dangerous because it makes it harder for your body to fight infections and to get well after you're sick.

People with HIV often do not eat enough for the following reasons:

- HIV and HIV medicines may reduce your appetite, make food taste bad, and prevent the body from absorbing food in the right way.

- Symptoms like a sore mouth, nausea, and vomiting make it difficult to eat.

- Fatigue from HIV or the medicines may make it hard to prepare food and eat regularly.

To keep your weight up, you will need to take in more protein and calories. What follows are ways to do that.

Adding Protein to Your Diet

Protein-rich foods include meats, fish, beans, dairy products, and nuts. To boost the protein in your meals try the following things:

- Spread nut butter on toast, crackers, fruit, or vegetables.

- Add cottage cheese to fruit and tomatoes.

- Add canned tuna to casseroles and salads.

- Add shredded cheese to sauces, soups, omelets, baked potatoes, and steamed vegetables.

- Eat yogurt on your cereal or fruit.

- Eat hard-boiled (hard-cooked) eggs. Use them in egg-salad sandwiches or slice and dice them for tossed salads.

- Add diced or chopped meats to soups, salads, and sauces.

- Add dried milk powder or egg white powder to foods (like scrambled eggs, casseroles, and milkshakes).

Adding Calories to Your Diet

The best way to increase calories is to add carbohydrates and some extra fat to your meals.

Carbohydrates include both starches and simple sugars.

Starches are in the following foods:

- Breads, muffins, biscuits, crackers

- Oatmeal and cold cereals

- Pasta

- Potatoes

- Rice

Simple sugars are in the following foods:

- Fresh or dried fruit (raisins, dates, apricots, etc.)

- Jelly, honey, and maple syrup added to cereal, pancakes, and waffles

Fats are more concentrated sources of calories. Add moderate amounts of the following to your meals:

- Butter, margarine, sour cream, cream cheese, peanut butter

- Gravy, sour cream, cream cheese, grated cheese

- Avocados, olives, salad dressing

How Can I Maintain My Appetite?

When you become ill, you often lose your appetite. This can lead to weight loss, which can make it harder for your body to fight infection.

Here are some tips for increasing your appetite:

- Try a little exercise, like walking or doing yoga. This can often stimulate your appetite and make you feel like eating more.

- Eat smaller meals more often. For instance, try to snack between meals.

- Eat whenever your appetite is good.

- Don't drink too much right before or during meals. This can make you feel full.

- Avoid carbonated (fizzy) drinks and foods such as cabbage, broccoli, and beans. These foods and drinks can create gas in your stomach and make you feel full and bloated.

- Eat with your family or friends.

- Choose your favorite foods, and make meals as attractive to you as possible. Try to eat in a pleasant location.

How Much Water Do I Need?

Drinking enough liquids is very important when you have HIV. Fluids transport the nutrients you need through your body.

Extra water can do the following things:

- Reduce the side effects of medications

- Help flush out the medicines that have already been used by your body

- Help you avoid dehydration (fluid loss), dry mouth, and constipation

- Make you feel less tired

Many of us don't drink enough water every day. You should be getting at least eight to ten glasses of water (or other fluids, such as juices or soups) a day.

Here are some tips on getting the extra fluids you need:

- Drink more water than usual. Try other fluids, too, like Gatorade or Sprite.

- Avoid colas, coffee, tea, and cocoa. These may contain caffeine and can actually dehydrate you. Read the labels on drinks to see if they have caffeine in them.

- Avoid alcohol.

- Begin and end each day by drinking a glass of water.

- Suck on ice cubes and popsicles.

Note: If you have diarrhea or are vomiting, you will lose a lot of fluids and will need to drink more than usual.

Do I Need Supplements?

Our bodies need vitamins and minerals, in small amounts, to keep our cells working properly. They are essential to our staying healthy. People with HIV need extra vitamins and minerals to help repair and heal cells that have been damaged.

Even though vitamins and minerals are present in many foods, your healthcare provider may recommend a vitamin and mineral supplement (a pill or other form of concentrated vitamins and minerals). While vitamin and mineral supplements can be useful, they can in no way replace eating a healthy diet.

If you are taking a supplement, here are some things to remember:

- Always take vitamin pills on a full stomach. Take them regularly.

- Some vitamins and minerals, if taken in high doses, can be harmful. Talk with your healthcare provider before taking high doses of any supplement.

What Should I Know about Food Safety?

Paying attention to food and water safety is important when you have HIV, because your immune system is already weakened and working hard to fight off infections.

If food is not handled or prepared in a safe way, germs from the food can be passed on to you. These germs can make you sick.

You need to handle and cook food properly to keep those germs from getting to you.

Here are some food safety guidelines:

- Keep everything clean! Clean your counters and utensils often.

- Wash your hands with soap and warm water before and after preparing and eating food.

- Check expiration dates on food packaging. Do not eat foods that have a past expiration date.

- Rinse all fresh fruits and vegetables with clean water.

- Thaw frozen meats and other frozen foods in the refrigerator or in a microwave. Never thaw foods at room temperature. Germs that grow at room temperature can make you very sick.

- Clean all cutting boards and knives (especially those that touch chicken and meat) with soap and hot water before using them again.

- Make sure you cook all meat, fish, and poultry "well-done." You might want to buy a meat thermometer to help you know for sure that it is done. Put the thermometer in the thickest part of the meat and not touching a bone. Cook the meat until it reaches 165 to 212 degrees Fahrenheit on your thermometer.

- Do not eat raw, soft-boiled, or "over easy" eggs, or Caesar salads with raw egg in the dressing.

- Do not eat sushi, raw seafood, or raw meats, or unpasteurized milk or dairy products.

- Keep your refrigerator cold, set no higher than 40 degrees. Your freezer should be at 0 degrees.

- Refrigerate leftovers at temperatures below 40 degrees F. Do not eat leftovers that have been sitting in the refrigerator for more than three days.

- Keep hot items heated to over 140 degrees F, and completely re-heat leftovers before eating.

- Throw away any foods (like fruit, vegetables, and cheese) that you think might be old. If food has a moldy or rotten spot, throw it out. When in doubt, throw it out.

- Some germs are spread through tap water. If your public water supply isn't totally pure, drink bottled water.

Can Diet Help Ease Side Effects and Symptoms?

Many symptoms of HIV, as well as the side effects caused by HIV medicines, can be helped by using (or avoiding) certain types of foods and drinks.

Below are some tips for dealing with common problems people with HIV face.

Nausea

- Try the BRATT diet (bananas, rice, applesauce, tea, and toast).

- Try some ginger—in tea, ginger ale, or ginger snaps.

- Don't drink liquids at the same time you eat your meals.

- Eat something small, like crackers, before getting out of bed.

- Keep something in your stomach; eat a small snack every one to two hours.

Avoid foods like the following:

- Fatty, greasy, or fried foods
- Very sweet foods (candy, cookies, or cake)

- Spicy foods
- Foods with strong odors

Mouth and Swallowing Problems

- Avoid hard or crunchy foods such as raw vegetables.
- Try eating cooked vegetables and soft fruits (like bananas and pears).
- Avoid very hot foods and beverages. Cold and room-temperature foods will be more comfortable to your mouth.
- Do not eat spicy foods. They can sting your mouth.
- Try soft foods like mashed potatoes, yogurt, and oatmeal.
- Also try scrambled eggs, cottage cheese, macaroni and cheese, and canned fruits.
- Rinse your mouth with water. This can moisten your mouth, remove bits of food, and make food taste better to you.
- Stay away from oranges, grapefruit, and tomatoes. They have a lot of acid and can sting your mouth.

Diarrhea

- Try the BRATT diet (bananas, rice, applesauce, tea, and toast).
- Keep your body's fluids up (hydrated) with water, Gatorade, or other fluids (those that don't have caffeine).
- Limit sodas and other sugary drinks.
- Avoid greasy and spicy foods.
- Avoid milk and other dairy products.
- Eat small meals and snacks every hour or two.
- Try taking glutamine protein powder to help repair the intestinal lining.

Points to Remember

You may feel that many things are out of your control if you have HIV. But you can control what you eat and drink, and how much. Good nutrition is an important part of your plan to stay well.

Eating right can make your body and your immune system stronger.

When you are HIV-positive, you may need to eat more. Be sure to eat a diet that is high in proteins and calories.

Exercise can stimulate your appetite and make you feel like eating more.

Drink plenty of liquids to help your body deal with any medications you are taking.

If you are vomiting or have diarrhea, you will need to drink more than usual.

Practice food safety. Keep your kitchen clean, wash foods, and be careful about food preparation and storage. If your tap water isn't pure, drink bottled water.

You can use certain foods and beverages to help you deal with symptoms and side effects.

Before taking vitamin and mineral supplements, check with your healthcare provider.

Remember, there is no one "right" way to eat. Eating well means getting the right amount of nutrients for your particular needs. Your healthcare provider can refer you to a dietitian or nutritionist who can help design a good diet for you.

Section 41.2

HIV and Exercise

What Is Exercise?

Exercise is activity that you do on a regular basis (every day, or several times a week) for the purpose of improving your health. Keep in mind that if it's something you do every day as part of your job, it's probably not exercise. Exercise needs to be outside of your daily routine.

That doesn't mean that increasing your normal activities during the day can't be helpful. Some studies have shown that adding small amounts of activity throughout the day can improve your health. This might mean taking the stairs instead of the elevator, parking farther back in the parking lot, or walking to places less than a mile or two away.

Benefits of Exercise

Everyone knows that exercise can make you stronger, give you endurance, and strengthen your heart. But there are many benefits of exercise that are especially helpful for people living with human immunodeficiency virus (HIV). An exercise routine can:

- increase muscle mass;
- reduce fat around the waist (lipohypertrophy);
- lower total cholesterol and low-density lipoprotein (LDL; the bad cholesterol);
- raise high-density lipoprotein (HDL; the good cholesterol);
- lower triglycerides;
- help control blood sugars;
- strengthen bones (help prevent bone disease);
- strengthen your immune system;
- reduce stress;

- give you more energy throughout the day.

There is also a strong connection between muscle mass and immunity. By increasing the size of your muscles, you may be able to slow the progression of your HIV. People who exercise often have higher CD4 cell counts and fewer side effects from HIV and HIV drugs.

What Type of Exercise Is Right for You?

There are several different types of exercise, all of which are important to try to include in an exercise routine. Some types of exercise to consider are as follows.

Aerobic (or Cardiovascular) Exercise

Aerobic exercise uses oxygen to burn fat in your body. This is why people who are trying to lose weight often do a lot of aerobic exercise. It is also called cardiovascular exercise, because it raises your heart rate and makes your heart stronger. Besides burning fat, it can increase your endurance, meaning that you don't get tired as quickly when you use energy.

Aerobic exercises can also lower cholesterol and triglycerides, or lower blood sugars. (In some HIV-positive people, exercise may not lower cholesterol and triglycerides enough. If this is the case, speak to your healthcare provider about lipid-lowering drugs.)

Some HIV-positive people should not do aerobic exercise, such as those who are wasting or have very little body fat. Ask your healthcare provider if you have any conditions that might keep you from doing aerobic exercise.

Good aerobic exercises:

- fast walking;
- jogging;
- stair-climbing;
- bicycling;
- swimming.

Weight-Bearing Exercise

Weight-bearing exercise (also called resistance or strength training) is when you move weight with your muscles. When you do this, your muscles tear, but when they heal they are bigger and stronger. It is important that when you do weight-bearing exercise, you wait until that part of the body is not sore anymore before you exercise it again. Your body needs plenty of time to heal the muscles.

Weight-bearing exercise can be helpful for most HIV-positive people and can help prevent or fight wasting. If you have had muscle loss, weight-bearing exercise is probably good for you. However, if you have osteoporosis (bone disease) or if you have been hurt recently, weight-bearing exercise could be dangerous, and you may need a physical therapist. Ask your healthcare provider if weight-bearing exercise is okay for you.

Good weight-bearing exercises:

- lifting weights with machines;

- push-ups;

- pull-ups;

- squats or lunges;

- dumbbells.

Mind-Body Exercise

Mind-body exercise such as yoga can improve physical qualities such as strength, flexibility, balance, and endurance. It can also improve mental health and help with anxiety and depression (which is very common in HIV-positive women). As with all new exercise routines, it is important to start slowly with yoga and take beginner classes. Many community centers (i.e., YMCA) offer low-cost or free yoga classes.

Good mind-body exercise:

- yoga;

- martial arts;

- tai chi;

- meditation.

Tips for Starting a New Exercise Routine

Speak to your healthcare provider about what types of exercise are okay for you.

Record your weight and the measurements of your arms, legs, chest, stomach, and hips before starting your exercise program. If possible, also check your body composition with a bio-electrical impedance analysis (BIA). A BIA can be done by your healthcare provider or by a fitness trainer at the gym.

Set realistic goals for yourself, such as increasing or decreasing some of your body measurements.

Find an exercise buddy. Setting up an exercise routine with a friend can keep you motivated and less likely to skip workouts!

Start slowly. Do what you can, but don't overdo it. Be patient with your body and your workout.

When starting aerobic exercise, walk or jog at a pace where you can talk but are not out of breath. Try to work up to thirty minutes three times a week. You may start out walking/jogging for ten minutes and slowly add five minutes to your workout until you are up to thirty minutes or more at least three times a week.

When starting weight-bearing exercise, use slow, controlled movements. Dropping the weights quickly can be dangerous and will not help build muscle. Try to work up to weight-bearing exercise at least three times a week for thirty minutes or more.

Stay hydrated! Remember to drink a lot of water before, during, and after your workout.

Eat well! Good nutrition is important to staying healthy and can help you exercise better. Wait two hours after a full meal before exercising.

Don't exercise when you're feeling sick (feverish, vomiting, dizzy, diarrhea, etc.)

Starting an exercise routine requires commitment. It may take a while for you to get used to your routine, but don't give up! If you are able, try hiring or talking to a certified fitness trainer to help you develop a good routine. Keep your healthcare provider informed about all forms of exercise you are doing.

Chapter 42

Avoiding Infections When You Have HIV/AIDS

Chapter Contents

Section 42.1

Preventing Infection from Pets

Reprinted from Centers for Disease Control and Prevention, June 21, 2007.

- You do not have to give up your pet.
- Although the risks are low, you can get an infection from pets or other animals.
- Several simple precautions are all you need to take with pets or other animals.
- Human immunodeficiency virus (HIV) cannot be spread by, or to, cats, dogs, birds, or other pets.

Should I keep my pets?

Yes. Most people with human immunodeficiency virus (HIV) can and should keep their pets. Owning a pet can be rewarding. Pets can help you feel psychologically and even physically better. For many people, pets are more than just animals—they are like members of the family. However, you should know the health risks of owning a pet or caring for animals. Animals may carry infections that can be harmful to you. Your decision to own or care for pets should be based on knowing what you need to do to protect yourself from these infections.

What kinds of infections could I get from an animal?

Animals can have cryptosporidiosis ("crypto"), toxoplasmosis ("toxo"), *Mycobacterium avium* complex ("MAC"), and other diseases. These diseases can give you problems like severe diarrhea, brain infections, and skin lesions.

What can I do to protect myself from infections spread by animals?

Always wash your hands well with soap and water after playing with or caring for animals. This is especially important before eating or handling food.

Be careful about what your pet eats and drinks. Feed your pet only pet food or cook all meat thoroughly before giving it to your pet. Don't give your pet raw or undercooked meat. Don't let your pets drink from toilet bowls or get into garbage. Don't let your pets hunt or eat another animal's stool (droppings).

Don't handle animals that have diarrhea. If the pet's diarrhea lasts for more than one or two days, have a friend or relative who does not have HIV take your pet to your veterinarian. Ask the veterinarian to check the pet for infections that may be the cause of diarrhea.

Don't bring home an unhealthy pet. Don't get a pet that is younger than six months old—especially if it has diarrhea. If you are getting a pet from a pet store, animal breeder, or animal shelter (pound), check the sanitary conditions and license of these sources. If you are not sure about the animal's health, have it checked out by your veterinarian.

Don't touch stray animals because you could get scratched or bitten. Stray animals can carry many infections.

Don't ever touch the stool of any animal.

Ask someone who is not infected with HIV and is not pregnant to change your cat's litter box daily. If you must clean the box yourself, wear vinyl or household cleaning gloves and immediately wash your hands well with soap and water right after changing the litter.

Have your cat's nails clipped so it can't scratch you. Discuss other ways to prevent scratching with your veterinarian. If you do get scratched or bitten, immediately wash the wounds well with soap and water. If you are bitten, you may need to seek medical advice.

Don't let your pet lick your mouth or any open cuts or wounds you may have.

Don't kiss your pet.

Keep fleas off your pet.

Avoid reptiles such as snakes, lizards, and turtles. If you touch any reptile, immediately wash your hands well with soap and water.

Wear vinyl or household cleaning gloves when you clean aquariums or animal cages and wash your hands well right after you finish.

Avoid exotic pets such as monkeys and ferrets, or wild animals such as raccoons, lions, bats, and skunks.

I have a job that involves working with animals. Should I quit?

Jobs working with animals (such as jobs in pet stores, animal clinics, farms, and slaughterhouses) carry a risk for infections. Talk with your doctor about whether you should work with animals. People who work with animals should take these extra precautions:

- Follow your worksite's rules to stay safe and reduce any risk of infection. Use or wear personal protective gear, such as coveralls, boots, and gloves.

- Don't clean chicken coops or dig in areas where birds roost if histoplasmosis is found in the area.

- Don't touch young farm animals, especially if they have diarrhea.

Can someone with HIV give it to their pets?

No. HIV cannot be spread to, from, or by cats, dogs, birds, or other pets. Many viruses cause diseases that are like acquired immunodeficiency syndrome (AIDS), such as feline leukemia virus, or FeLV, in cats. These viruses cause illness only in a certain animal and cannot infect other animals or humans. For example, FeLV infects only cats. It does not infect humans or dogs.

Are there any tests a pet should have before I bring it home?

A pet should be in overall good health. You don't need special tests unless the animal has diarrhea or looks sick. If your pet looks sick, your veterinarian can help you choose the tests it needs.

What should I do when I visit friends or relatives who have animals?

When you visit anyone with pets, take the same precautions you would in your own home. Don't touch animals that may not be healthy. You may want to tell your friends and family about the need for these precautions before you plan any visits.

Should children with HIV handle pets?

The same precautions apply for children as for adults. However, children may want to snuggle more with their pets. Some pets, like cats, may bite or scratch to get away from children. Adults should be extra watchful and supervise an HIV-infected child's hand washing to prevent infections.

Section 42.2

Safe Food and Water

Reprinted from Centers for Disease
Control and Prevention, June 21, 2007.

- You can protect yourself from many infections by preparing food and drinks properly.

- Meat, poultry (such as chicken or turkey), and fish can make you sick if they are raw, undercooked, or spoiled.

- Raw fruits and vegetables are safe to eat if you wash them carefully first.

- Don't drink water straight from lakes, rivers, streams, or springs.

Why should I be careful about food and water?

Food and water can carry germs that cause illness. Germs in food or water may cause serious infections in people with human immuno-deficiency virus (HIV).

You can protect yourself from many infections by preparing food and drinks properly.

What illnesses caused by germs in food and water do people with HIV commonly get?

Germs in food and water that can make someone with HIV ill include *Salmonella*, *Campylobacter*, *Listeria*, and *Cryptosporidium*. They can cause diarrhea, upset stomach, vomiting, stomach cramps, fever, headache, muscle pain, bloodstream infection, meningitis, or encephalitis.

Do only people with HIV get these illnesses?

No, they can occur in anyone. However, these illnesses are much more common in people with HIV.

Are these illnesses the same in people with HIV as in other people?

No. The diarrhea and nausea are often much worse and more difficult to treat in people with HIV. These illnesses are also more likely to cause serious problems in people with HIV, such as bloodstream infections and meningitis. People with HIV also have a harder time recovering fully from these illnesses.

If I have HIV, can I eat meat, poultry, and fish?

Yes. Meat, poultry (such as chicken or turkey), and fish can make you sick only if they are raw, undercooked, or spoiled.

To avoid illness, do the following:

- Cook all meat and poultry until they are no longer pink in the middle. If you use a meat thermometer, the temperature inside the meat or poultry should be over 165° F. Fish should be cooked until it is flaky, not rubbery.

- After handling raw meat, poultry, and fish, wash your hands well with soap and water before you touch any other food.

- Thoroughly wash cutting boards, cooking utensils, and countertops with soap and hot water after they have had contact with raw meat, poultry, or fish.

- Do not let uncooked meat, poultry, or fish or their juices touch other food or each other.

- Do not let meat, poultry, or fish sit at room temperature for more than a few minutes. Keep them in the refrigerator until you are ready to cook them.

- Eat or drink only pasteurized milk or dairy products.

Can I eat eggs if I have HIV?

Yes. Eggs are safe to eat if they are well cooked. Cook eggs until the yolk and white are solid, not runny. Do not eat foods that may contain raw eggs, such as hollandaise sauce, cookie dough, homemade mayonnaise, and Caesar salad dressing. If you prepare these foods at home, use pasteurized eggs instead of eggs in the shell. You can find pasteurized eggs in the dairy case at your supermarket.

Can I eat raw fruits and vegetables?

Yes. Raw fruits and vegetables are safe to eat if you wash them carefully first. Wash, then peel fruit that you will eat raw. Eating raw alfalfa sprouts and tomatoes can cause illness, but washing them well can reduce your risk of illness.

How can I make my water safe?

Don't drink water straight from lakes, rivers, streams, or springs.

Because you cannot be sure if your tap water is safe, you may wish to avoid tap water, including water or ice from a refrigerator ice-maker, which is made with tap water. Always check with the local health department and water utility to see if they have issued any special notices for people with HIV about tap water.

You may also wish to boil or filter your water, or to drink bottled water. Processed carbonated (bubbly) drinks in cans or bottles should be safe, but drinks made at a fountain might not be because they are made with tap water. If you choose to boil or filter your water or to drink only bottled water, do this all the time, not just at home.

Boiling is the best way to kill germs in your water. Heat your water at a rolling boil for one minute. After the boiled water cools, put it in a clean bottle or pitcher with a lid and store it in the refrigerator. Use the water for drinking, cooking, or making ice. Water bottles and ice trays should be cleaned with soap and water before use. Don't touch the inside of them after cleaning. If you can, clean your water bottles and ice trays yourself.

What should I do when shopping for food?

Read food labels carefully. Be sure that all dairy products that you purchase have been pasteurized. Do not buy any food that contains raw or undercooked meat or eggs if it is meant to be eaten raw. Be sure that the "sell by" date has not passed.

Put packaged meat, poultry, or fish in separate plastic bags to prevent their juices from dripping onto other groceries or each other.

Check the package that the food comes in to make sure that it isn't damaged.

Do not buy food that has been displayed in unsafe or unclean conditions. Examples include meat that is allowed to sit without refrigeration or cooked shrimp that is displayed with raw shrimp.

After shopping, put all cold and frozen foods into your refrigerator or freezer as soon as you can. Do not leave food sitting in the car. Keeping cold or frozen food out of refrigeration for even a couple of hours can give germs a chance to grow.

Is it safe for me to eat in restaurants?

Yes. Like grocery stores, restaurants follow guidelines for cleanliness and good hygiene set by the health department. However, you should follow these general rules in restaurants:

- Order all food well done. If meat is served pink or bloody, send it back to the kitchen for more cooking. Fish should be flaky, not rubbery, when you cut it.

- Order fried eggs cooked on both sides. Avoid eggs that are "sunny-side up." Scrambled eggs should be cooked until they are not runny. Do not order foods that may contain raw eggs, such as Caesar salad or hollandaise sauce. If you aren't sure about the ingredients in a dish, ask your waiter before you order.

- Do not order any raw or lightly steamed fish or shellfish, such as oysters, clams, mussels, sushi, or sashimi. All fish should be cooked until done.

Should I take special measures with food and water in other countries?

Yes. Not all countries have high standards of food hygiene. You need to take special care abroad, particularly in developing countries. Follow these rules when in other countries:

- Do not eat uncooked fruits and vegetables unless you can peel them. Avoid salads.

- Eat cooked foods while they are still hot.

- Boil all water before drinking it. Use only ice made from boiled water. Drink only canned or bottled drinks or beverages made with boiled water.

- Steaming-hot foods, fruits you peel yourself, bottled and canned processed drinks, and hot coffee or tea should be safe.

- Talk with your healthcare provider about other advice on travel abroad.

Section 42.3

Staying Healthy while Traveling

"Preventing Infections During Travel" is reprinted from Centers for Disease Control and Prevention, June 21, 2007. "Travel Abroad" is excerpted from AIDS.gov, October 2010.

Preventing Infections During Travel

In the United States or abroad? For business or pleasure? When you travel, you risk coming into contact with germs you might not find at home. Many of these germs can make you very sick.

For people with special health needs, travel can be risky to their health. If you have human immunodeficiency virus (HIV)—the virus that causes acquired immunodeficiency syndrome (AIDS)—you should have all the facts. Travel, especially to developing countries, can increase your risk of getting opportunistic infections. (They are called "opportunistic" because a person may get the infection when their weakened immune system gives it the opportunity to develop.) The best thing you can do when you travel is to know the medical risks and to take steps to protect yourself.

Before You Travel

Talk to your doctor or an expert in travel medicine about health risks in the area you plan to visit. They can tell you how to keep yourself healthy when you travel to places where certain illnesses are a problem. They also can tell you about places that might not be safe for you to visit. Ask them if they know of doctors who treat people with HIV in the region you plan to visit.

Plan in advance for problems that might come up.

Traveler's diarrhea is a common problem. Carry a three- to seven-day supply of medicine (antibiotics) to treat it. A common drug for traveler's diarrhea is ciprofloxacin. If you are pregnant, your doctor may suggest you take TMP- SMX (trimethoprim-sulfamethoxazole) instead.

Insect-borne diseases are also a major problem in many areas. Take a good supply of an insect repellent that contains 30 percent or less "Deet" with you. Plan to sleep under a mosquito net, preferably one treated with permethrin, in places where there is malaria or dengue fever. Unless you need to go there, avoid areas where yellow fever is found.

Ask your doctor if you need to take medicine or get special vaccinations before you travel. He or she will know which vaccines are safe for you. Your doctor will also know the best ways to protect you from such things as malaria, typhoid fever, and hepatitis. Make sure all your routine vaccinations are up to date. This is very important for HIV-infected children who are traveling.

If you are leaving the United States, make sure you know if the countries you plan to visit have special health rules for visitors. These rules can include vaccinations that may not be safe for HIV-infected people to take. Your doctor or local health department can help you with this.

If you have medical insurance, check to see what it covers when you are away from home. Many insurance plans have limited benefits outside the United States. Very few plans cover the cost of flying you back to the United States if you become very sick. Make sure your paperwork is in order, and take along proof of insurance when you travel.

When You Travel

Food and water in developing countries may not be as clean as they are at home. These items might contain bacteria, viruses, or parasites that could make you sick.

Do not eat raw fruit and vegetables that you do not peel yourself, raw or undercooked seafood or meat, unpasteurized dairy products, or anything from a street vendor. Also, do not drink tap water, drinks made with tap water, or with ice made from tap water, or unpasteurized milk.

Food and drinks that are generally safe include steaming-hot foods, fruits that you peel yourself, bottled (especially carbonated) drinks, hot coffee or tea, beer, wine, and water that you bring to a rolling boil for one full minute. If you can't boil your water, you can filter and treat it with iodine or chlorine, but this will not work as well as boiling.

Tuberculosis, or "TB," is very common worldwide, and can be severe in people with HIV. Avoid hospitals and clinics where coughing TB patients are treated. When back in the United States, have your doctor test you for TB.

In many places, animals may roam more freely than they do in the area where you live. If you think animals have left droppings on beaches or other areas, always wear shoes and protective clothing and sit on a towel to avoid direct contact with the sand or soil.

Swimming can make you sick if you swallow water. You should never swim in water that might contain even very small amounts of sewage or animal waste. To make sure that you get the most fun from your trip, protect your health (and the health of others) just as you do at home.

Take all medications as prescribed by your doctor.

If your doctor has you on a special diet, stick with it.

Take the same precautions that you take at home to prevent giving HIV to others.

Travel Abroad

Restrictions on Traveling with HIV/AIDS

Some countries, including the United States, restrict visitors who are HIV-positive from entering their borders. (U.S. restrictions apply only to individuals who are not American citizens.) Before you travel internationally, you should check to see if the country or countries you plan to visit have those restrictions.

Before You Travel

Talk to your healthcare provider or an expert in travel medicine about health risks in the area you plan to visit—especially if it is in a developing country. There are places where it is simply not safe for people living with HIV/AIDS to travel. If possible, get the names of doctors who treat people with HIV in the region you plan to visit.

Infectious diseases are a big problem in certain parts of the world—and you may be especially vulnerable if you have HIV disease. Before you travel outside the United States, ask your healthcare provider if you should be immunized against certain diseases or take medications before you leave. You want to protect yourself from infectious diseases that are found in other areas of the world (including malaria, dengue, polio, and yellow fever), and lower your risk of opportunistic infections.

Staying Healthy While Traveling

Be aware that food and water in some countries may not be as clean and safe as they are in the United States. If you eat raw or undercooked food, or drink contaminated water, you could get sick from bacteria, viruses, or parasites.

Insurance Outside of the United States

U.S. health insurance is generally not accepted in other countries, nor do the Medicare and Medicaid programs provide coverage for hospital or medical costs outside the United States. If your health insurance policy does not cover you abroad, it is a good idea to consider purchasing a short-term policy that does.

Bringing Medications or Filling Prescriptions Abroad

Before traveling outside of the United States., the Department of State recommends that you get a letter from your doctor listing your prescription medications. Any medications being carried overseas should be left in their original containers and be clearly labeled. When checking your personal belongings for air travel, you should inform officials if you have needles or syringes in your luggage for your medication. In addition, you should carry one week's worth of medications in your carry-on baggage in case your luggage is lost.

You should check with the foreign embassy of the country or countries you plan to visit to make sure that your required medications are not considered to be illegal narcotics.

Section 42.4

Vaccinations

This section begins with "What Do I Need to Know about Immunizations," reprinted from AIDSinfo.gov, June 2009. It concludes with "If You Have HIV Infection, Which Vaccinations Do You Need?" © 2010 Immunization Action Coalition (www.immunize.org). Reprinted with permission.

What Do I Need to Know about Immunizations?

I Am HIV Positive. Why Do I Need Immunizations?

When you have HIV you are at increased risk for certain infections. Some of these infections can be prevented with vaccines.

I Am Not Sure Which Immunizations I Have Had. What Should I Do?

Your doctor can help you determine which immunizations you have had. There are several blood tests that may also help determine if you have already had an immunization or the disease itself:

- **Hepatitis A:** An antibody test will determine if you have had this immunization series or if you have had hepatitis A.

- **Hepatitis B:** An antibody test will help determine if you have received this immunization series and if it was effective or if you have had hepatitis B.

- **Measles:** If you were born before 1957 you will not need this immunization. An antibody test will help determine if you have received this immunization or if you have had measles.

- **Mumps:** If you were born before 1957 you will not need this immunization. An antibody test will help determine if you have received this immunization or if you have had the mumps.

- **Rubella:** If you were born before 1957 you will not need this immunization. An antibody test will help determine if you have received this immunization or if you have had rubella. If the test results are unclear and you are a woman of child-bearing age, you may need to have this immunization.

- **Measles, Mumps, Rubella (MMR):** If you were born before 1957 you will not need this immunization. If you weren't previously immunized, have a CD4 count higher than 200, and have no or only mild HIV symptoms, you will need at least one dose of MMR. If you have moderate or severe symptoms from HIV, you should not receive MMR due to the risk of severe complications.

- **Varicella:** If you were born before 1980 you will not need this immunization. If you have had chicken pox or shingles, have documentation of two doses of varicella vaccine, or have laboratory evidence of immunity you will not need this vaccine. If your CD4 count is below 200 you should not have this immunization.

Are There Side Effects from Immunizations?

Side effects may or may not occur:

- Swelling, redness, and soreness at the injection site are common with any injection.

- Moderate side effects such as fever, headache, and muscle aches may also occur.

- Severe side effects such as an allergic reaction are possible and usually occur immediately or within several hours after the injection.

- Certain immunizations, such as for pneumonia and influenza, may increase your viral load for several weeks.

- If any side effects persist or become severe, contact your doctor.

When Should I Get Immunized?

It is suggested that you begin getting the recommended immunizations as soon as possible after you are diagnosed with HIV.

Some immunizations are more effective if your CD4 count is higher than 200 cells/mm^3 when you receive them. Your doctor will decide when you should receive these immunizations.

For the influenza vaccine, it is best for your CD4 count to be greater than 100 cells/mm^3 and your viral load to be less than 30,000 copies/ mL

Do Any of the Immunizations Need to Be Given Again?

Some immunizations may need to be repeated:

- After receiving the hepatitis B series, an antibody test may indicate that you have not developed antibodies in response to the immunization. You should then receive additional doses to be sure the immunization will be effective.

- Influenza immunization should be repeated in the fall of every year when the vaccine becomes available.

- Pneumococcal immunization is recommended to be repeated one time after five years, or if your CD4 count was lower than 200 cells/mm^3 when you received the first dose.

- Tetanus and diphtheria (Td) immunization should be repeated every ten years. Tetanus, diphtheria, and pertussis (TDap) immunization should replace your next Td booster. Once you have received one Tdap immunization, you will only need to receive the Td booster in the future because there is no need for repeated pertussis immunization.

- Meningococcal immunization is recommended to be repeated after five years if you remain at risk for infection. You are considered at risk for infection if you are a college student, military recruit, do not have a spleen, or travel to certain parts of the world.

Are There Any Other Immunizations I Should Have?

If you travel outside of the United States, you may need additional immunizations for some countries.

Certain people, such as military personnel and healthcare workers, are advised to have specific immunizations.

Talk with your doctor to determine whether you need other immunizations.

Are There Any Immunizations I Should Not Have?

HIV-positive people should usually avoid getting immunized with live vaccines because their immune systems may have been weakened by HIV. A weakened immune system might not be strong enough to fight off the viral/bacterial infection that may result from a live vaccine. MMR and varicella immunizations are an exception to this recommendation.

If You Have HIV Infection, Which Vaccinations Do You Need?

The following information shows which vaccinations you should have to protect your health. Make sure you and your healthcare provider keep your vaccinations up to date.

Influenza

Yes! You should get vaccinated against influenza each fall (or winter).

Pneumococcal

Yes! This vaccine is specifically recommended for you because of your HIV infection. If you haven't been vaccinated, you should get one dose now. If you were vaccinated when you were younger than age sixty-five and you are sixty-five years or older now, you should get another dose now, provided at least five years have passed since your first dose.

Tetanus, Diphtheria, Pertussis (Td, Tdap)

Yes! If you haven't had at least three doses of tetanus-and-diphtheria-containing shots sometime in your life, you need to start or complete a three-dose series now. Start with dose #1, followed by dose #2 in one month, and dose #3 in six months. You'll also need a Td booster dose every ten years. If you're younger than sixty-five years, your next booster dose should also contain pertussis (whooping cough) vaccine—known as Tdap. Be sure to consult your healthcare provider any time you get a deep or dirty wound.

Hepatitis A (Hep A)

Maybe. You may be at higher risk for hepatitis A virus infection if you meet certain criteria (e.g., plan to travel outside the United States [except for Canada, Japan, Australia, New Zealand, and Western Europe], are a man who has sex with men, are an injecting drug user). If you have any of the risk factors listed above or, if you simply want the assurance of being protected against hepatitis A, you'll need two doses of this vaccine, spaced six to eighteen months apart. Discuss your need for a screening blood test with your healthcare provider.

Hepatitis B (Hep B)

Yes. Because you are HIV-positive, you are at higher risk for hepatitis B virus infection. If you haven't had a series of hepatitis B vaccinations, you need three doses of this vaccine. Start with dose #1 now, followed by dose #2 in one month, and dose #3 approximately five months later. If you started the three-dose series earlier but didn't complete it, you can simply continue from where you left off. Discuss your need for screening blood tests with your healthcare provider.

Human Papillomavirus (HPV)

Yes (for some)! If you are a young woman age twenty-six years or younger, you should get HPV vaccine to prevent cervical cancer and genital warts. One brand, Gardasil®, can be given to men age twenty-six years or younger to prevent genital warts. The vaccine is given in three doses over six months.

Measles, Mumps, Rubella (MMR)

Maybe. Most adults are already protected because they got MMR vaccine as children or had measles, mumps, and rubella. If you weren't previously protected, were born in 1957 or later, and have no HIV symptoms or only mild symptoms, you need at least one dose of MMR. If you have moderate or severe symptoms from HIV, you should not receive MMR. If you are exposed to measles, call your healthcare provider right away. If you get measles, you are at risk of developing severe complications because of your HIV infection.

Meningococcal

Maybe. Because of your HIV infection, you may be at increased risk for meningococcal disease, a rare but sometimes fatal bacterial infection. Talk to your healthcare provider about getting vaccinated against this disease.

Varicella

Maybe. Most adults are already protected because they had chickenpox as children. However, if you are an adult born in the United States in 1980 or later, have no HIV symptoms or only mild symptoms, and have never had chickenpox or the vaccine, you can be vaccinated with this two-dose series. Talk to your healthcare provider.

Zoster (Shingles)

Maybe. This vaccine is recommended for adults ages sixty years and older to prevent shingles. If you have any symptoms of HIV, you should not be vaccinated. Talk to your healthcare provider.

Chapter 43

Life Issues When You Have HIV/AIDS

Chapter Contents

Section 43.1

Dating and HIV

© 2010 The Well Project (www.thewellproject.org).
Reprinted with permission.

Meeting Someone

Dating can be tricky for anyone, but if you're human immunodeficiency virus (HIV)–positive, you have some extra things to think about. Two important things to consider are:

- Who do I date (positive or negative person)?

- When do I tell?

If you are looking for a positive partner, consider going to places (online and in person) where you will meet other HIV-positive people. These include HIV-focused support groups, conferences, or dating websites such as www.hivnet.com, www.pozmatch.com, http://personals .poz.com, www.positivesingles.com, and www.hivpoz.net.

If it does not matter to you whether your partner is positive or negative, you can focus more on traditional methods—singles events, places of worship, dating websites like www.match.com, online dating/ personals ads, or networking through friends.

Disclosure

For many positive women, the big issue is disclosure. How and when do you tell? There is no one easy or perfect way to tell someone you are HIV-positive. As HIV-positive educator and humorist River Huston puts it, "Unless he's in a coma or you have a gun, there is no right time!"

Often, it's not how or when you tell, it's who. If a potential partner is going to find your status unacceptable, it may not matter when you tell. Similarly, if a person is going to accept you and the diagnosis, timing of disclosure may not matter either (as long as you tell before having sex).

There are two main approaches to when to tell.

Tell and Kiss

Tell before the first kiss, often before the first date:

- **Plus side:** Less emotional attachment before a possible rejection
- **Minus side:** More people find out that you have HIV

Kiss and Tell

Wait until after a few dates when you feel comfortable with the person:

- **Plus side:** No need to disclose to every date; more privacy
- **Minus side:** The "Why didn't you tell me before?" reaction

Is one of these more "right" than the other? Not really; it's a personal choice.

Tell Before Sex

Although you might be tempted to wait to disclose your status until after a sexual encounter for fear of rejection or embarrassment, there are several major reasons *not* to do this:

- You can expose your partner to HIV.
- Even if you have safe sex, and even if the partner is not infected by the contact, it is illegal in many states and countries to engage in sex without disclosing!
- If you have unprotected sex, you're in danger, too. You can still catch other sexually transmitted diseases (STDs), hepatitis C, or another strain of HIV.
- Most people lose their trust in sexual partners who conceal important information. How would you feel if a date waited until after the two of you had sex to mention that he or she was married?
- Several studies show that telling after sex leads to an increased risk of violence.

HIV Dating Tips

- Have "the talk" well before you wind up in the bedroom.
- Have the discussion when you're both sober.

- Read up on HIV and safe sex and HIV transmission. It will make it easier for you to talk about.

- If you date an HIV-positive person, don't spend so much time caring for him or her that you neglect to care for yourself.

- If you are concerned about a really negative or possibly violent reaction, consider disclosing in a public place or with an HIV advocate present.

- Get advice from those who have gone before. Attend a support group for HIV-positive people and ask others how they handle disclosure and dating.

- Be prepared for rejection. Just remember that dating is a process of finding the right person for you. Whether or not you are HIV-positive, most everyone has to go through some trial runs before finding that special person!

Other Positive Dating Issues

Some HIV-positive people find it hard to contemplate dating because they feel less desirable or less appealing than HIV-negative people. Remember that there is much more to you than just HIV. Don't let your status rob you of your self-esteem or your standards. You don't have to settle for being alone because no one will want you, and you don't have to settle for the wrong person.

Don't be afraid to have love in your life. Look for a loving relationship with a person who wants to be with you for you. Sex can also be an important and exciting part of your relationship. If you feel worried or guilty about the possibility of infecting your partner, make sure you know how to protect him or her by practicing safer sex.

It can be normal to feel ashamed of or embarrassed by your HIV status when dating. But if these feelings persist and prevent you from dating, or lead to depression or isolation, seek help. Find a support group or therapist; you'll probably begin to feel more enthusiastic about dating and romance before too long.

Section 43.2

Having Children

Excerpted from AIDS.gov, October 2010.

"Positive" Parenting

If you want to be a parent, having human immunodeficiency virus (HIV) shouldn't stop you. There a number of options for both HIV-positive women and men who want to be parents.

If you are an HIV-positive woman and you are pregnant—or want to become pregnant—the first thing you should do is talk with your health-care provider. There are medications you can take during pregnancy, labor, and delivery to help prevent your baby from being infected with HIV.

If you are an HIV-positive man, sperm washing may be an option for you and your partner. Artificial insemination with donor sperm and adoption services are additional options to help HIV-positive men and women to become parents.

Pregnancy and Transmission

If you are an HIV-positive woman and you become pregnant, you should be evaluated by your healthcare provider as soon as possible. If you have not been taking antiretroviral medications (ARVs), you can start taking them safely at the beginning of your second trimester of pregnancy (twelve weeks).

If you are already on ARVs and become pregnant, you should talk to your healthcare provider immediately to make sure you are taking the safest ARVs during your pregnancy. In most cases, women continue on the medications they were taking before becoming pregnant—but you and your healthcare provider should discuss your options and make the decision that fits your situation best.

It is better to be treated with ARVs throughout your pregnancy, but you can still receive treatment even during labor and delivery. It's important to tell medical staff at the hospital or clinic where you go to deliver that you are HIV-positive, so that they can give you medication to protect your baby.

Sperm Washing

Sperm are carried in seminal fluid, which contains some of the highest concentrations of HIV of any bodily fluid. Sperm washing involves taking a sample of semen and washing the seminal fluid away in a laboratory, so that only uninfected sperm are left.

This process appears to significantly decrease the risk of HIV infection from HIV-positive males to HIV-negative females. The process is still controversial, however. In 1990, the Centers for Disease Control and Prevention (CDC) issued a recommendation against sperm washing, citing a case in which a previously HIV-negative woman was found to be HIV-positive after she was inseminated with "washed" sperm from her HIV-positive husband. That recommendation has never been revised.

More recent studies have found sperm washing to be a safe way for serodiscordant couples to conceive, as long as the washing is done by qualified medical personnel. For more information, see the September 2007 edition of *AIDS: Official Journal of the International AIDS Society.*

The process can be time-consuming and very expensive, and it is rarely covered by insurance. Consult with your healthcare provider for more information.

Artificial Insemination

Female partners of HIV-positive men have the option of artificial insemination using donor sperm from a sperm bank in order to get pregnant. By law, donor sperm samples are tested for HIV, so women who are artificially inseminated with donor sperm are protected against HIV infection.

Adoption

Adoption is another option for people living with HIV/AIDS who want to have children. The Americans with Disabilities Act (ADA) prohibits adoption agencies from discriminating against couples or individuals living with HIV/AIDS.

Your HIV/AIDS service providers may be able to refer your to the proper agencies or organizations and help you begin the adoption process.

Section 43.3

Aging with HIV/AIDS

Excerpted from "Aging and HIV," *PI Perspective*, February 2010. © 2010 Project Inform. Reprinted with permission. For more information, contact the National HIV/AIDS Treatment Hotline, 800-822-7422, or visit www .projectinform.org.

Our society is aging. Baby boomers are reaching their senior years and the impact on our healthcare infrastructure is being felt. In California, half of the state's population will reach sixty-five years old or older in the next ten years.

Due to the success of antiretroviral therapy, people with human immunodeficiency virus (HIV) are also living longer and into their senior years. Today in the United Kingdom, nearly one-third of people with HIV are more than forty-five years old. In the United States, it's predicted that by 2015 half of people with HIV will be over fifty. In San Francisco, 27 percent of people with HIV were over fifty in 2003, but by 2008 40 percent were older than fifty. This growing number will impact social service delivery and affect our already fragile healthcare system. Providers are generally not sensitive to the concerns and needs of an aging HIV population.

Fifteen percent of newly diagnosed people with HIV are over fifty years old. Since this population is mostly heterosexual, it raises many concerns over the lack of targeted prevention for older people in a society that stigmatizes them as a population of people who don't or shouldn't have sex.

The remaining aging population has been on HIV treatment for a long time and is generally healthier, having returned to work or at least maintained a reasonable quality of life. We know that the cumulative survival rate is going up due to this success, but it is also an odd paradox that many who have been successfully treated and reached undetectability are also now at increased risk for certain diseases commonly seen in the elderly.

The fact remains that life expectancy is lower for those who started HIV treatment late or their CD4 cells never increased as a result of therapy. The Antiviral Therapy Collaborative Cohort Study showed life expectancy has increased due to therapy but has not reached the same level seen in the HIV-negative population. Our work is cut out for us.

The physical effects of aging are well known. However, the consequences of aging and HIV are interrelated. But it is still not completely understood if HIV causes premature aging or if aging makes HIV disease worse. Researchers are looking for answers in ongoing and planned laboratory and clinical research.

Non-AIDS (Acquired Immunodeficiency Syndrome) Events

Today, a third or more of deaths most common in older people with HIV are not caused by AIDS. Most of these clinical issues are known as non-AIDS events, which are illnesses not related to HIV. These events are also being seen more often than in the earlier days of the epidemic. Before highly active antiretroviral therapy (HAART), the biggest cause of mortality was due to opportunistic infections in people with severe CD4 loss. Non-AIDS events such as cardiovascular disease and malignancies are most often caused by direct viral infection, a suboptimal CD4 response to therapy and by inflammation.

Despite effective HAART, there remains a low level of latent virus that leads to inflammation, which causes some of the non-AIDS events such as heart disease. Also, many of the non-AIDS conditions are also common in older people in general, so as HIV-positive people grow older the risks become greater.

Heart disease has long been a concern in HIV, and especially in recent years as the HIV population ages and cumulative data on different markers for heart disease, including heart attacks, are growing. Heart disease is the most important cause of death in the general population and is higher in people with HIV. Heart attack risk is increased with Ziagen® or Epzicom® although the reason has not been established. Protease inhibitors increase lipids that are associated with heart disease, however newer drugs may be less of a problem. Other lipid-friendly regimens exist, so providers should individualize therapy based on risk factors for heart disease.

More long-term research is needed in people with HIV to understand the cumulative effect of HIV therapy as they grow older.

The liver is the body's critical filtering mechanism. It makes sense that, over time, the liver wears down, especially in co-infection with HIV and hepatitis B or C. Inflammation and low CD4s are related to liver disease. In aging populations of people with HIV, alcohol, obesity, and poly-pharmacy, or the use of many drugs together, are also factors related to liver disease.

AIDS-related cancers such as non-Hodgkin lymphoma and Kaposi sarcoma have declined in the HAART era. However, most malignancies occur as people age, and as time passes older people with HIV will be at a higher risk for cancer. In HIV, Hodgkin lymphoma, anal, throat, liver, and head and neck cancers are the most common malignancies. These cancers are most often caused by an infectious agent such as hepatitis B or C, or human papillomavirus. Low CD4 cells and inflammation are also related. Today, AIDS dementia is also less common due to HAART because neurocognitive decline is greatly slowed with effective HAART. But some are concerned that many effective HIV drugs do not penetrate the central nervous system, which may lead to mild neurocognitive symptoms that are quite common in older people with HIV. Alzheimer disease and senility have been a big concern in the general aging population, but persistent HIV and inflammation are contributing to these already debilitating and frustrating conditions in older people with HIV.

Bone fractures and osteoporosis (loss of bone density) are also common in older people. Yet, osteoporosis is three times higher in people with HIV. Osteopenia (thinning of the bone mass) is even higher. Long-term HIV disease, inflammation, and non-HIV-related factors such as alcohol use are all risks to good bone health in older people with HIV. There has been some concern regarding Viread® (tenofovir) causing bone disease, however this has not been borne out in studies thus far. Doctors suggest using vitamin D supplements and calcium where appropriate.

Frailty is characterized as unintentional weight loss, exhaustion, low physical activity, weakness, and slowness. It includes poor general health, risk of falling, poor appetite, loss of muscle mass, and bone demineralization. It is a common geriatric condition but is now being seen in older people with HIV. Again, persistent inflammation and low CD4 counts are related to this condition.

The Consequences of Low-Level, Persistent HIV

Despite effective treatment, HIV persists in small amounts (millions of copies) in various "reservoirs" in the body where it can lay silent in cells that are "asleep." These cells must be activated to release new virus, which in turn starts a normal immune response. Since this is an ongoing low-level response, inflammation can remain as long as virus is present. This low level is not detected by standard tests, but researchers detect it in highly sensitive assays that reach below one copy.

Viral proteins released by this persistent virus in the latent reservoir can be toxic to the body and also cause immune activation. HIV persistence is being researched and may lead to what is being called "functional cure."

Inflammation is a normal immune process involving specific cells and cytokines that in HIV are switched on due to chronic immune responses (either due to suboptimal treatment or low level persistent HIV). Inflammation does decrease w/ HAART but never returns to normal.

A process called microbial translocation is seen within a few weeks of HIV infection and can weaken a person's immune capacity, possibly never being fully restored. After infection, HIV targets CD4 cells in the gut, demolishing a large part of the body's important immune reserves. Then, bacterial microbes travel outside of the gut and enter the bloodstream where the immune system responds to them, activating T cells that are infected with HIV. More HIV is produced, leading to further immune damage. This is one of the most important physiological reasons for stopping the virus as soon as possible after infection.

Aging and HIV and the Immune System

As we grow older certain aging processes are similar to what chronic HIV does to our bodies. Apoptosis is our natural mechanism to rid our bodies of unnecessary, weak, or damaged cells. Apoptosis can lead to suppression of the immune system, which can also lead to cancers. It is a process that most likely occurs more often in older people with HIV.

HIV damages lymph node structure and causes thymic dysfunction, and there is a cumulative effect as people with HIV grow older. Over long-term HIV infection, the thymus loses its function and fewer crucial T cells are produced, causing low CD4 and CD8 ratios and low memory to naive cell ratios. This leads to further immune system damage.

Another process that becomes dysregulated in aging and HIV is called immunosenescence. This is another word for "immunologic aging" or "exhaustion" of T cells. This can cause a destructive high T cell turnover and may be part of premature "aging" of the immune system.

In HIV disease and in older people the immune system's functional capacity decreases. This is what causes a poor response to vaccines and the tuberculosis (TB) skin test. Oxidative stress occurs in both the elderly and people with HIV. Over time this can further suppress the immune system.

Research Is Needed

Although we have made huge progress with HIV therapy, the effects of living longer with HIV despite viral control are still not completely understood. It is clear that this issue requires more research, although it's hard to know if there will be clear answers anytime soon. There are still many unknowns in HIV pathogenesis, technical laboratory issues, new assays needing development, and clinical studies will be challenging to design and recruit. Much that scientists are learning about aging and HIV is daunting and most of the news is sobering. Yet people with HIV are gaining years on their lives, and surviving despite critical odds. People with HIV can maintain health through a few practical management tips such as monitoring for and treating underlying cardiovascular disease, screening and reducing risk for cancers, individualizing HIV treatment, appropriate exercise, healthy diets, and stress reduction. Importantly, research is promising on immune-related therapies and better, less toxic HIV drugs that have the potential to take us into a different paradigm of living with HIV.

Chapter 44

HIV/AIDS Status Disclosure

Chapter Contents

Section 44.1

Do You Have to Tell? Legal Disclosure Requirements and Other Considerations

Excerpted from "Do You Have to Tell?" and "Legal Disclosure,"
AIDS.gov, October 2010.

Do You Have to Tell?

Sharing Your Human Immunodeficiency Virus (HIV) Status

After you are diagnosed with HIV, you will have to decide whether to share that information with other people, and—if so—whom you should tell.

It is very important that you talk to your current and past sexual partners about your HIV status. If you have shared needles with others to inject drugs, you need to tell them too. If you are afraid or embarrassed to tell them yourself, the health department in your area can notify your sexual or needle-sharing partners that they may have been exposed to HIV without giving your name.

Disclosure can be a tough process, but you don't have to face it alone. Talk to your healthcare provider and ask for help in finding support groups or other individuals who can help you in the disclosure process.

Sharing your HIV status with those you trust—such as family members, friends, and children—can help with the stresses of having HIV, and can actually improve your overall health. Disclosing your status to your healthcare provider is important to make sure that you receive the best care for your HIV.

In most cases, sharing your HIV status is a personal choice—but it may also be a legal requirement. Many states have laws that require you to tell specific people about your HIV status.

Before you decide to tell people that you are HIV-positive, here are some things to consider:

- Think about the people you rely on for support, like family, friends, or co-workers.

- What kind of relationship do you have with these people? What are the pros and cons of telling them you are living with HIV?

- Are there particular issues a person might have that will affect how much he or she can support you?

- What is that person's attitude and knowledge about HIV?

- Why do you want to disclose to this person? What kind of support can this person provide?

- For each person you want to tell, ask yourself if the person needs to know now—or if it's better to wait.

Legal Disclosure

HIV Disclosure Policies and Procedures

If your HIV test is positive, the clinic or other testing site will report the results to your state health department. They do this so that public health officials can monitor what's happening with the HIV epidemic in your city and state. (It's important for them to know this, because federal and state funding for HIV and acquired immunodeficiency syndrome (AIDS) services is often targeted to areas where the epidemic is strongest.)

Your state health department will then remove all of your personal information (name, address, etc.) from your test results and send the information to the U.S. Centers for Disease Control and Prevention (CDC). CDC is the federal agency responsible for tracking national public health trends. CDC does not share this information with anyone else, including insurance companies.

Many states and some cities have partner-notification laws—meaning that, if you test positive for HIV, you (or your healthcare provider) may be legally obligated to tell your sex or needle-sharing partner(s). In some states, if you are HIV-positive and don't tell your partner(s), you can be charged with a crime. Some health departments require healthcare providers to report the name of your sex and needle-sharing partner(s) if they know that information—even if you refuse to report that information yourself.

Some states also have laws that require clinic staff to notify a "third party" if they know that person has a significant risk for exposure to HIV from a patient the staff member knows is infected with HIV. This is called duty to warn. The Ryan White HIV/AIDS Program requires that health departments receiving money from the Ryan White program show "good faith" efforts to notify the marriage partners of a patient with HIV/AIDS.

Disclosure Policies in Correctional Facilities

If you are serving time in a jail or prison, your HIV status may be disclosed legally under the Occupational Safety and Health Administration's (OSHA) Standard for Occupational Exposure to Bloodborne Pathogens. State or local laws may also require that your HIV status be reported to public health authorities, parole officers, spouses, or sexual partners.

Section 44.2

Telling Your Spouse or Sexual Partners

Excerpted from "Partner/Spouse" and "Sexual Partners,"
AIDS.gov, October 2010.

Partner/Spouse

How Should You Tell Your Intimate Partner You Have Human Immunodeficiency Virus (HIV)?

Many people worry that they will lose an important—or even their only—support system when they tell their intimate partners that they are HIV-positive. It's perfectly normal to feel nervous, embarrassed, or even fearful of your partner's reaction, which may be verbal or even physical.

Disclosure is a process, so it may take you several conversations. It's possible that your spouse or partner's reactions to learning your status may change as time goes by. To make the disclosure process as open as possible, do the following things:

- Have your conversations in a safe and secure place. Choose a space that provides privacy, yet offers comfort and familiarity.

- Tell your spouse or partner that you have some important news to share.

- Be prepared to talk about your diagnosis in a clear way and provide basic information about what it means to live with HIV.

- Do not attempt to discuss your diagnosis if you feel you do not have a clear sense about what it means.

- It may be helpful to have some information, (printed material or websites) available to help with any questions your spouse or partner may have.

- Be prepared to explain that HIV can be contracted during unprotected sex and provide your partner with information about HIV testing and where he or she can get tested.

Do I Have to Tell My Spouse or Partner?

Though each state has different policies and procedures related to partner notification, each does require that all past, present, and future sex and needle-sharing partners be notified of a potential exposure to HIV. Health departments can assist with the notifications.

Sexual Partners

Partner Counseling and Referral Services (PCRS)

Once you have been diagnosed, you will be asked to identify your sexual and needle-sharing partners, so that they can be told that they have been exposed to HIV and need to be tested. Partner notification is one of the most important ways to prevent the spread of HIV. (It's also important, of course, that you use a condom during sex and don't share needles.)

The Partner Counseling and Referral Service (PCRS) can help you with notifying your partner(s). Most state public health departments have a PCRS program. PCRS can also help your partner(s) get counseling, a medical evaluation, treatment, and any other services they may need.

Notifying and Testing Partners

Once you have identified your partners, they should be notified as soon as possible. This gives them an opportunity to protect themselves from infection if they don't have HIV—or, if they are having sex or sharing needles with others—to take steps to protect or notify those partners.

Notification can happen in four ways:

- Provider referral means that your healthcare provider notifies your partner(s) for you.

- Self-referral means that you notify your partner(s) yourself.

- Contract referral means that you make a "contract" to notify your partner(s) by a particular date. If, by the contract date, your partners have not come in for counseling and testing, the health department will contact them.

- Dual referral means that you and the health department will notify your partner(s) together.

If your partner(s) are notified by your healthcare provider or the health department, they will also be given information about where they can get tested for HIV and where they can find treatment if they need it. Healthcare officials would prefer that people get tested for HIV at the same time they're notified because not everyone follows through on going to the testing sites.

It's possible for your partner(s) to test negative for HIV even when they are already infected if they take the test during the window period. That's the time between when a person is infected with HIV and the time that the body develops antibodies to the virus. Partners are advised to be retested three months after the date of their last known exposure.

Disclosing without Patient Consent

A physician or HIV counselor may disclose a patient's HIV status without his or her consent only under the following conditions:

- The physician or counselor has made a reasonable effort to counsel and encourage the patient to voluntarily provide this information to the spouse or sexual partner.

- The physician or counselor reasonably believes the patient will not provide the information to the spouse or sexual partner.

- Disclosure is necessary to protect the health of the spouse or sexual partner.

Section 44.3

Telling Your Family and Friends

Reprinted from "Family," "Children," and "Friends," AIDS.gov, October 2010.

Family

Telling Your Family

There is no right or wrong way to talk to your family about your human immunodeficiency virus (HIV) status. Every family has a different style of communicating and a different way of handling challenges.

If your family responds in a way that hurts, or doesn't seem supportive, try to remember that first reactions are not permanent. The way that your family responds to your news can—and probably will—change over time, as they learn more about what it means to live with HIV. One of the best things you can do is to acknowledge your family members' feelings about your diagnosis because, in a way, they now have to live with the realities of HIV too.

While telling your family that you have HIV may seem difficult, you should know that disclosure actually has many benefits—studies have shown that people who disclose their HIV status respond better to treatment than those who don't.

That may be because people who disclose their HIV status are more likely to have a good support system—it's hard to have "real" relationships with your family when you are hiding a big secret like HIV. Disclosing may provide a greater degree of closeness within your family, and promote understanding and acceptance—and it may keep you healthier too!

You may find it easier, and possibly more effective, to have a third party, such as a counselor or a family member who already knows about your diagnosis, to help you tell your family.

Children

How Do You Tell Your Child You Have HIV?

There is no "right" way to talk to your children about having HIV. Every child will react differently to the news.

Some studies show that being open about your HIV diagnosis with your children is better than not telling them. Your kids may already know something is wrong, especially if you have been ill. Keeping your diagnosis a secret from them can confuse them and make them feel anxious.

Secrets can be stressful in another way too. If you tell your children about your HIV diagnosis, it may not be the best idea to ask them to keep your HIV status a secret from other family or friends. Several studies have shown that this can be very stressful to children and can bring on behavior problems.

Some children have a hard time learning that their parent has HIV. They may react by developing behavior issues or difficulties at school, and some start taking sexual risks themselves. Other kids may not react much at all.

Disclosure as Prevention

Whether you have HIV or not, it is never too early to talk about HIV with your children. By third grade, up to 93 percent of children have heard about HIV—but not enough children have accurate information about HIV and other sexually transmitted diseases (STDs).

If you decide to tell your kids that you have HIV, you can use that opportunity to talk with them about how they can protect themselves from HIV in the future. It could be a golden opportunity to talk with them about the need to avoid risky sexual and drug-taking behaviors themselves.

Friends

Your Friends and Your HIV Status

Your friends know lots of things about you. Should you tell them that you have IIIV?

Friends can be a significant source of support as you are learning to live with HIV. You may even find that your friendship actually becomes stronger once you've confided in them—but only you can decide whether and to whom you will disclose your HIV status.

When you are deciding which of your friends to tell, first ask yourself why you want them to know. Have they trusted you with deeply personal information in the past? Do you have reason to believe that they will provide you with the support you need? If the answer to these questions is "Yes," then you may want to disclose.

There is no "right" way to talk to a friend about HIV. You've probably had confidential conversations and shared experiences with this person in the past. Think about those interactions and approach your HIV disclosure conversations in the same way.

Talk to your friend about HIV at a familiar and comfortable place, and be sure that you have plenty of privacy. Be prepared for your friend to show a range of emotions and reactions at first, and to go through stages of dealing with the news—probably similar to the ones you experienced when you were first told of your diagnosis.

You will want to be prepared to answer your friend's questions about your HIV status. Your friend will probably have concerns about your health and may also be concerned about whether or not he or she could get HIV from you. This is a chance to educate your friend about HIV basics—transmission, prevention, and treatment—and to eliminate those fears.

It's a good idea to have printed or online information ready for your friend in case you're not prepared to answer every question. You might also consider inviting your friend to the clinic or doctor's office where you took your test, got your results, or are being treated. This offers an opportunity for your friend to ask questions and learn more about living with HIV.

Section 44.4

Workplace Disclosure

Excerpted from "Co-Workers/Workplace,"
AIDS.gov, October 2010.

Weighing the Decision

The decision to disclose your human immunodeficiency virus (HIV) status at work is a deeply personal choice that can have both positive and negative outcomes, so think carefully about the pros and cons before you act.

One benefit of disclosing at work is that it can create supportive relationships with your co-workers. On the other hand, telling people that you are living with HIV may have the opposite effect and cause your colleagues to treat you differently. You have to be the judge of which outcome is more likely.

If you decide to disclose to one or more of your co-workers, think carefully about which individuals to tell and how to tell them. Should you tell your boss or the Human Resources Department before you talk to your co-workers? Should you tell your entire work team about your diagnosis or just disclose to individuals?

It's good to have a plan in mind before you start telling your colleagues.

Help in Your Workplace

If you aren't sure how to handle disclosing your HIV status at work, many employers offer an Employee Assistance Program (EAP) intended to help employees deal with personal issues that affect their work performance, health, or wellbeing. EAP services are free of charge and usually available for an employee's immediate family as well. Issues and information that you discuss with an EAP provider remain confidential from your employer, unless the service is mandated by your employer for corrective purposes (such as dealing with substance abuse issues).

Discrimination Is Illegal

Although there are pros and cons to disclosing your HIV status to your co-workers, it's important to keep in mind that workplace discrimination based on HIV status is illegal.

The following laws may apply to people living with HIV and acquired immunodeficiency syndrome (AIDS):

- Americans with Disabilities Act (ADA)

- Occupational Safety and Health Act (OSHA) and the OSHA Bloodborne Pathogens Standards

- Family Medical Leave Act (FMLA)

- Health Insurance Portability and Accountability Act (HIPAA)

- Consolidated Omnibus Budget Reconciliation Act (COBRA)

- State, county, and municipal laws on HIV testing, discrimination, etc.

If you are experiencing discrimination after disclosing your status, there are resources available to assist you.

Section 44.5

Disclosure to Healthcare Providers

Excerpted from "Other Providers," AIDS.gov, October 2010.

Requirements and Benefits of Disclosing to Healthcare Providers

Your healthcare providers (doctors, clinical workers, dentists, etc.) have to know about your human immunodeficiency virus (HIV) status in order to be able to give you the best possible care. It's also important that healthcare providers know your HIV status so that they don't prescribe medication for you that may be harmful when taken with your HIV medications.

Some states require you to disclose your HIV-positive status before you receive any healthcare services from a physician or dentist. For this reason, it's important to discuss the laws in your state about disclosure in medical settings with the healthcare provider who gave you your HIV test results.

Your HIV test result will become part of your medical records so that your doctor or other healthcare providers can give you the best care possible. All medical information, including HIV test results, falls under strict confidentiality laws such as the Health Insurance Portability and Accountability Act's (HIPAA) Privacy Rule and cannot be released without your permission.

Medical Discrimination

It is against the law for a healthcare provider to refuse to treat you because you have HIV. Both the Rehabilitation Act of 1973 (Section 504) and the Americans with Disabilities Act of 1990 prohibit discrimination against qualified persons with HIV and other disabilities.

If you believe that you have been discriminated against because of your HIV status, you can file a complaint with the Office for Civil Rights (OCR) in the U.S. Department of Health and Human Services (HHS). The deadline for filing a complaint is 180 days from the date the discrimination occurred.

Chapter 45

HIV/AIDS Patients and Legal Rights

Chapter Contents

Section 45.1

Your Rights in the Workplace

Can I be fired or denied a job because I have human immunodeficiency virus (HIV)?

Probably not. The national law protects anyone with acquired immunodeficiency syndrome (AIDS) or HIV, but only applies to businesses with more than fourteen workers. Many state or local laws cover smaller businesses, but some only cover people who are sick.

How can I find out for sure if I can be fired or denied a job?

First, contact your nearest AIDS service organization. They may know. More likely, they might be able to find someone who can tell you. If not, look in the phone book under "AIDS" or search the internet for "AIDS legal" to see if you can find an agency that can tell you.

Can a boss or company change my job or put me in a new job because I have AIDS or HIV?

Probably not. First, find out if your job is covered (see the question just before this one). If it is, your company or boss can't change your job just because they're afraid of people with HIV. They can't change your job just because they think customers or co-workers are afraid of HIV. But they can change your job if it's dangerous for you to do it. That means if you could infect other people, or if you could get hurt because of your HIV. But there aren't many jobs like that.

Can a boss or company force me to tell them if I have AIDS or HIV?

Probably not before you have been offered a job. Until you've been offered a job, a boss or company can only ask questions about whether you can do the job. So they can't ask unless your HIV or AIDS makes you unable to do parts of the job. But this is true only if the law where you live covers you and the job (see the second question).

What about after I've been offered a job?

Your company or boss can make everyone take a general medical exam. As part of the exam, they can ask you what illnesses you have and what medications you take. You then have to tell them about your HIV. But they can't take the job back because of your answer as long as you can do the job safely, so don't lie. If you lie and they find out, they can take your job away for lying.

If I tell my boss or company that I have AIDS or HIV, do they have to keep it a secret?

Sometimes. If your company is covered by the national law, and your boss asks you about your medical condition, they have to keep anything you tell them confidential. But if you tell them for some other reason, they may or may not have to keep it a secret. And if your company is smaller than fifteen people, whether they have to keep your HIV status private depends on the law in your state. It is always a good idea, if you tell your boss or company that you have AIDS or HIV, to say that you don't want them to tell anyone else. You'll have better legal protection. And many people will respect your privacy.

Does my boss or company have to give me different hours or special treatment if I have AIDS or HIV?

Probably, but the more special treatment you need, the tougher it is to get. Your boss or company has to make small changes to your job as long as you can still do the important parts of the job. So, for example, if you need to see your doctor at what is usually work time, your boss has to let you unless the job has to be done at that particular time. The bigger your company, the more likely it is that the company will have to adjust. The bigger the changes you need, the more likely it is that the company won't have to adjust.

To get time off, do I have to tell my boss or company I have AIDS or HIV?

Maybe not. You can say you have a medical condition, and that your doctor will back you up in a note. Lots of companies don't want more information. Some laws say that they can't ask for more.

What if I am so sick I can't do the job?

Your company or boss doesn't have to give you a job or keep you in a job if you can't do that job. The Family Medical Leave Act, a national law covering many employers, might require the company to keep the job open for you until you can return to work, at least for a few months. In some places, the company may have to keep paying you for a while. If you can't work, you should consider applying for disability. Some jobs have private disability insurance. Many states do, and you should apply for Social Security. Your nearest HIV/AIDS agency should be able to help you figure this out.

What if my partner, someone I live with, or someone in my family has AIDS or HIV? Can I be fired, denied a job, or have my job changed?

Probably not. Again, first find out if your job is covered by the law (see the answer to the second question). If it is, you can't be fired, denied a job, or have your job changed because you have a partner, friend, or family member with AIDS or HIV.

Can I take time off to help take care of my partner or family member with AIDS or HIV?

Many employers will let you do this, at least for a while. Many won't pay you while you are off, although some will let you use your sick leave. If an employer lets other people use sick leave or take unpaid leave to take care of partners and family members who are sick, they can't refuse because the family member has AIDS or HIV. But the rules on same-sex and unmarried opposite-sex partners can be a little tricky. In most places, even though a company lets you take time off to take care of a husband or wife, the company doesn't have to let you take time off to care for your partner.

Section 45.2

Fair Housing Act: Frequently Asked Questions

Reprinted from "Housing and Civil Enforcement Section: Frequently Asked Questions," U.S. Department of Justice, July 25, 2008.

What is the Fair Housing Act?

The Fair Housing Act prohibits discrimination in housing on the basis of race, color, religion, sex, national origin, familial status, or disability by housing providers, such as landlords and real estate companies as well as other entities, such as municipalities, banks or other lending institutions, and homeowners insurance companies.

How does the Department of Justice enforce the Fair Housing Act?

Under the Fair Housing Act, the Department of Justice may start a lawsuit where it has reason to believe that a person or entity is engaged in a "pattern or practice" of discrimination or where a denial of rights to a group of persons raises an issue of general public importance. Through these lawsuits, the department can obtain money damages, both actual and punitive damages, for those individuals harmed by a defendant's discriminatory actions as well as preventing any further discriminatory conduct. The defendant may also be required to pay money penalties to the United States. If you have information that suggests a pattern or practice of discrimination in housing, please contact us.

The Department of Housing and Urban Development (HUD) investigates individual cases of discrimination in housing. If HUD determines that reasonable cause exists to believe that a discriminatory housing practice has occurred, then either the complainant or the respondent (the person against whom the complaint was filed) may elect to have the case heard in federal court. In those instances, the Department of Justice will bring the case on behalf of the individual complainant.

In addition, where force or a threat of force is used to deny or interfere with fair housing rights, the Department of Justice may begin criminal proceedings.

Finally, in cases involving discrimination in home mortgage loans or home improvement loans, the department may file suit under both the Fair Housing Act and the Equal Credit Opportunity Act.

What do I do if I believe I have been the victim of illegal discrimination in housing?

Individuals who believe that they have been victims of an illegal housing practice may file a complaint with the Department of Housing and Urban Development (HUD) or file their own lawsuit in federal or state court. You must file the complaint with HUD within one year of the incident you believe to be housing discrimination. If you choose to file your own lawsuit in federal or state court, the Act requires that you do so within two years of the incident.

Does the Fair Housing Act prohibit discrimination on the basis of a person's sexual orientation?

When sexual orientation is the only basis of discrimination, no. However, we evaluate these complaints on a case-by-case basis to determine whether any other form of discrimination is present (such as sex or disability, for example). In addition, many state and local laws prohibit discrimination in housing based on sexual orientation. You should consult with your local or state civil rights enforcement agency to determine whether discrimination on this basis is protected.

What is the Equal Credit Opportunity Act?

Under the Equal Credit Opportunity Act, a creditor may not discriminate on the basis of sex, race, color, religion, national origin, marital status, age, or source of income in any credit transaction.

How does the Department of Justice enforce the Equal Credit Opportunity Act?

The Department of Justice may start a lawsuit where it has reason to believe that a creditor is engaged in a "pattern or practice" of discrimination. Through these lawsuits, the department can obtain money damages, both actual and punitive damages, for those individuals harmed by a defendant's discriminatory actions as well as preventing further discrimination by the defendant. Each year, the department files a report with Congress on its activities under the statute. If you have information that suggests a pattern or practice of discrimination in credit, please contact us.

Individual complaints of discrimination are handled by the creditor's federal regulatory agency. The agencies and the types of financial institutions that they regulate are as follows:

- **Office of Thrift Supervision [OTS]:** Savings associations and federally chartered savings banks (the word "federal" or the initials "F.S.B." appear in a federal institution's name)

- **Comptroller of Currency [OCC]:** National banks, federal branches/agencies of foreign banks (the word "national" or the initials "N.A." appear in or after the bank's name)

- **Federal Reserve Board [FRB]:** Financial institutions that are members of the Federal Reserve System, except national banks and federal branches/agencies of foreign banks

- **Federal Deposit Insurance Corporation [FDIC]:** State chartered banks that are not members of the Federal Reserve System

- **National Credit Union Association [NCUA]:** Federal credit unions (the words "federal credit union" appear in the institution's name)

- **Federal Trade Commission [FTC]:** Retailers, finance companies, creditors (including most mortgage companies) that are not assigned to another agency

What do I do if I believe that I have been the victim of an unfair credit transaction involving residential property?

Individuals who believe that they have been victims of an illegal housing practice, such as the denial of a mortgage that involved credit, may file a complaint with the Department of Housing and Urban Development (HUD).

What is Title II of the Civil Rights Act of 1964?

This law prohibits discrimination because of a person's race, color, religion, or national origin in certain places of public accommodation, such as hotels, restaurants, and places of entertainment.

How does the Department of Justice enforce Title II?

When there is reason to believe that a person or entity has engaged in a "pattern or practice" of discrimination, which violates Title II, the Department of Justice can bring a lawsuit. However, unlike lawsuits enforcing the Fair Housing Act or the Equal Credit Opportunity Act, the department cannot obtain monetary damages for individuals in Title II cases.

What do I do if I believe that I have been the victim of discrimination under Title II?

Individuals who believe that a place of public accommodation has violated Title II may file their own lawsuit in federal court. In addition, you may have some rights under other federal laws, state laws, or local ordinances and should consult with your local or state civil rights enforcement agency.

What is the Religious Land Use and Institutionalized Persons Act (RLUIPA)?

This law prohibits local governments from adopting or enforcing land use regulations that discriminate against religious assemblies and institutions or which unjustifiably burden religious exercise.

How does the Department of Justice enforce the Religious Land Use and Institutionalized Persons Act (RLUIPA)?

The department can investigate and bring suit to enforce the statute on behalf of individuals, houses of worship, or other religious institutions. The department may obtain injunctive, but not monetary, relief. Individuals may file their own lawsuit in federal or state court.

Section 45.3

How the Laws Apply to Persons with HIV

Reprinted from "HIV and the Law: ADA," "HIV and the Law: OSHA," "HIV and the Law: FMLA," "HIV and the Law: HIPAA," and "HIV and the Law: COBRA," Centers for Disease Control and Prevention. The full text of these documents is available online at http://www.hivatwork.org/law/laws.cfm; accessed May 23, 2010.

Americans with Disabilities Act (ADA)

The Americans with Disabilities Act of 1990 (ADA) prohibits discrimination in employment on the basis of a person's disability, including human immunodeficiency virus (HIV) and acquired immunodeficiency syndrome (AIDS). The ADA, which covers employers of fifteen or more people, applies to employment decisions at all stages. To apply the ADA to everyday employment situations, employers must remember four key points:

- The definition of disability

- The importance of knowing the essential functions of jobs

- The concept of reasonable accommodation

- Preserving confidentiality of medical information and limiting medical inquiries within the boundaries of the law

An individual with a disability is a person who:

- has a physical or mental impairment that substantially limits one or more major life activities;

- has a record of such an impairment;

- is regarded as having such an impairment.

A qualified employee or applicant with a disability is an individual who, with or without reasonable accommodation, can perform the essential functions of the job in question.

Reasonable accommodation may include, but is not limited to the following:

- Making existing facilities used by employees readily accessible to and usable by persons with disabilities

- Job restructuring, modifying work schedules, reassignment to a vacant position

- Acquiring or modifying equipment or devices; adjusting or modifying examinations, training materials, or policies; and providing qualified readers or interpreters

As more effective drug therapies are extending the lives of HIV-positive people—and improving their quality of life—more workers are returning to the workforce and staying productive. Lawsuits filed by HIV-infected workers continue under the ADA. Most of these lawsuits are preventable through training and education.

For example, on June 25, 1998, the Supreme Court decided a case with major impact when it determined in Bragdon v. Abbott, 1998 U.S. LEXIS 4212 (1998), that, in this case, the individual plaintiff who is HIV-positive but asymptomatic is protected as an individual with a disability under the Americans with Disabilities Act of 1990. The Court remanded on the issue of whether individual healthcare providers could determine the extent of direct threat of patients with HIV.

Bragdon v. Abbott

Bragdon v. Abbott, 1998 U.S. LEXIS 4212 (1998), involves Sidney Abbott, a woman with no symptoms of HIV, but who disclosed that she was HIV-positive when seeking dental treatment from Randon Bragdon, a dentist in Maine. Dr. Bragdon examined her in his dental office but refused to fill her cavity in his dental office; he indicated that he would fill her cavity only in a hospital and that she would be required to bear additional hospital expenses. She brought suit under Title III of the Americans with Disabilities Act of 1990, which prohibits private providers of public accommodations (such as a private dentist) from discriminating against otherwise qualified individuals with disabilities on the basis of their disabilities. The same definition of "disability" applies in Title I cases under the ADA, governing employment.

On the issue of whether being HIV-positive but asymptomatic qualifies an individual as being substantially limited in one or more major life activities, the Court held in this case that she was covered. It looked to reproduction as a major life activity and held that Sidney Abbott had demonstrated that her ability to reproduce and to bear children was substantially limited by her HIV infection.

To be protected under the ADA, an individual must have a physical or mental impairment that substantially limits one or more major life activities, must have a record of such an impairment, or be regarded as having such an impairment. The ADA also permits differing treatment in cases where the individual seeking protection is not considered to be otherwise qualified, or because the individual poses a "direct threat" to himself or herself or others that cannot be eliminated through a reasonable accommodation.

Occupational Safety and Health Administration (OSHA)

The mission of the Occupational Safety and Health Administration (OSHA) is to save lives, prevent injuries, and protect the health of America's workers. To accomplish this, federal and state governments must work in partnership with the more than one hundred million working men and women and their six-and-one-half million employers who are covered by the Occupational Safety and Health Act of 1970.

Employers have certain responsibilities under OSHA, including the following:

- Providing a workplace free from serious recognized hazards and complying with standards, rules, and regulations issued under the OSHA Act

- Examining workplace conditions to make sure they conform to applicable OSHA standards

- Making sure employees have and use safe tools and equipment and properly maintain this equipment

- Establishing or updating operating procedures and communicating them so that employees follow safety and health requirements

- Not discriminating against employees who exercise their rights under the Act

The Occupational Safety and Health Administration released its blood-borne pathogens standards intended to protect millions of workers across the nation from workplace exposure to HIV and hepatitis. These standards cover employees exposed to blood and other infectious materials, including but not limited to employees in hospitals, health-care facilities, nursing homes, and research laboratories. The standard requires employers to (1) develop a written exposure control plan, (2) establish a Hepatitis B vaccination program, (3) provide employees with hazard information and training, (4) maintain certain medical records surrounding exposure incidents, and (5) implement certain work practice controls, such as protective clothing and puncture-proof receptacles for tainted needles and other medical wastes.

OSHA says the rules will protect approximately 5.6 million employees in hospitals, doctors' offices, dentists' offices, nursing homes, funeral homes, linen services, medical equipment-repair companies, correctional facilities, emergency-response agencies, and law enforcement agencies. OSHA projects that the new restrictions will prevent 200 deaths and 9,200 blood-borne infections annually.

Family Medical Leave Act (FMLA)

The Family Medical Leave Act of 1993 (FMLA) applies to private-sector employers with fifty or more employees within seventy-five miles of the worksite. Eligible employees may take leave for serious health conditions or to provide care for an immediate family member with a serious health condition—including HIV/AIDS. Eligible employees are entitled to a total of twelve weeks of job-protected, unpaid leave during any twelve-month period.

During this leave, an eligible employee is entitled to continued group health plan coverage as if the employee had continued to work.

Upon return from leave, the law generally requires that employees be restored to the same or an equivalent position with equivalent pay, benefits, and working conditions.

In order for individuals with HIV or AIDS to invoke FMLA protection, the disclosure of medical information to the employer may be required. Employers are not required to provide unpaid medical leave under FMLA if they are not informed that a disability or serious health condition exists.

If an employee makes an employer aware of his or her AIDS or HIV infection, laws such as the ADA require that information to be held in strict confidence.

Unpaid leaves of absence in addition to leave under the FMLA (or for employees covered by the ADA but not necessarily eligible under FMLA) may also be required as a "reasonable accommodation" under the ADA.

Health Insurance Portability and Accountability Act (HIPAA)

The Health Insurance Portability and Accountability Act of 1996 (HIPAA) attempts to address some of the barriers to healthcare

610

coverage and related job mobility impediments facing people with HIV as well as other vulnerable populations.

HIPAA has three main goals:

- It provides persons with group coverage new protections from discriminatory treatment.

- It enables small groups (such as businesses with a small number of employees) to obtain and keep health insurance coverage more easily.

- It gives persons losing/leaving group coverage new options for obtaining individual coverage.

This law provides several protections important to people with HIV/AIDS:

- It limits (but does not wholly eliminate) the use of preexisting condition exclusions.

- It prohibits group health plans from discriminating by denying you coverage or charging additional fees for coverage based on an employee's family member's past or present poor health.

- It guarantees certain small employers, and certain individuals who lose job-related coverage, the right to purchase individual health insurance.

- It guarantees, in most cases, that employers or individuals who purchase health insurance can renew the coverage regardless of any health conditions of individuals covered under the insurance policy.

Consolidated Omnibus Budget Reconciliation Act (COBRA)

The Consolidated Omnibus Budget Reconciliation Act of 1986 (COBRA) allows employees to continue their health insurance coverage at their own expense for a period of time after their employment ends. For most employees ceasing work for health reasons, the period of time to which benefits may be extended ranges from eighteen to thirty-six months.

Qualifying events determine how long COBRA coverage will be extended, such as:

- Termination of employment—eighteen months of coverage

- Disability—eighteen to twenty-nine months of coverage (coinciding with the Medicare waiting period)

- Reduction of work hours with loss of benefits—eighteen months of coverage

- Death of covered employee—coverage can be continued indefinitely for an eligible spouse, or until age twenty-three or marriage for dependents

- Divorce or legal separation from covered employee—thirty-six months of coverage

Medical benefits provided under the terms of the plan and available to COBRA beneficiaries may include the following:

- Inpatient and outpatient hospital care

- Physician care

- Surgery and other major medical benefits

- Prescription drugs

- Any other medical benefits, such as dental and vision care

If an employee is entitled to COBRA benefits, the employer must give the employee notice of his or her right to continue benefits provided by the plan. The employee must reply within sixty days to accept coverage or forfeit his or her right to continued coverage.

Note: Life insurance is not a benefit that must be offered to individuals for purposes of health continuation coverage.

Chapter 46

Public Benefits, Insurance, and Housing Options for Persons with HIV

Chapter Contents

Section 46.1

Social Security for People Living with HIV/AIDS

Reprinted from "Social Security for People Living with HIV/AIDS," Social Security Administration, February 2005. The full text of this document is available online at http://www.ssa.gov/pubs/10019.html; accessed May 23, 2010.

If you have human immunodeficiency virus (HIV) or acquired immunodeficiency syndrome (AIDS) and cannot work, you may qualify for disability benefits from the Social Security Administration. Your disability must be expected to last at least a year or end in death, and must be serious enough to prevent you from doing substantial gainful work.

If your child has HIV/AIDS, he or she may be able to get Supplemental Security Income (SSI) if your household income is low enough.

We pay disability benefits under two programs: the Social Security disability insurance program for people who paid Social Security taxes; and the Supplemental Security Income program for people who have little income and few resources. If your Social Security benefits are very low and you have limited other income and resources, you may qualify for benefits from both programs.

How do I qualify for Social Security disability benefits?

When you work and pay Social Security taxes, you earn Social Security credits. (Most people earn the maximum of four credits a year.) The number of years of work needed for disability benefits depends on how old you are when you become disabled. Generally, you need five years of work in the ten years before the year you become disabled. Younger workers need fewer years of work. If your application is approved, your first Social Security disability benefit will be paid for the sixth full month after the date your disability began.

What will I get from Social Security?

The amount of your monthly benefits depends on how much you earned while you were working. You also will qualify for Medicare after you have been getting disability benefits for twenty-four months. Medicare helps pay for hospital and hospice care, lab tests, home health care, and other medical services.

How do I qualify for SSI disability payments?

If you have not worked long enough to get Social Security or your Social Security benefits are low, you may qualify for SSI payments if your total income and resources are low enough.

If you get SSI, you most likely will be eligible for food stamps and Medicaid. Medicaid takes care of your medical bills while you are in the hospital or receiving outpatient care. In some states, Medicaid pays for hospice care, a private nurse, and prescription drugs used to fight HIV disease. For more information about Medicaid, contact your local social services office.

How do I file for benefits?

You can apply for Social Security disability benefits online at www.socialsecurity.gov, or you can call our toll-free number, 1-800-772-1213 (for the deaf or hard of hearing, call our TTY number, 1-800-325-0778), to ask for an appointment. We can answer specific questions and provide information by automated phone service twenty-four hours a day.

We treat all calls confidentially. We also want to make sure you receive accurate and courteous service. That is why we have a second Social Security representative monitor some telephone calls.

How do you decide my claim?

All applications we receive from people with HIV/AIDS are processed as quickly as possible. Social Security works with an agency in each state called the Disability Determination Services.

The state agency will look at the information you and your doctor give us and decide if you qualify for benefits.

We can pay you SSI benefits right away for up to six months before we make a final decision on your claim if the following are true:

- You are not working

- You meet the SSI rules about income and resources

- Your doctor or other medical source certifies that your HIV infection is severe enough to meet our medical eligibility rules

How can I help speed up my claim?

You can help speed up the processing of your claim by having certain information when you apply. This includes the following:

- Your Social Security number and birth certificate and the Social Security numbers and birth certificates of any family members who may be applying for benefits

- A copy of your most recent W-2 form. (If you are applying for SSI, we also will need information about your income and resources; for example, bank statements, unemployment records, rent receipts, and car registration.)

We also need information about the following things:

- The names and addresses of any doctors, hospitals, or clinics you have been to for treatment

- How HIV/AIDS has affected your daily activities, such as cleaning, shopping, cooking, taking the bus, etc.

- The kinds of jobs you have had during the past fifteen years

Additionally, we will ask your doctor to complete a form telling us how your HIV infection has affected you. Call the 800 number to ask for form "SSA-4814" for adults or "SSA-4815" for children.

You should take the form to your doctor to complete and bring or send the completed form to us.

What happens if I go back to work?

If you return to work, there are special rules that let your benefits continue while you work. These rules are important for people with HIV/AIDS who may be able to go back to work when they are feeling better.

Section 46.2

Insurance Options for People with HIV

Excerpted from "Insurance," AIDS.gov, October 2010.

Insurance Options for People with Human Immunodeficiency Virus (HIV)

Because it can be very expensive to treat HIV, it's important to know what your health insurance options are if you are living with HIV disease. Some of the options are as follows.

Group Health Insurance Plans

Group health insurance is private insurance that often comes with employment. Many of these programs cover comprehensive medical care, including hospital visits, outpatient care (clinic settings), prescription coverage, and specialist visits. In some cases, however, you may still have to pay for some of your healthcare costs, even if you have private insurance. Some of these costs might include co-pays or premiums.

Individual Health Insurance Policies

You may be able to buy an individual health insurance policy, but they tend to be more expensive and require a pre-screening application that may exclude coverage for preexisting conditions, like HIV disease.

Public Healthcare Programs

If you don't have health insurance—or you need help because your insurance doesn't pay for the care you need—the programs listed below can help by paying for care that is delivered by local and state agencies:

- **Ryan White HIV/AIDS Program:** Funds outpatient primary care, HIV/AIDS drugs, and supportive services only when other public or private sources are not available.

- **Medicaid:** Supports healthcare for low-income individuals who meet eligibility requirements. Medicaid is administered by states, and each state sets its own guidelines for eligibility and services.

- **Medicare:** Federal health insurance program that supports medical care for those who qualify based on work history, age, and disability status.

- **Other programs that pay for HIV/AIDS medications:** These include: the Ryan White AIDS Drug Assistance Program (ADAP); Medicare Part D; patient assistance programs; and clinical trials.

Health Insurance Portability and Accountability Act (HIPAA)

The Health Insurance Portability and Accountability Act of 1996 (HIPAA) is not a type of insurance—but it was designed to make it easier for people to get and keep health insurance.

HIPAA has three main functions:

- It protects people with group insurance coverage from discriminatory treatment.

- It enables small groups (such as businesses with a small number of employees) to get, and keep, health insurance coverage more easily.

- It gives people new options for getting individual coverage when they lose or leave their group insurance (because of a job change or being fired/laid off, etc.).

This law provides several protections important to people with HIV/AIDS:

- It limits (but doesn't eliminate) the ability of insurance companies to exclude you from coverage if you have a preexisting condition.

- If you have a family member who has had health problems in the past, or is having them now, HIPAA keeps group health plans from denying you coverage or charging additional fees for coverage because of your family member's health.

- It guarantees certain small business employers (and certain individuals who lose job-related coverage) the right to purchase individual health insurance.

- HIPAA guarantees, in most cases, that employers or individuals who purchase health insurance can renew the coverage, regardless of any health conditions of individuals covered under the insurance policy.

Section 46.3

Housing Options for People with HIV

"Housing Options for HIV-Positive People," © 2010 The Well Project (www.thewellproject.org). Reprinted with permission.

Getting Started

Having a safe and affordable place to live is important to everyone's quality of life. When you are human immunodeficiency virus (HIV)–positive, it is also an important part of taking care of your overall health. One reason for this is that taking your HIV drugs can be hard without access to stable housing, clean water, bathrooms, refrigeration, and food.

Finding affordable housing can sometimes be difficult. A good place to begin is a housing assistance program or acquired immunodeficiency syndrome (AIDS) service organization (ASO) in your area. The Housing Opportunities for Persons Living with AIDS (HOPWA) is a housing resource for HIV-positive people and has programs in many U.S. cities.

Once you find a housing program or ASO, call and ask to speak with the "housing search advocate" or "someone to help me look for housing." The housing advocate can explain the different options available to you and help you with applications.

General Information

Different housing programs help people in different situations. For example, some only help single people and some help only families. Ask your housing advocate what the eligibility requirements are for the programs in your area.

Other examples of eligibility requirements include:

- income level;

- HIV status and/or the stage of your illness;

- age;

- gender;

- other health problems, disabilities, mental illness, or substance abuse problems;

- criminal record.

What you pay in rent depends on what type of housing you find. If you get housing through a government program, the program will provide some kind of help with rent. Generally you will pay about one-third of your household income toward rent and utilities and the program will pay the rest.

Sometimes people are discriminated against when they are looking for housing because of things like race, sexual orientation, physical disability (including HIV), or source of income. If you think this is the case, let your housing advocate know and ask about assistance from a legal advocate.

Unless you are applying for housing specifically for HIV-positive people, you are not required to disclose your HIV status to the housing agency. You may need a letter from a public agency or your healthcare provider stating you have a disability, but it does not need to state your HIV diagnosis.

Housing Options

Different housing options are available in different places. Check to see what is available in your community.

Emergency Housing

- Provided by shelters, churches, community groups, YMCAs

- Allow you to stay for thirty to ninety days

- May be able to find you more permanent housing

- Sometimes do not allow you to stay in shelter during the day

Transitional Housing

- Housing you can stay in for a short period of time (up to three years), so it's important to have a plan in place for moving on to a more permanent residence.

- These programs can help you find permanent housing while you are living there.
- Sometimes you have to share an apartment or share a kitchen and bathroom.
- Some programs are just for HIV-positive people and/or people in recovery from drugs and alcohol.

HIV Residential Program

- Permanent housing for HIV-positive people
- You can stay there as long as you pay your rent and follow the rules
- Some programs provide you with your own apartment
- Some programs provide you with your own bedroom and you have to share a bathroom and a kitchen
- A residential program is suitable if you are looking for a lot of support and help

HIV Scattered-Site Housing

HIV-specific housing programs called "scattered-site housing" are agencies that refer you to a building or help you find an apartment in the community:

- A social service agency rents the apartment to you or you may have the lease in your name.
- Sometimes can assist with telephone, heating, electric, and moving costs.
- May provide HIV/AIDS case management services You can stay in your apartment as long as you pay the rent and follow the program rules.

Public Housing Authorities

Public housing authorities offer several different housing assistance programs for low-income people and persons living with disabilities (including HIV). Not every community has a housing authority; however, many larger cities do.

Housing authorities provide multiple types of assistance:

- Housing in buildings they own—"public housing."

- Rental assistance subsidies (help paying rent). Subsidies are not attached to a particular apartment or building. You need to find an apartment in the community and the subsidy helps to pay the rent and utilities.

- Project-based units are set aside in buildings.

Eligibility for these programs is based on your family's household size and income, and in some cases, your current living status (if homeless) and age (for senior housing). If social security is your only source of income, you are probably eligible.

Some agencies have special housing available for the elderly and disabled. If you are disabled, let the housing authority know when you apply. However, you don't have to let them know what your specific disability is.

There may be more than one housing authority in the area where you want to live, especially if you are looking in a large city. You will need to contact each housing authority to find out where they take applications, what is available, and how long you will be on the waiting list. In many cases, you will be on the waiting list for months or even years, so apply as soon as possible. Fill out applications at as many authorities as you can, even places that might not be your first choice.

You can find housing authority contact information for your state by going to the U.S. Department of Housing and Urban Development (HUD) website at http://www.hud.gov/offices/pih/pha/contacts/index.cfm.

Private Rental Market

You can try and find an apartment through the newspapers or a realtor. If you do this you will have to pay full rent. However, you may be able to find a program that will assist you with the rent through a subsidy (financial assistance). Ask your housing advocate about this option.

If you rent an apartment and get a subsidy, you will pay a portion of your household income toward rent and utilities. The housing agency or program will pay the rest directly to the landlord. You do not need to tell your landlord why you are receiving a subsidy—that information is confidential.

Homelessness

Homelessness is a problem that affects many people in the United States, including many HIV-positive people. Treating your HIV and taking care of your overall health can be difficult if you are homeless.

If you are homeless there are programs that provide a range of services, including shelter, food, counseling, and jobs-skills training. For help and resource information contact a local homeless assistance agency or go to the HUD website at http://www.hud.gov/homeless/index.cfm or the National Coalition for the Homeless website at http://www.nationalhomeless.org.

If you fear you could become homeless, it may be possible to avoid it by finding emergency assistance programs in your area that can help pay rent or bills. Some programs are run by the state, county, or local division of housing assistance, or by the division of social/human services. Try looking in the government listings in your phone book for these agencies. Churches and nonprofit organizations also offer emergency help.

Homeowners with problems that could result in losing their homes can contact a HUD-approved, housing-counseling agency for advice on defaults, foreclosures, and credit issues. Renters can also call for advice. For an agency near you, contact 800-569-4287.

Special Considerations for Women

Finding the right housing for women with HIV can have its own set of challenges. Many HIV-positive women do not earn enough money to afford a decent place to live because they are taking care of children, spouses, and other family members. Women may find that they qualify for housing, but their loved ones (especially male partners and teen-age sons) don't.

It can be helpful to look beyond HIV-related housing for women and families. There may be housing and shelter options available for battered women, for pregnant women, for women coming out of jail, and for women needing substance abuse treatment. Talk to your case manager or housing advocate about the people you are caring for and your housing needs in order to find the best program for you.

Chapter 47

Caring for Someone with AIDS at Home

How to Get Ready to Take Care of Someone at Home

Every situation is different, but here are some tips to get you started:

- Take a home care course, if possible. Learn the skills you need to take care of someone at home and how to manage special situations. Your local Red Cross chapter, Visiting Nurses Association, state health department, or HIV/AIDS service organization can help you find a home care course.

- Talk with the person you will be caring for. Ask them what they need. If you are nervous about caring for them, say so. Ask if it is OK for you to talk to their doctor, nurse, social worker, case manager, other healthcare professional, or lawyer when you need to. Together you can work out what is best for both of you.

- Talk with the doctor, nurse, social worker, case manager, and other healthcare workers who are also providing care. They may need the patient's permission, sometimes in writing, to talk to you, but you need to talk to these people to find out how you can help. Work with them and the person you are caring for to develop a plan for who does what.

- Get clear, written information about medicines and other care you'll give. Ask what each drug does and what side effects to look out for.

Excerpted from the Centers for Disease Control and Prevention, June 21, 2007.

- Ask the doctor or nurse what changes in the person's health or behavior to watch for. For example, a cough, fever, diarrhea, or confusion may mean an infection or problem that needs a new medicine or even putting the person in the hospital.

- You also need to know whom to call for help or information and when to call them. Make a list of doctors, nurses, and other people you might need to talk to quickly, their phone numbers, and when they are available. Keep this list by the phone.

- Talk to a lawyer or AIDS support organization. For some medical care or life support decisions, you may need to be legally named as the care coordinator. If you are going to help file insurance claims, apply for government aid, pay bills, or handle other business for the person with AIDS, you may also need a power of attorney. There are many sources of help for people with AIDS, and you can help the person with AIDS get what they are entitled to.

- Think about joining a support group or talking to a counselor. Taking care of someone who is sick can be hard emotionally as well as physically. Talking about it with people with the same kind of worries helps sometimes. You can learn how other people cope and realize that you are not alone.

- Take care of yourself. You can't take care of someone else if you are sick or upset. Get the rest and exercise you need to keep going. You also need to do some things you enjoy, such as visit your friends and relatives. Many AIDS service organizations can help with "respite care" and send someone to be with the person you're caring for while you get out of the house for awhile.

Giving Care

People living with AIDS should take care of themselves as much as they can for as long as they can. They need to be and feel as independent as possible. They need to control their own schedules, make their own decisions, and do what they want to do as much as they are able.

There are some simple things you can do to help someone with AIDS feel comfortable at home:

- Respect their independence and privacy.

- Give them control as much as possible. Ask to enter their room, ask permission to sit with them, etc. Saying "Can I help you with that?" lets them keep control.

- Ask them what you can do to make them comfortable. Many people feel shy about asking for help, especially help with things like using the toilet, bathing, shaving, eating, and dressing.

- Keep the home clean and looking bright and cheerful.

- Let the person with AIDS stay in a room that is near a bathroom.

- Leave tissues, towels, a trash basket, extra blankets, and other things the person might need close by so these things can be reached from the bed or chair.

If the person you care for has to spend most of their time in bed, be sure to help them change position often. If possible, a person with AIDS should get out of bed as often as they can. A nurse can show you how to help someone move from a bed to a chair without hurting yourself or them. This helps prevent stiff joints, bedsores, and some kinds of pneumonia. They may also need your help to turn over or to adjust the pillows or blankets. A medical "trapeze" over the bed can help the person shift position by themselves if they are strong enough. If they are so weak they can't turn over, have a nurse show you how to use a sheet to help roll the person in bed from side to side. Usually a person in bed needs to change position at least every four hours.

Bedsores

Bedsores or other broken skin can be serious problems for someone with AIDS. In addition to changing position in bed often, to help keep skin healthy, put extra-soft material (sheepskin, "egg crate" foam, or water mattresses) under the person, keep the sheets dry and free from wrinkles, and massage the back and other parts of the body (like hips, elbows, and ankles) that press down on the bed. Report any red or broken areas on the skin to the doctor or nurse right away.

Exercises

Even in bed, a person can do simple arm, hand, leg, and foot exercises. These are usually called "range of motion" exercises. These exercises help prevent stiff, sore points and help keep the blood moving. A doctor, nurse, or physical therapist can show you how to help.

Breathing

If someone is having trouble breathing, sitting them up may help. Raise the head of a hospital-type bed or use extra pillows or some other soft back support. If they have severe trouble breathing, they need to see a doctor.

Providing Emotional Support

You are caring for a person, not just a body; their feelings are important too. Since every person is different, there are no rules about what to do or say, but here are some ideas that may help:

- Keep them involved in their care. Don't do everything for them or make all their decisions. Nobody likes feeling helpless.

- Have them help out around the house if they can. Everybody likes to feel useful. They want to be part of the group, contributing what they can.

- Include them in the household. Make them part of normal talk about books, TV shows, music, what is going on in the world, and so on. Many people will want to feel involved in the things that are happening around them. But you don't always have to talk; just being there is sometimes enough. Just watching TV together or sitting and reading in the same room is often comforting.

- Talk about things. Sometimes they may need to talk about AIDS or talk through their own situation as a way to think out loud. Having AIDS can make a person angry, frustrated, depressed, scared, and lonely, just like any other serious illness. Listening, trying to understand, showing you care, and helping them work through their emotions is a big part of home care. A support group of other people with AIDS can also be a good place for them to talk things out. Contact the National Association of People with AIDS for information about support groups in your area. If they want professional counseling, help them get it.

- Invite their friends over to visit. A little socializing can be good for everyone.

- Touch them. Hug them, kiss them, pat them, hold their hands to show that you care. Some people may not want physical closeness, but if they do, touch is a powerful way of saying you care.

- Get out together. If they are able, go to social events, shopping, riding around, walking around the block, or just into the park, yard, or porch to sit in the sun and breath fresh air.

Guarding Against Infections

People living with AIDS can get very sick from common germs and infections. Hugging, holding hands, giving massages, and many other types of touching are safe for you, and needed by the person with AIDS. But you have to be careful not to spread germs that can hurt the person you are caring for.

Wash Your Hands

Washing your hands is the single best way to kill germs. Do it often! Wash your hands after you go to the bathroom and before you fix food. Wash your hands again before and after feeding them, bathing them, helping them go to the bathroom, or giving other care. Wash your hands if you sneeze or cough; touch your nose, mouth, or genitals; handle garbage or animal litter; or clean the house. If you touch anybody's blood, semen, urine, vaginal fluid, or feces, wash your hands immediately. If you are caring for more than one person, wash your hands after helping one person and before helping the next person. Wash your hands with warm, soapy water for at least fifteen seconds. Clean under your fingernails and between your fingers. If your hands get dry or sore, put on hand cream or lotion, but keep washing your hands frequently.

Cover Your Sores

If you have any cuts or sores, especially on your hands, you must take extra care not to infect the person with AIDS or yourself. If you have cold sores, fever blisters, or any other skin infection, don't touch the person or their things. You could pass your infection to them. If you have to give care, cover your sores with bandages, and wash your hands before touching the person. If the rash or sores are on your hands, wear disposable gloves. Do not use gloves more than one time; throw them away and get a new pair. If you have boils, impetigo, or shingles, if at all possible, stay away from the person with AIDS until you are well.

Keep Sick People Away

If you or anybody else is sick, stay away from the person with AIDS until you're well. A person with AIDS often can't fight off colds, flu, or other common illnesses. If you are sick and nobody else can do what needs to be done for the person with AIDS, wear a well-fitting, surgical-type mask that covers your mouth and nose and wash your hands before coming near the person with AIDS.

Watch Out for Chickenpox

Chickenpox can kill a person with AIDS. If the person you are caring for has already had the chickenpox, they probably won't get it again. But, just to be on the safe side:

- Never let anybody with chickenpox in the same room as a person with AIDS, at least not until all the chickenpox sores have completely crusted over.

- Don't let anybody who recently has been near somebody with chickenpox in the same room as a person who has AIDS. After three weeks, the person who was exposed to the chickenpox can visit, if they aren't sick. Most adults have had chickenpox, but you have to be very careful about children visiting or living in the house if they have not yet had chickenpox. If you are the person who was near somebody with chickenpox and you have to help the person with AIDS, wear a well-fitting, surgical-type mask, wash your hands before doing what you have to do for the person with AIDS, and stay in the room as short a time as you can. Tell the person with AIDS why you are staying away from them.

- Don't let anybody with shingles (herpes zoster) near a person with AIDS until all the shingles have healed over. The germ that causes shingles can also cause chickenpox. If you have shingles and have to help the person with AIDS, cover all the sores completely and wash your hands carefully before helping the person with AIDS.

- Call the doctor as soon as possible if the person with AIDS does get near somebody with chickenpox or shingles. There is a medicine that can make the chickenpox less dangerous, but it must be given very soon after the person has been around someone with the germ.

Get Your Shots

Everybody living with or helping take care of a person with AIDS should make sure they took all their "childhood" shots (immunizations). This is not only to keep you from getting sick, but also to keep you from getting sick and accidentally spreading the illness to the person with AIDS. Just to be sure, ask your doctor if you need any shots or boosters for measles, mumps, or rubella, since these shots may not have been available when you were a child. Discuss any vaccinations with your doctor and the doctor of the person with AIDS before you get the shot. If the person with AIDS is near a person with measles, call the doctor that day. There is a medicine that can make the measles less dangerous, but it has to be given very soon after the person is around the germ.

Children or adults who live with someone with AIDS and who need to get vaccinated against polio should get an injection with "inactivated virus" vaccine. The regular oral polio vaccine has weakened polio virus that can spread from the person who got the vaccine to the person with AIDS and give them polio.

Everyone living with a person with AIDS should get a flu shot every year to reduce the chances of spreading the flu to the person with AIDS. Everyone living with a person with AIDS should be checked for tuberculosis (TB) every year.

Be Careful with Pets and Gardening

Pets can give love and companionship. Having a pet around can make a person with AIDS feel better and enjoy life more. However, people with HIV or AIDS should not touch pet litter boxes, feces, bird droppings, or water in fish tanks. Many pet animals carry germs that don't make healthy people sick, but can make the person with AIDS very sick. A person with AIDS can have pets, but must wash their hands with soap and water after handling the pet. Someone who does not have HIV infection must clean the litter boxes, cages, fish tanks, pet beds, and other things. Wear rubber gloves when you clean up after pets and wash your hands before and after cleaning. Empty litter boxes every day, don't just sift. Just like the people living with AIDS, pets need yearly checkups and current vaccinations. If the pet gets sick, take it to the veterinarian right away. Someone with AIDS should not touch a sick animal.

Gardening can also be a problem. Germs live in garden or potting soil. A person with AIDS can garden, but they must wear work gloves while handling dirt and must wash their hands before and after handling dirt. You should do the same.

Personal Items

A person with HIV infection should not share razors, toothbrushes, tweezers, nail or cuticle scissors, pierced earrings or other "pierced" jewelry, or any other item that might have their blood on it.

Laundry

Clothes and bed sheets used by someone with AIDS can be washed the same way as other laundry. If you use a washing machine, either hot or cold water can be used, with regular laundry detergent. If clothes or sheets have blood, vomit, semen, vaginal fluids, urine, or feces on them, use disposable gloves and handle the clothes or sheets as little as possible. Put them in plastic bags until you can wash them. You can but you don't need to add bleach to kill HIV; a normal wash cycle will kill the virus. Clothes may also be dry cleaned or hand-washed. If stains from blood, semen, or vaginal fluids are on the clothes, soaking them in cold water before washing will help remove the stains. Fabrics and furniture can be cleaned with soap and water or cleansers you can buy in a store; just follow the directions on the box. Wear gloves while cleaning.

Cleaning House

Cleaning kills germs that may be dangerous to the person with AIDS. You may want to clean and dust the house every week. Clean tubs, showers, and sinks often; use household cleaners, then rinse with fresh water. You may want to mop floors at least once a week. Clean the toilet often; use bleach mixed with water or a commercial toilet bowl cleaner. You may clean urinals and bedpans with bleach after each use. Replace plastic urinals and bedpans every month or so. About one-quarter cup of bleach mixed with one gallon of water makes a good disinfectant for floors, showers, tubs, sinks, mops, sponges, etc. (Or one tablespoon of bleach in one quart of water for small jobs). Make a new batch each time because it stops working after about twenty-four hours. Be sure to keep the bleach and the bleach and water mix, like other dangerous chemicals, away from children.

Food

Someone with AIDS can eat almost anything they want; in fact, the more the better. A well-balanced diet with plenty of nutrients, fiber, and liquids is healthy for everybody. Fixing food for a person with AIDS takes a little care, although you should follow these same rules for fixing food for anybody:

- Don't use raw (unpasteurized) milk.

- Don't use raw eggs. Be careful: raw eggs may be in home-made mayonnaise, hollandaise sauce, ice cream, fruit drinks (smoothies), or other homemade foods.

- All beef, pork, chicken, fish, and other meats should be cooked well done, with no pink in the middle.

- Don't use raw fish or shellfish (like oysters).

- Wash your hands before handling food and wash them again between handling different foods.

- Wash all utensils (knives, spatulas, mixing spoons, etc.) before reusing them with other foods. If you taste food while cooking, use a clean spoon every time you taste; do not stir with the spoon you taste with.

- Don't let blood from uncooked beef, pork, or chicken or water from shrimp, fish, or other seafood touch other food.

- Use a cutting board to cut things on and wash it with soap and hot water between each food you cut.

- Wash fresh fruits and vegetables thoroughly. Cook or peel organic fruits and vegetables because they may have germs on the skins. Don't use organic lettuce or other organic vegetables that cannot be peeled or cooked.

A person living with AIDS does not need separate dishes, knives, forks, or spoons. Their dishes don't need special cleaning either. Just wash all the dishes together with soap or detergent in hot water.

A person with AIDS can fix food for other people. Just like everybody else who fixes food, people with AIDS should wash their hands first and not lick their fingers or the utensils while they are cooking. However, no one who has diarrhea should fix food.

To keep food from spoiling, serve hot foods hot and cold foods cold. Cover leftover food and store it in the refrigerator as soon as possible.

Protect Yourself

A person who has AIDS may sometimes have infections that can make you sick. You can protect yourself, however. Talk to the doctor or nurse to find out what germs can infect you and other people in the house. This is very important if you have HIV infection yourself.

For example, diarrhea can be caused by several different germs. Wear disposable gloves if you have to clean up after or help a person with diarrhea and wash your hands carefully after you take the gloves off. Do not use disposable gloves more than one time.

Another cause of diarrhea is the cryptosporidiosis parasite. It is spread from the feces of one person or animal to another person or animal, often by contaminated water, raw food, or food that isn't cooked well enough. Again, wash your hands after using the bathroom and before fixing food. You can check with your local health department to see if cryptosporidiosis is in the water. If you hear that the water in your community may have cryptosporidiosis parasites, boil your drinking water for at least one minute to kill the parasite, then let the water cool before drinking. You may want to buy bottled (distilled) water for cooking and drinking if the cryptosporidiosis parasite or other organisms that might make a person with HIV infection sick could be in the tap water.

If the person with AIDS has a cough that lasts longer than a week, the doctor should check them for TB. If they do have TB, then you and everybody else living in the house should be checked for TB infection, even if you aren't coughing. If you are infected with TB germs, you can take medicine that will prevent you from developing TB.

If the person with AIDS gets yellow jaundice (a sign of acute hepatitis) or has chronic hepatitis B infection, you and everybody else living in the house and any people the person with AIDS has had sex with should talk to their doctor to see if anyone needs to take medicine to prevent hepatitis. All children should get hepatitis B vaccine whether or not they are around a person with AIDS.

If the person with AIDS has fever blisters or cold sores (herpes simplex) around the mouth or nose, don't kiss or touch the sores. If you have to touch the sores to help the person, wear gloves and wash your hands carefully as soon as you take the gloves off. This is especially important if you have eczema (allergic skin) since the herpes simplex virus can cause severe skin disease in people with eczema. Throw the used gloves away; never use disposable gloves more than once.

Many persons with or without AIDS are infected with a virus called cytomegalovirus (CMV), which can be spread in urine or saliva. Wash your hands after touching urine or saliva from a person with AIDS. This is especially important for someone who may be pregnant because a pregnant woman infected with CMV can also infect her unborn child. CMV causes birth defects such as deafness.

Remember, to protect yourself and the person with AIDS from these diseases and others, be sure to wash your hands with soap and water before and after giving care, when handling food, after taking gloves off, and after going to the bathroom.

Gloves

Because the virus that causes AIDS is in the blood of infected persons, blood or other body fluids (such as bloody feces) that have blood in them could infect you. You can protect yourself by following some simple steps. Wear gloves if you have to touch semen, vaginal fluid, cuts or sores on the person with AIDS, or blood or body fluids that may have blood in them. Wear gloves to give care to the mouth, rectum, or genitals of the person with AIDS. Wear gloves to change diapers or sanitary pads or to empty bedpans or urinals. If you have any cuts, sores, rashes, or breaks in your skin, cover them with a bandage. If the cuts or sores are on your hands, use bandages and gloves. Wear gloves to clean up urine, feces, or vomit to avoid all the germs, HIV and other kinds, that might be there.

There are two types of gloves you can use. Use disposable, hospital-type latex or vinyl gloves to take care of the person with AIDS if there is any blood you might touch. Use these gloves one time, then throw them away. Do not use latex gloves more than one time even if they are marked "reusable." You can buy hospital-type gloves by the box at most drugstores, along with urinals, bedpans, and many other medical supplies. Many insurance companies and Medicaid will pay for these gloves if the doctor writes a prescription for them. For cleaning blood or bloody fluids from floors, bed, etc., you can use household rubber gloves, which are sold at any drug or grocery store. These gloves can be cleaned and reused. Clean them with hot, soapy water and with a mixture of bleach and water (about one-quarter cup bleach to one gallon of water). Be sure not to use gloves that are peeling, cracked, or have holes in them. Don't use the rubber gloves to take care of a person with AIDS; they are too thick and bulky.

To take gloves off, peel them down by turning them inside out. This will keep the wet side on the inside, away from your skin and other people. When you take the gloves off, wash your hands with soap and water right away. If there is a lot of blood, you can wear an apron or smock to keep your clothes from getting bloody. (If the person with AIDS is bleeding a lot or very often, call the doctor or nurse.) Clean up spilled blood as soon as you can. Put on gloves, wipe up the blood with paper towels or rags, put the used paper towels or rags in plastic bags to get rid of later, then wash the area where the blood was with a mix of bleach and water.

Since HIV can be in semen, vaginal fluid, or breast milk just as it can be in blood, you should be as careful with these fluids as you are with blood.

If you get blood, semen, vaginal fluid, breast milk, or other body fluid that might have blood in it in your eyes, nose, or mouth, immediately pour as much water as possible over where you got splashed, then call the doctor, explain what happened, and ask what else you should do.

Needles and Syringes

A person with AIDS may need needles and syringes to take medicine for diseases caused by AIDS or for diabetes, hemophilia, or other illnesses. If you have to handle these needles and syringes, you must be careful not to stick yourself. That is one way you could get infected with HIV.

Use a needle and syringe only one time. Do not put caps back on needles. Do not take needles off syringes. Do not break or bend needles. If a needle falls off a syringe, use something like tweezers or pliers to pick it up; do not use your fingers. Touch needles and syringes only by the barrel of the syringe. Hold the sharp end away from yourself.

Put the used needle and syringe in a puncture-proof container. The doctor, nurse, or an AIDS service organization can give you a special container. If you don't have one, use a puncture-proof container with a plastic top, such as a coffee can. Keep a container in any room where needles and syringes are used. Put it well out of the reach of children or visitors, but in a place you can easily and quickly put the needle and syringe after they are used. When the container gets nearly full, seal it and get a new container. Ask the doctor or nurse how to get rid of the container with the used needles and syringes.

If you get stuck with a needle used on the person with AIDS, don't panic. The chances are very good (better than 99 percent) that you will not be infected. However, you need to act quickly to get medical care. Put the needle in the used needle container, then wash where you stuck yourself as soon as you can, using warm, soapy water. Right after washing, call the doctor or the emergency room of a hospital, no matter what time it is, explain what happened, and ask what else you should do. Your doctor may want you to take medicine, such as azidothymidine (AZT). If you are going to take AZT, you should begin taking it as soon as possible, certainly within a few hours of the needle stick.

Wastes

Flush all liquid waste (urine, vomit, etc.) that has blood in it down the toilet. Be careful not to splash anything when you are pouring liquids into the toilet. Toilet paper and tissues with blood, semen, vaginal fluid, or breast milk may also be flushed down the toilet.

Paper towels, sanitary pads and tampons, wound dressings and bandages, diapers, and other items with blood, semen, or vaginal fluid on them that cannot be flushed should be put in plastic bags. Put the items in the bag, then close and seal the bag. Ask the doctor, nurse, or local health department about how to get rid of things with blood, urine, vomit, semen, vaginal fluid, or breast milk on them. If you can't have plastic bags handy, wrap the materials in enough newspaper to stop any leaks. Wear gloves when handling anything with blood, semen, vaginal fluids, or breast milk on it.

Sex

If you used to or still do have sex with a person with HIV infection, and you didn't use latex condoms the right way every time you had sex, you could have HIV infection, too. You can talk to your doctor or a counselor about taking an HIV antibody test. The idea of being tested for HIV may be scary. But if you are infected, the sooner you find out and start getting medical care, the better off you will be. Talk to your sex partner about what will need to change. It is very important that you protect yourself and your partner from transmitting HIV infection and other sexually transmitted diseases. Talk about types of sex that don't risk HIV infection. If you decide to have sexual intercourse (vaginal, anal, or oral), use condoms. Latex condoms can protect you from HIV infection if they are used the right way every time you have sex.

Other Help You Can Give

Dealing with hospitals or insurance companies, filling out forms, and looking up records can be difficult even if you are well. Many people with AIDS need help with these tasks:

- Getting a ride to the doctor's office, clinic, drugstore, or other places can be a problem. Don't wait to be asked; offer to help.

- Keeping a diary of medical events and other information for the person you are taking care of can help them and any other people who are helping. Be sure the person you are caring for knows what you are writing and helps keep the diary if they can.

- Keeping a record of medicine and other care for the doctor or the other people providing care can help a lot. Make sure you know what drugs the person is taking, how often they should take them, and what side effects to watch out for. The doctor, nurse, or pharmacist can tell you what to do. People who are sick sometimes forget to take medicine or take too much or too little. Divided pillboxes or a chart showing what medicines to take, when to take them, and how much of each to take can help.

- If the person you are caring for has to go into the hospital, you can still help. Take a special picture or other favorite things to the hospital. Tell the hospital staff of any special needs or habits the person has or if you see any problems. Most of all, visit often.

Children with AIDS

Infants and children with HIV infection or AIDS need the same things as other children—lots of love and affection. Small children need to be held, played with, kissed, hugged, fed, and rocked to sleep. As they grow, they need to play, have friends, and go to school, just like other kids. Kids with HIV are still kids, and need to be treated like any other kids in the family.

Kids with AIDS need much of the same care that grown-ups with AIDS need, but there are a few extra things to look out for:

- Watch for any changes in health or the way the child acts. If you notice anything unusual for that child, let the doctor know. For a child with AIDS, little problems can become big problems very quickly. Watch for breathing problems, fever, unusual sleepiness, diarrhea, or changes in how much they eat. Talk to the child's doctor about what else to look for and when to report it.

- Talk to the doctor before the child gets any immunizations (including oral polio vaccine) or booster shots. Some vaccines could make the child sick. No child with HIV or anyone in the household should ever take oral polio vaccine.

- Stuffed and furry toys can hold dirt and might hide germs that can make the child sick. Plastic and washable toys are better. If the child has any stuffed toys, wash them in a washing machine often and keep them as clean as possible.

- Keep the child away from litter boxes and sandboxes that a pet or other animal might have been in.

- Ask the child's doctor what to do about pets that might be in the house.

- Try to keep the child from getting infectious diseases, especially chickenpox. If the child with HIV infection gets near somebody with chickenpox, tell the child's doctor right away. Chickenpox can kill a child with AIDS.

- Bandage any cuts or scrapes quickly and completely after washing with soap and warm water. Use gloves if the child is bleeding.

Taking care of a child who is sick is very hard for people who love that child. You will need help and emotional support. You are not alone. There are people who can help you get through this.

Changing Symptoms

People with AIDS seem to get very sick, then get better, then get very sick, then better, and so on. Sometimes they get sicker and sicker. You can't always tell if they are going to live through a particular illness or not. These times are very rough on everyone involved. If you know what to expect, you can deal with these rough times better.

Dementia (having trouble thinking) can be a problem for a person with AIDS. AIDS can affect the brain and cause poor memory; short attention span; trouble moving, speaking, or thinking; less alertness; loss of interest in things; and wide mood swings. These problems can upset the person with AIDS as well as the people around them. Mental problems can make it hard to follow the planned routines for care and make it difficult to protect the person with AIDS from infections. Be prepared to recognize these problems, understand what is happening, and talk to the doctor, nurse, social worker, or mental health worker about what to do.

If the person you are caring for does develop mental problems, you can help:

- Keep important things in the same place all the time, a place that is easy to reach and easy to see.

- If you need to, remind the person you are caring for where they are and who you are.

- Put a clock and a calendar where the person you are caring for can see them. Mark off the days on the calendar. Write in what will happen each day.

- Put up pictures of people who might be in the house with their names on the pictures where the person with AIDS can see them.

- Speak in short, simple sentences.

639

- Don't be afraid to be firm. Remove things like dangerous objects from reach.

- Keep the sound from TVs, radios, and other noises down so the person doesn't get confused by unexpected sounds.

- Talk to a healthcare worker who deals with people with dementia about how to handle problems.

As AIDS Progresses

Here are some of the things to expect as AIDS enters its final stages and ways to try to cope. Like other people nearing death, a person with AIDS who is near death does the following things:

- Sleeps more and more and is hard to wake up. Try to talk to them and do things during those times when they do seem alert.

- Becomes confused about where they are, the time or date, or who people are. Tell them where they are, what time and day it is, and who people are. Don't scold them for forgetting, just tell them.

- Begins to wet their pants or lose bowel control. Clean them, using gloves, and use powder or lotion to prevent rashes. A catheter for passing urine may become necessary.

- Has skin that feels cool to the touch and may turn darker on the side of their body touching the bed as the circulation slows down. Keep them covered with warm blankets, but don't use electric blankets because they can burn a person with poor circulation.

- May have trouble seeing or hearing. Even so, never talk to other people as if the person with AIDS can't hear you. Always talk to the person with AIDS or anyone else in the room as if the person with AIDS hears you.

- May seem restless, pulling at the sheets on the bed or acting as if they see things that you don't. Stay calm, speak slowly, and reassure the person. Comfort them with gentle reminders about who you are and where they are.

- May stop eating and drinking. Wipe their mouth often with a wet cloth. Keep their lips wet with lip moisturizer.

- May almost stop urinating. If there is a catheter, it may need to be rinsed or flushed to keep it from getting blocked. A nurse can show you how to do this.

- Has noisy breathing because they can't cough up the fluids that collect in the back of their throat. Talk to their doctor; the doctor may suggest raising the head of the bed or putting extra pillows under their head. Turning them on their side may also help. If they can swallow, feed them some ice chips. If they have trouble swallowing, a cool, wet washcloth on the lips can keep their mouth and lips moist and may satisfy their thirst. If they begin to have irregular breathing or seem to stop breathing for a minute, call the doctor.

Hospice Care

Many people have found hospice care (programs for people who are dying and their caregivers) for adults and children a big help. Others feel that hospice care isn't right for them. Hospice services can help caregivers, family, and other loved ones, as well as help the dying person deal with the concerns and fears that may come near the end of their life. You should be able to find hospice organizations listed in your local phone book.

Final Arrangements

A person with AIDS, like every other adult, should have a will. This can be a difficult subject to discuss, but a will may need to be written before there is any question of the mental competence of the person with AIDS. You may want to be sure the person you are caring for has a will and that you know where it is.

Living wills, which specify what medical care the person with AIDS wants or does not want, also have to be written before their mental competence could be questioned. You, as the caregiver, may be the person asked to see that the doctors follow the wishes of the person with AIDS. This can be a very hard experience to deal with, but is another way of showing respect for a dying person. You may want to be sure the person you are caring for knows that they can control their medical care through living wills.

Often, people who know that they will die soon choose to make their own funeral or memorial arrangements. This helps make sure that the funeral will be done the way they want it done. It also makes things easier for those left behind. They no longer have to guess what their friend or loved one would have wanted. You may be asked to help the person with AIDS plan the funeral, make arrangements with the funeral home, and select a cemetery plot or mausoleum. You may be able to help the person with AIDS decide how they wish to be buried or if they want to be cremated.

After the death, there will still be things to do. Programs that have been providing help, such as Supplemental Security Income, will have to be officially informed of the death. Some money already sent or received may have to be returned. The will may name you, a relative, or another person as the one to handle these tasks.

Dying at Home

Whether or not to die at home is a big decision, but it may not have to be made right away. As the health of the person with AIDS changes, you and they may change your minds several times. However, it is something you should talk about with the person with AIDS ahead of time. Plans should be made; legal papers may need to be signed. What the dying person wants and needs, the needs and abilities of the caregivers and other loved ones, the advice of the doctors and other medical professionals, the advice of clergy or other spiritual leaders, may all need to be considered in deciding what is best. Consideration must be given to everyone living in the home. Small children and others may not be ready to cope with death in their home. Others in the home may prefer to face the final moments of the person with AIDS in familiar surroundings. Just be sure the person with AIDS knows that they will not die alone, that the people they love will try to be with them, wherever they choose to die. You also should get help to deal with your own grief after the death.

Help for You

Taking care of someone who is very sick is hard. It wears you down physically and emotionally and creates stress. You can get very angry watching a person you love get sicker and sicker no matter how hard you work or how much you care. You have to do something with this anger. Many people can talk out their anger with other people who have the same problems or with counselors, ministers, rabbis, friends, family, or health workers. Many AIDS service organizations can help you find people to talk to.

You should not try to be the only person taking care of someone with AIDS. You need some time for yourself. The sicker the person you are taking care of becomes, the more important this is. If you try to do everything yourself, you will wear yourself out and not be able to go on. You are not alone. Other people have done this before. Learn from them.

Part Seven

Additional Help and Information

Chapter 48

Glossary of HIV/AIDS-Related Terms

acquired immunodeficiency syndrome (AIDS): A disease of the body's immune system caused by the human immunodeficiency virus (HIV). AIDS is characterized by the death of CD4 cells (an important part of the body's immune system), which leaves the body vulnerable to life-threatening conditions, such as infections and cancers.

acute HIV infection: The period of rapid HIV replication that occurs two to four weeks after infection by HIV. Acute HIV infection is characterized by a drop in CD4 cell counts and an increase in HIV levels in the blood. Some, but not all, individuals experience flu-like symptoms during this period of infection.

adherence: Closely following (adhering to) a prescribed treatment regimen. Requires a patient to take the correct dose of a drug at the correct time, exactly as prescribed. Failure to adhere to an anti-HIV treatment regimen can lead to virologic failure and drug resistance.

AIDS-defining condition: Any of a list of illnesses that, when occurring in an HIV-infected person, leads to a diagnosis of AIDS, the most serious stage of HIV infection. AIDS is also diagnosed if an HIV-infected person has a CD4 count less than 200 cells/mm³, whether or not that person has an AIDS-defining condition.

antiretroviral therapy (ART): Treatment with drugs that inhibit the ability of retroviruses, such as HIV, to multiply in the body. The

---

Excerpted from "AIDS Glossary," AIDSinfo.gov, August 2010.

antiretroviral therapy recommended for HIV infection is referred to as highly active antiretroviral therapy (HAART), which uses a combination of drugs to attack HIV at different points in its life cycle.

B lymphocyte: Infection-fighting white blood cell that develops in the bone marrow and spleen. B lymphocytes produce antibodies. In people with HIV, the ability of B lymphocytes to do their job may be damaged.

baseline: An initial measurement (for example, CD4 count or viral load) made before starting treatment or therapy for a disease or condition. In people infected with HIV, the baseline measurement is used as a reference point to monitor HIV infection.

CD4 cell: A type of infection-fighting white blood cell that carries the CD4 receptor on its surface. CD4 cells coordinate the immune response, which signals other cells in the immune system to perform their special functions. The number of CD4 cells in a sample of blood is an indicator of the health of the immune system. HIV infects and kills CD4 cells, which leads to a weakened immune system.

CD4 cell count: A measurement of the number of CD4 cells in a sample of blood. The CD4 count is one of the most useful indicators of the health of the immune system and the progression of HIV/AIDS. A normal CD4 cell count is between 500 and 1,400 cells/mm^3 of blood, but an individual's CD4 count can vary. In HIV-infected individuals, a CD4 count at or below 200 cells/mm^3 is considered an AIDS-defining condition.

class-sparing regimen: An anti-HIV drug regimen that purposefully does not include one or more classes of anti-HIV drugs. A class-sparing regimen may be prescribed to save certain classes of drugs for later use or to avoid side effects specific to a class.

clinical failure: The occurrence or recurrence of HIV-related infections or a decline in physical health despite taking an HIV treatment regimen for a minimum of three months. Clinical failure may occur as a result of virologic or immunologic failure.

clinical progression: A term for the overall progression of a disease as measured by deterioration of clinical outcomes. In an HIV-infected person, clinical progression may be defined as the occurrence or recurrence of HIV-related events (after at least three months on an antiretroviral regimen), excluding immune reconstitution syndromes. HIV-infected patients who have a CD4 T-cell count less than 100 cells/mm^3 are considered to have a high likelihood of clinical progression.

co-infection: Infection with more than one virus, bacterium, or other microorganism at a given time. For example, an HIV-infected individual may be co-infected with hepatitis C virus (HCV) or tuberculosis (TB).

combination therapy: Two or more drugs used together to achieve optimal results in controlling HIV infection. Combination therapy has proven more effective in decreasing viral load than monotherapy, which is no longer recommended for the treatment of HIV.

discordant couple: A pair of long-term sexual partners in which one person is infected with a sexually transmitted infection (such as HIV) and the other is not.

drug resistance: The ability of some microorganisms to adapt so that they can multiply even in the presence of drugs that would normally kill them.

enzyme-linked immunosorbent assay (ELISA): A highly sensitive laboratory test used to determine the presence of antibodies to HIV in the blood or saliva.

false negative: A test or procedure result that incorrectly indicates a negative or normal result when an abnormal condition is actually present.

false positive: A test or procedure result that incorrectly indicates a positive or abnormal result when no abnormal condition is actually present.

genotypic assay: Also known as: Genotypic antiretroviral resistance test. A test that determines if HIV is resistant to particular anti-HIV drugs. The test analyzes a sample of the virus from an individual's blood to identify any genetic mutations that are associated with resistance to specific drugs.

highly active antiretroviral therapy (HAART): The name given to treatment regimens that aggressively suppress HIV replication and progression of HIV disease. The usual HAART regimen combines three or more anti-HIV drugs from at least two different classes.

human immunodeficiency virus (HIV): The virus that causes acquired immunodeficiency syndrome (AIDS). HIV is in the retrovirus family, and two types have been identified: HIV-1 and HIV-2. HIV-1 is responsible for most HIV infections throughout the world, whereas HIV-2 is found primarily in West Africa.

immune reconstitution syndrome (IRS): Also known as immune restoration disease (IRD) or immune reconstitution inflammatory syndrome (IRIS). An inflammatory reaction that can occur when an immunocompromised person's immune system improves, such as when a person with HIV disease begins anti-HIV treatment and experiences an increase in CD4 cell count. Fever, along with swelling, redness, or discharge at the site of an injury or infection, may signal that an infection that was previously unnoticed by a weak immune system is now a target of a stronger immune system. Although IRS indicates that a person's immune system has grown healthier, it can be a serious, sometimes fatal condition and must be treated aggressively.

immunocompromised: Unable to mount a normal immune response because of an impaired immune system.

immunodeficiency: Inability to produce normal amounts of antibodies, immune cells, or both.

immunologic failure: Occurs when an HIV-infected individual's CD4 count decreases below the baseline count or does not increase above the baseline count within the first year of anti-HIV treatment.

incubation period: The period between infection with a microorganism and the development of symptoms.

latency: The time period when an infectious organism is in the body but is not producing any noticeable symptoms. In HIV disease, latency usually occurs in the early years of infection. Also refers to the period when HIV has integrated its genome into a cell's deoxyribonucleic acid (DNA) but has not yet begun to replicate.

latent HIV reservoir: A collection of resting cells (such as T cells) in the body that are infected with HIV. The virus is spread within the body when these host cells become active.

maintenance therapy: A treatment to prevent an infection from coming back after it has been brought under control.

monotherapy: The use of only one drug to treat a disease. For HIV, combination therapy with three or more active anti-HIV drugs has proven to be more effective than monotherapy.

non-nucleoside reverse transcriptase inhibitor (NNRTI): A class of anti-HIV drugs that bind to and disable HIV-1's reverse transcriptase enzyme, a protein that HIV needs to make more copies of itself. Without functional reverse transcriptase, HIV replication is halted. Current NNRTI drugs are only effective against HIV-1 and not against HIV-2.

nucleoside analogue reverse transcriptase inhibitor (NRTI): A class of anti-HIV drug. Nucleoside analogues are faulty versions of the building blocks necessary for HIV reproduction. When HIV's reverse transcriptase enzyme uses a nucleoside analogue instead of a normal nucleoside, reproduction of the virus's genetic material is halted. Also called nucleoside analogues or nukes.

opportunistic infection (OI): An illness caused by any one of various organisms that occur in people with weakened immune systems, including people with HIV/AIDS.

post-exposure prophylaxis (PEP): Administration of anti-HIV drugs within seventy-two hours of a high-risk exposure, including unprotected sex, needle sharing, or occupational needle stick injury, to help prevent development of HIV infection.

pre-exposure prophylaxis (PrEP): The use of antiretroviral drugs as a preventive measure to potentially decrease the risk of HIV transmission.

rapid test: A type of HIV-1 enzyme-linked immunosorbent assay (ELISA) that can detect antibodies to HIV in the blood in less than thirty minutes with greater than 99 percent sensitivity and specificity. A positive rapid test result should be confirmed by an HIV Western blot test.

salvage therapy: Also known as rescue therapy. An HIV treatment regimen designed for people who have used many different anti-HIV drugs in the past, have failed at least two anti-HIV regimens, and have extensive drug resistance.

seroconversion: The process by which a newly infected person develops antibodies to HIV. These antibodies are then detectable by an HIV test. Seroconversion may occur anywhere from days to weeks or months following HIV infection.

superinfection: A new infection acquired on top of an existing infection. For example, a person infected with one strain of HIV-1 can, if exposed to a different strain, become infected with the new strain in addition to the existing strain. Superinfection can complicate HIV treatment by requiring additional drugs to target the newly introduced HIV strain.

T cell: A type of lymphocyte (disease-fighting white blood cell). The T stands for the thymus, the organ in which T cells mature. T cells include CD4 cells and CD8 cells, which are both critical components of the body's immune system.

therapeutic HIV vaccine: Any HIV vaccine used for the treatment of an HIV-infected person. Therapeutic HIV vaccines are designed to boost an individual's immune response to HIV infection to better control the virus. This therapeutic approach is currently being tested in clinical trials.

treatment failure: A broad term that describes failure of an anti-HIV treatment to adequately control HIV infection. The three types of HIV treatment failure are virologic, immunologic, and clinical failure. Factors that contribute to treatment failure include poor adherence, drug resistance, and drug toxicity.

undetectable viral load: The point at which levels of HIV RNA in the blood are too low to be detected with a viral load test. This does *not* mean that the virus has stopped replicating or has been removed from the body entirely, only that the small amount of virus remaining is below the test's ability to measure it.

viral load (VL): The amount of HIV RNA in a blood sample, reported as number of HIV RNA copies per milliliter of blood plasma. The VL provides information about the number of cells infected with HIV and is an important indicator of HIV progression and of how well treatment is working.

Western blot: A laboratory technique used to detect a specific protein. A Western blot test to detect HIV proteins in the blood is used to confirm a positive HIV antibody test (ELISA).

window period: The time period between a person's infection with HIV and the appearance of detectable anti-HIV antibodies. The time delay typically ranges from fourteen to twenty-one days, but varies for different people. Nearly everyone infected with HIV will have detectable antibodies by three to six months after infection.

Chapter 49

Directory of Organizations for People with HIV/AIDS and Their Families and Friends

AIDS.gov
Website: http://www.aids.gov

AIDSInfo (AIDS Information Service)
P.O. Box 6303
Rockville, MD 20849-6303
Toll-Free: 800-HIV-0440
(448-0440)
Phone: 301-315-2816
Fax: 301-315-2818
TTY: 888-480-3739
Website:
http://www.aidsinfo.nih.gov
E-mail: ContactUs@aidsinfo.gov

AIDS InfoNet
P.O. Box 810
Arroyo Seco, NM 87514
Website:
http://www.aidsinfonet.org

AIDS Vaccine Advocacy Coalition (AVAC)
101 West 23rd Street, #2227
New York, NY 10011
Phone: 212-367-1279
Fax: 646-365-3452
Website: http://www.avac.org
E-mail: avac@avac.org

AIDSmeds.com
462 Seventh Avenue, 19th Floor
New York, NY 10018-7424
Website:
http://www.aidsmeds.com

American Academy of Family Physicians
P.O. Box 11210
Shawnee Mission, KS 66207-1210
Toll-Free: 800-274-2237
Phone: 913-906-6000
Fax: 913-906-6075
Website: http://www.aafp.org

Resources in this chapter were compiled from several sources deemed reliable. All contact information was verified and updated in November 2010.

AVERT
4 Brighton Road
Horsham
West Sussex
RH13 5BA
United Kingdom
Website: http://www.avert.org/

The Body.com
250 West 57th Street,
Suite 1614
New York, NY 10107
Phone: 212-541-8500
Website: http://www.thebody.com

Canadian AIDS Treatment Information Exchange (CATIE)
555 Richmond Street West
Suite 505
Box 1104
Toronto, Ontario M5V 3B1
Canada
Toll-Free: 800-263-1638
Phone: 416-203-7122
Fax: 416-203-8284
Website: http://www.catie.ca

Canadian Federation for Sexual Health
2197 Riverside Drive
Suite 403
Ottawa, Ontario K1H 7X3
Canada
Phone: 613-241-4474
Fax: 613-241-7550
Website: http://www.cfsh.ca
E-mail: admin@cfsh.ca

Center for AIDS Information and Advocacy
P.O. Box 66306
Houston, Texas 77266-6306
Toll-Free: 800-341-1788
Phone: 713-527-8219
Fax: 713-521-3679
Website:
http://www.centerforaids.org
E-mail: info@centerforaids.org

Center for AIDS Prevention Studies—University of California at San Francisco
AIDS Research Institute
University of California at
San Francisco
50 Beale Street, Suite 1300
San Francisco, CA 94105
Phone: 415-597-9100
Fax: 415-597-9213
Website:
http://www.caps.ucsf.edu
E-mail: CAPS.Web@ucsf.edu

Centers for Disease Control and Prevention
1600 Clifton Road
Atlanta, GA 30333
Toll-Free: 800-232-4636
TTY: 888-232-6348
Website: http://www.cdc.gov

CDC National Prevention Information Network
P.O. Box 6003
Rockville, Maryland 20849-6003
Toll-Free: 800-458-5231
TTY: 800-243-7012
Website: http://www.cdcnpin.org

Foundation for AIDS Research (amfAR)
120 Wall Street, 13th Floor
New York, NY 10005-3908
Phone: 212-806-1600
Fax: 212-806-1601
Website: http://www.amfar.org
E-mail: information@amfar.org

Elizabeth Glaser Pediatric AIDS Foundation
1140 Connecticut Avenue, NW
Suite 200
Washington, DC 20036
Toll-Free: 888-499-HOPE (-4673)
Phone: 202-296-9165
Fax: 202-296-9185
Website: http://www.pedaids.org
E-mail: info@pedaids.org

HIV InfoSource
NYU School of Medicine
550 First Avenue, Old Bellevue
C&D Bldg., Room 558
New York, NY 10016
Website:
http://www.hivinfosource.org

International AIDS Vaccine Initiative (IAVI)
110 William Street, Floor 27
New York, NY 10038-3901
Phone: 212-847-1111
Website: http://www.iavi.org

Elton John AIDS Foundation
584 Broadway, Suite 906
New York, NY 10012
Website: http://www.ejaf.org

National Association of People with AIDS (NAPWA)
8401 Colesville Road
Suite 505
Silver Spring, MD 20910
Toll-Free: 866-846-9366
Phone: 240-247-0880
Fax: 240-247-0574
Website: http://www.napwa.org

National Cancer Institute
NCI Office of Communications and Education
Public Inquiries Office
6116 Executive Boulevard
Suite 300
Bethesda, MD 20892-8322
Toll-Free: 800-4-CANCER
(800-422-6237)
Website: http://www.cancer.gov

National Institute of Allergy and Infectious Diseases
6610 Rockledge Drive
MSC 6612
Bethesda, MD 20892-6612
Toll-Free: 866-284-4107
Phone: 301-496-5717
TDD: 800-877-8339
Website:
http://www.niaid.nih.gov

National Institute on Aging
Information Center
P.O. Box 8057
Gaithersburg, MD 20898-8057
Toll-Free: 800-222-2225
TTY: 800-222-4225
Website: http://www.nia.nih.gov

National Minority AIDS Council

1931 13th Street NW
Washington, DC 20009
Phone: 202-483-6622
Website: http://www.nmac.org
E-mail: info@nmac.org

National NeuroAIDS Tissue Consortium

401 N. Washington Street
Suite 700
Rockville, MD 20850
Phone: 866-668-2272 or
301-251-1161
Fax: 301-576-4597
Website: http://www.
hivbrainbanks.org
E-mail: nntc@emmes.com

Office of AIDS Research

National Institutes of Health
5635 Fishers Lane MSC 9310
Bethesda, Maryland 20892-9310
Phone: 301-496-0357
Fax: 301-496-2119
Website: http://www.oar.nih.gov
E-mail: oartemp1
@od31em1.od.nih.gov

Project Inform

1375 Mission Street
San Francisco, CA 94103–2621
Phone: 415-558-8669
Fax: 415-558-0684
Website:
http://www.projectinform.org

Services & Advocacy for Gay, Lesbian, Bisexual & Transgender Elders (SAGE)

305 7th Avenue
6th Floor
New York, NY 10001
Phone: 212-741-2247
Website: http://www.sageusa.org

U.S. Department of Veterans Affairs

Clinical Public Health Programs:
HIV/AIDS
Website: http://www.hiv.va.gov

Well Project

Toll-Free: 888-616-WELL (9355)
Website:
http://www.thewellproject.org
E-mail: info@thewellproject.org

Index

Index

Health Reference Series